T0263626

.

Gastroenteropancreatic System and Its Tumors: Part 2

Guest Editor

AARON I. VINIK, MD, PhD

ENDOCRINOLOGY AND METABOLISM CLINICS OF NORTH AMERICA

www.endo.theclinics.com

Consulting Editor
DEREK LEROITH, MD, PhD

March 2011 • Volume 40 • Number 1

SAUNDERS an imprint of ELSEVIER, Inc.

W.B. SAUNDERS COMPANY
A Division of Elsevier Inc.

1600 John F. Kennedy Boulevard • Suite 1800 • Philadelphia, Pennsylvania 19103-2899

http://www.theclinics.com

ENDOCRINOLOGY AND METABOLISM CLINICS OF NORTH AMERICA Volume 40, Number 1
March 2011 ISSN 0889-8529, ISBN-13: 978-1-4557-0440-8

Editor: Rachel Glover
Developmental Editor: Donald Mumford

© **2011 Elsevier Inc. All rights reserved.**

This journal and the individual contributions contained in it are protected under copyright by Elsevier, and the following terms and conditions apply to their use:

Photocopying

Single photocopies of single articles may be made for personal use as allowed by national copyright laws. Permission of the Publisher and payment of a fee is required for all other photocopying, including multiple or systematic copying, copying for advertising or promotional purposes, resale, and all forms of document delivery. Special rates are available for educational institutions that wish to make photocopies for non-profit educational classroom use. For information on how to seek permission visit www.elsevier.com/permissions or call: (+44) 1865 843830 (UK)/(+1) 215 239 3804 (USA).

Derivative Works

Subscribers may reproduce tables of contents or prepare lists of articles including abstracts for internal circulation within their institutions. Permission of the Publisher is required for resale or distribution outside the institution. Permission of the Publisher is required for all other derivative works, including compilations and translations (please consult www.elsevier.com/permissions).

Electronic Storage or Usage

Permission of the Publisher is required to store or use electronically any material contained in this journal, including any article or part of an article (please consult www.elsevier.com/permissions). Except as outlined above, no part of this publication may be reproduced, stored in a retrieval system or transmitted in any form or by any means, electronic, mechanical, photocopying, recording or otherwise, without prior written permission of the Publisher.

Notice

No responsibility is assumed by the Publisher for any injury and/or damage to persons or property as a matter of products liability, negligence or otherwise, or from any use or operation of any methods, products, instructions or ideas contained in the material herein. Because of rapid advances in the medical sciences, in particular, independent verification of diagnoses and drug dosages should be made.

Although all advertising material is expected to conform to ethical (medical) standards, inclusion in this publication does not constitute a guarantee or endorsement of the quality or value of such product or of the claims made of it by its manufacturer.

Endocrinology and Metabolism Clinics of North America (ISSN 0889-8529) is published quarterly by Elsevier Inc., 360 Park Avenue South, New York, NY 10010-1710. Months of issue are March, June, September, and December. Periodicals postage paid at New York, NY and additional mailing offices. Subscription prices are USD 290.00 per year for US individuals, USD 503.00 per year for US institutions, USD 146.00 per year for US students and residents, USD 364.00 per year for Canadian individuals, USD 616.00 per year for Canadian institutions, USD 422.00 per year for international individuals, USD 616.00 per year for international institutions, and USD 216.00 per year for international and Canadian and foreign students/residents. To receive student/resident rate, orders must be accompanied by name of affiliated institution, date of term, and the signature of program/residency coordinator on institution letterhead. Orders will be billed at individual rate until proof of status is received. Foreign air speed delivery is included in all *Clinics* subscription prices. All prices are subject to change without notice. **POSTMASTER:** Send address changes to *Endocrinology and Metabolism Clinics of North America*, Elsevier Health Sciences Division, Subscription Customer Service, 3251 Riverport Lane, Maryland Heights, MO 63043. **Customer Service: Telephone: 1-800-654-2452** (U.S. and Canada); **1-314-447-8871** (outside U.S. and Canada). **Fax: 1-314-447-8029. E-mail: journalscustomerservice-usa@elsevier.com** (for print support); **journalsonlinesupport-usa@elsevier.com** (for online support).

Reprints. For copies of 100 or more, of articles in this publication, please contact the Commercial Rights Department, Elsevier Inc., 360 Park Avenue South, New York, NY 10010-1710; phone: (+1) 212-633-3813; fax: (+1) 212-462-1935; e-mail: reprints@elsevier.com.

Endocrinology and Metabolism Clinics of North America is covered in *MEDLINE/PubMed (Index Medicus)*, *EMBASE/Excerpta Medica*, *Current Contents/Clinical Medicine*, *Current Contents/Life Sciences*, *Science Citation Index*, *ISI/BIOMED*, *BIOSIS*, and *Chemical Abstracts*.

Printed and bound by CPI Group (UK) Ltd, Croydon, CR0 4YY

Transferred to Digital Print 2011

Contributors

CONSULTING EDITOR

DEREK LEROITH, MD, PhD
Chief, Division of Endocrinology, Metabolism, and Bone Diseases, Department
of Medicine, Mount Sinai School of Medicine, New York, New York

GUEST EDITOR

AARON I. VINIK, MD, PhD, FCP, MACP
Professor of Medicine, Pathology and Neurobiology, Director of Research and
Neuroendocrine Unit, Eastern Virginia Medical School, Strelitz Diabetes Center,
Norfolk, Virginia

AUTHORS

LOWELL B. ANTHONY, MD, FACP
Professor of Medicine, Sections of Hematology and Oncology and Medical Oncology,
Department of Medicine, Louisiana State University Health Sciences Center, New Orleans,
Louisiana

RICHARD P. BAUM, MD
Department of Nuclear Medicine/Center for Positron Emission Tomography, Zentralklinik
Bad Berka GmbH, Bad Berka, Germany

J. PHILIP BOUDREAUX, MD, FACS
Professor of Surgery, Sections of Endocrine Surgery, Surgical Oncology and Transplant
Surgery, Department of Surgery, Louisiana State University Health Sciences Center,
New Orleans, Louisiana

DAVID L. BUSHNELL, MD
Division of Nuclear Medicine, Department of Radiology, Roy J. and Lucille A. Carver
College of Medicine, University of Iowa; Diagnostic Imaging and Radioisotope Therapy
Service, Iowa City Veterans Administration Medical Center, Iowa City, Iowa

RICHARD CAMPEAU, MD
Clinical Professor of Radiology and Medicine, Section of Radiation Oncology,
Departments of Medicine and Radiology, Louisiana State University Health Sciences
Center, New Orleans, Louisiana

ANTHONY CHAN, MD
Gastrointestinal Pathobiology Research Group, Department of Surgery, Yale University
School of Medicine, New Haven, Connecticut

JASON CUNDIFF, MD
Section of Endocrine Surgery, Department of Surgery, Louisiana State University Health
Sciences Center, New Orleans, Louisiana

WOUTER W. DE HERDER, MD, PhD
Department of Internal Medicine, Erasmus Medical Center, Rotterdam, The Netherlands

FLAVIO FORRER, MD, PhD
Department of Radiology and Nuclear Medicine, University Hospital Basel, Basel,
Switzerland

GIAMPIERO GIOVACCHINI, MD, PhD
Department of Radiology and Nuclear Medicine, University Hospital Basel, Basel,
Switzerland

VAY LIANG GO, MD
Professor of Medicine, David Geffen School of Medicine at University of California
Los Angeles, University of California Los Angeles Center for Excellence in Pancreatic
Diseases, Los Angeles, California

MICHAEL RAYMUND C. GONZALES, MD
Fellow, Division of Endocrinology and Metabolism, Department of Internal Medicine,
Eastern Virginia Medical School, Norfolk, Virginia

BJORN I. GUSTAFSSON, MD, PhD
Department of Gastroenterology, St Olavs Hospital; Department of Cancer Research
and Molecular Medicine, Norwegian University of Science and Technology,
Trondheim, Norway

SAJU JOSEPH, MD
Assistant Professor of Surgery, Sections of Endocrine and Hepatobiliary Surgery,
Department of Surgery, Louisiana State University Health Sciences Center, New Orleans,
Louisiana

MARK KIDD, PhD
Gastrointestinal Pathobiology Research Group, Department of Surgery, Yale University
School of Medicine, New Haven, Connecticut

ERIC P. KRENNING, MD, PhD
Department of Nuclear Medicine, Erasmus Medical Center, Rotterdam, The Netherlands

DIK J. KWEKKEBOOM, MD, PhD
Department of Nuclear Medicine, Erasmus Medical Center, Rotterdam, The Netherlands

BEN LAWRENCE, MBChB, MSc
Gastrointestinal Pathobiology Research Group, Department of Surgery, Yale University
School of Medicine, New Haven, Connecticut

GREGG MAMIKUNIAN, MS
Chairman and CEO, Inter Science Institute, Inglewood, California

MARY ELIZABETH MASON, MD, FACE, FACP
Associate Professor, Department of Medicine, Eastern Virginia Medical School, Strelitz
Diabetes Center, Norfolk, Virginia

IRVIN M. MODLIN, MD, PhD, DSc, FRCS(Eng & Ed)
Professor, Gastrointestinal Pathobiology Research Group, Department of Surgery,
Yale University School of Medicine, New Haven, Connecticut

JAN MÜLLER-BRAND, MD
Department of Radiology and Nuclear Medicine, University Hospital Basel, Basel, Switzerland

GUILLAUME NICOLAS, MD
Department of Radiology and Nuclear Medicine, University Hospital Basel, Basel, Switzerland

M. SUE O'DORISIO, MD, PhD
Distinguished Professor, Department of Pediatrics, Roy J. and Lucille A. Carver College of Medicine, University of Iowa, Iowa City, Iowa

THOMAS O'DORISIO, MD
Professor of Internal Medicine, Roy J. and Lucille A. Carver College of Medicine, University of Iowa, University of Iowa Hospitals and Clinics, Iowa City, Iowa

MARIANNE PAVEL, MD
Professor, Med. Klinik m.S. Hepatologie und Gastroenterologie, Charité-Campus Virchow Klinikum, Universitätsmedizin Berlin, Berlin, Germany

DANIEL RAINES, MD
Assistant Professor of Clinical Medicine; Section Chief, Section of Gastroenterology, Department of Medicine, Louisiana State University Health Sciences Center, New Orleans, Louisiana

DONALD W. RICHARDSON, MD
Associate Professor, Department of Medicine, Eastern Virginia Medical School, Strelitz Diabetes Center, Norfolk, Virginia

MARIE-ELLEN SARVIDA, MD
Assistant Professor, Department of Pediatrics, Ronald McDonald Children's Hospital, Loyola University Medical Center, Maywood, Illinois

MARIA P. SILVA, MD
Neuroendocrine Unit, Eastern Virginia Medical School, Strelitz Diabetes Center, Norfolk, Virginia

BERNHARD SVEJDA, MD
Gastrointestinal Pathobiology Research Group, Department of Surgery, Yale University School of Medicine, New Haven, Connecticut

AARON I. VINIK, MD, PhD, FCP, MACP
Professor of Medicine, Pathology and Neurobiology, Director of Research and Neuroendocrine Unit, Eastern Virginia Medical School, Strelitz Diabetes Center, Norfolk, Virginia

ETTA VINIK, MA(Ed)
Associate Director of Education, Neuroendocrine Unit, Eastern Virginia Medical School, Strelitz Diabetes Center, Norfolk, Virginia

YI-ZARN WANG, MD, FACS
Professor of Surgery, Sections of Endocrine Surgery and Surgical Oncology, Department of Surgery, Louisiana State University Health Sciences Center, New Orleans, Louisiana

EUGENE A. WOLTERING, MD, FACS
The James D. Rives Professor of Surgery and Neuroscience, Sections of Surgical Oncology and Endocrine Surgery; Director of Surgical Research, Department of Surgery, Louisiana State University Health Sciences Center, New Orleans, Louisiana

Contents

Obesity is a disease state with polygenic inheritance, the phenotypic penetrance of which has been greatly expanded by the attributes of modern civilization. More than two-thirds of obese persons have comorbidities, many of which are characteristic of cardiometabolic risk syndrome (CMRS) in addition to other life-quality–reducing complaints. The CMRS is associated with increased cardiovascular events and mortality. Individuals with a body mass index greater than 35 infrequently achieve or maintain weight loss adequate to resolve these metabolic and anatomic issues by lifestyle or pharmacologic strategies. Data suggest that some of these patients may be better served by bariatric surgery.

The measurement of health-related quality of life (HRQOL) has become essential for evaluating the impact of neuroendocrine tumors (NETs) on symptoms and social, emotional, psychological, and physical functioning of patients who harbor these tumors. This article describes instruments that have been developed to capture the spectrum of symptoms and the impact of the disease on their overall well-being. The authors discuss the importance of adequate sensitivity, specificity, and reproducibility and the value of psychometric factor analysis to explore the domains that embrace the manifestations of these tumors as well as aspects of the instruments that reflect tumor burden, biochemical, and hormonal status.

Chromogranin A, although it exhibits limitations, is currently the most useful general tumor biomarker available for use in the diagnosis and management of gastroenteropancreatic neuroendocrine tumors (NETs). The value of the chromogranin A lies in its universal cosecretion by the majority of neuroendocrine cells that persists after malignant transformation. Clinicians aware of the physiologic role of chromogranin A and its secretion in a variety of non-NET–related pathologic conditions can use this protein as a moderately effective tumor biomarker in the management of GEP-NETs.

Modern medicine, and specifically clinical diagnosis, relies, among other diagnostic procedures, on the measurements of the biogenic analytes for elucidation and correlation of specific neuroendocrine markers. Tremendous advances have been made in imaging and radioactive uptake procedures to elucidate tumor presence and characterization. However, such advances only partially provide the fundamental degree of tumor activity and clinical confirmational validity. The author points out in some detail the problems that may arise when the methodological differences presented by each investigational study and investigators are not standardized. This variation causes a concern with the specific objectives of the investigator and the specific aims of the research project at hand, and ultimately for the validity of the published results.

Standard Imaging Techniques for Neuroendocrine Tumors

David L. Bushnell and Richard P. Baum

Several diagnostic imaging techniques have been used successfully for evaluating patients with neuroendocrine tumors (NETs). These techniques include computed tomography (CT), magnetic resonance imaging, positron emission tomography/CT, single-photon emission CT (SPECT), and SPECT/CT. This article reviews the various imaging methods and their respective advantages and limitations for use in different types of NETs, in particular carcinoid tumors.

Surgery for Gastroenteropancreatic Neuroendocrine Tumors (GEPNETS)

J. Philip Boudreaux

The only therapy with the potential for complete cure of patients with gastroenteropancreatic neuroendocrine tumors is complete surgical excision. Surgical options per se are often dictated by the tumor's site of origin, degree of tumor burden, and overall health or debility of the individual patient. This article considers different options based on the type of tumor and site of origin.

Somatostatin Receptor-Targeted Radionuclide Therapy in Patients with Gastroenteropancreatic Neuroendocrine Tumors

Dik J. Kwekkeboom, Wouter W. de Herder, and Eric P. Krenning

Treatment with radiolabeled somatostatin analogs is a promising tool in the management of patients with inoperable or metastasized neuroendocrine tumors. Symptomatic improvement may occur with all [111]Indium-, [90]Yttrium-, or [177]Lutetium-labeled somatostatin analogs used for peptide receptor radionuclide therapy. If kidney protective agents are used, the side-effects are few and mild, and the median duration of the therapy response is 30 and 40 months, respectively. Overall survival is several years from diagnosis. These data compare favorably with the limited number of alternative treatments. If more widespread use of PRRT can be guaranteed, such therapy may become the therapy of first choice.

Targeted Radiotherapy with Radiolabeled Somatostatin Analogs

Guillaume Nicolas, Giampiero Giovacchini, Jan Müller-Brand, and Flavio Forrer

Targeted radiopeptide therapy with [90]Yttrium- or [177]Lutetium-labeled somatostatin analogs has been proven to improve significantly quality of life and survival in patients suffering from metastatic or unresectable neuroendocrine tumors (NETs). Roughly 25% of patients achieve partial remission; progression-free survival is estimated to be 30 to 40 months.

A wide range of protocols using different somatostatin analogs, isotopes, injected activity per cycle of administration, and number of cycles are reported. More patient-based therapy protocols are under development, taking into consideration the complexity of NET cell biology, dosimetric issues, and the availability of different radiolabeled analogs. This article reviews the effectiveness and safety of the different protocols and discusses several clinical algorithms used in an attempt to optimize targeted radio-peptide therapy.

Neuroendocrine tumors (NETs) are rare neoplasms found in diverse locations within the body. These tumors are commonly classified by the primary tumor's location, further subclassified by their differentiation, and finally segregated by their ability to hypersecrete peptides or amines. A number of groups have summarized their recommendations for diagnosis and therapy; however, the rarity of these lesions makes prospective randomized multiinstitutional trials difficult. Thus, these "consensus statements" often remain opinion-based. The authors have collaboratively developed a consensus on the current diagnostic work-up necessary for patients with NETs to help clinicians with this confusing field and followed this with some of the more advanced surgical techniques and considerations that are currently only available in specialty centers to show the evolving management of NETs.

VISIT US ONLINE!
Access your subscription at:
www.theclinics.com

Foreword

Gastroenteropancreatic System and Its Tumors: Part 2

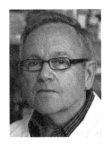

Derek LeRoith, MD, PhD
Consulting Editor

This second issue opens with an article on the epidemiology of gastroenteropancreatic neuroendocrine tumors (GEP-NETs) by Drs Lawrence, Gustafsson, Chan, Svejda, Kidd, and Modlin. As discussed by the authors, there is an apparent increased incidence of GEP-NETs. Further, each anatomical site retains its own unique epidemiological profile; for example, rectal neuroendocrine tumors (NETs) are diagnosed at a younger age compared to colonic NETs, which are detected at an older age and have a worse prognosis.

In an extremely detailed article, Drs Vinik and Gonzales describe new and emerging syndromes due to NET. As they discuss, these tumors are fairly uncommon and often slow growing. Many of the biochemical markers are nonspecific and it behooves the clinician to be aware of the symptoms that may be the clue to the disorder. Dry flushing is almost always due to a NET, such as a phaechromocytoma. Flushing may also be a symptom of carcinoids. Diarrhea may be caused by different hormones or biogenic amines released by NETs. Other clinical clues include peptic ulcer, hypoglycemia, and bronchoconstriction, all associated with different tumors. The article also describes provocative tests to help in the diagnosis, and pathological and genetic diagnostic tools used in cases of NETs and pancreatic NETs. The article covers all the NETs and the various combinations of multiple endocrine tumors and should be "the" resource for this field.

While neuroendocrine tumors are uncommon in children, pediatric endocrinologists and colleagues need to be aware of their occurrence and presentations, as diagnosis can be readily made using the same techniques used in adult patients. Because they are uncommon, diagnoses are often made late. Drs Sarvida and O'Dorisio also describe the treatment for these neuroendocrine tumors, treatment specific for this population.

Bariatric surgery has become a very important surgical procedure in the management of morbid obesity and also for obese uncontrolled type 2 diabetic patients. In

Endocrinol Metab Clin N Am 40 (2011) xiii–xv
doi:10.1016/j.ecl.2011.01.002
0889-8529/11/$ – see front matter © 2011 Elsevier Inc. All rights reserved.

this article Drs Richardson, Mason, and Vinik discuss the obesity epidemic, the cardiovascular risks associated with obesity, and the various nonsurgical therapies, most of which are totally inadequate. Therefore as surgical procedures become more available and have fewer complications, they may help in reducing cardiovascular complications of obesity and associated disorders.

In diagnosing and treating neuroendocrine tumors, the health care professional should always be cognizant of the patient's well-being, commonly forgotten while investigating these tumors and considering therapies. Ms Vinik, and Drs Silva and Vinik have devised a quality of life (QOL) questionnaire that covers all aspects of symptomatology, including psychometric analyses. While a similar European QOL questionnaire is available, the Norfolk questionnaire is more comprehensive and has proven to enhance the health care provider's ability to identify areas of patients' needs more appropriately.

Chromogranin A (CgA) has been suggested as a biochemical marker to be used in the diagnosis of GEP-NETS. Initially discovered in secretory granules in the adrenal, CgA apparently is widely expressed in neuroendocrine cells and therefore in these tumors; indeed, even after malignant transformation, the cells still secrete CgA. As Drs Lawrence, Gustafsson, Kidd, Pavel, Svejda, and Modlin point out in their article, there are some limitations to the use of CgA measurements for the diagnosis and as a prognostic indicator.

NETs classically express and secrete hormones and biogenic amines, substances that often are the cause of the symptomatology, specific for that tumor. Measurements of these amines would greatly enhance our diagnostic ability; however, as discussed by Dr Mamikunian, there remain numerous problems. While the technology has greatly advanced over many years, especially in the use of radioimmunoassay, the variability in levels that are found are so great that results need to be interpreted cautiously.

As described by Drs Bushnell and Baum, most neuroendocrine tumors and metastases are detected by CT scanning and MRI technology during the arterial phase of delivery of the contrast material. Other techniques include single-photon emission computed tomography, isotopic labeled MIBG scanning, Octreoscans, F-18 FDG PET scanning, and numerous other functional imaging techniques. While the article focused primarily on imaging of carcinoids, the authors suggest that for all NETs, using various combinations of the technology gives maximum results.

Surgery is a potential "cure" for GEP-NETS and includes resection of the primary tumor or the metastases. Dr Boudreaux discusses the experience with various tumors in this class, focusing particularly on carcinoids. Interestingly, while hepatic metastases can sometimes be resected, if the liver metastases are inoperable, this may be an indication for liver transplantation, one of the few indications for metastatic disease.

When neuroendocrine tumors are inoperable as in the case of metastases, there are limited options. One new technique that has been used successfully is radiolabeled somatostatin analogs, ie, octreotide or octreotate. As discussed by Kwekkeboom, de Herder, and Krenning, who have pioneered these therapies, survival compared to historical controls is increased, often by years, and the QOL is also improved significantly.

Drs Nicolas, Giovacchini, Müller-Brand, and Forrer use radioactive peptide therapy in treating these tumors. Numerous protocols are in use in Europe with substantial success, with the most commonly used peptide being radioactive somatostatin analogs. The side effects are often minimal and the acute side effects include nausea, vomiting, and pain at the tumor sites. More substantial side effects include hematological, renal, and, to a lesser extent, liver. Outcomes are quite impressive with partial remissions in up to 25% of cases and progression-free survival up to 30–40 months.

Drs Joseph, Wang, Boudreaux, Anthony, Campeau, Raines, O'Dorisio, Go, Vinik, Cundiff, and Woltering in their article present clinical recommendations for diagnosis and surgical management for cases with suspected NETS. As they discuss, since these tumors are rare, one can only make recommendations, because no controlled trials can be undertaken. Thus this group, that represents many of the leaders in the field, has convened to help those of us with less experience in dealing with those patients presenting with vague signs and symptoms. The article also discusses the advances in diagnostic radiological techniques and aggressive surgical techniques once a diagnosis is made, overall a very useful guide for the practicing endocrinologist.

Once again, Dr Vinik and his fellow authors have presented us with important information on the endocrine aspect of the gastrointestinal tract and disorders emanating from this system.

Derek LeRoith, MD, PhD
Division of Endocrinology, Metabolism, and Bone Diseases
Department of Medicine
Mount Sinai School of Medicine
One Gustave L. Levy Place
Box 1055, Altran 4-36
New York, NY 10029, USA

E-mail address:
derek.leroith@mssm.edu

Preface

Gastroenteropancreatic System and Its Tumors: Part 2

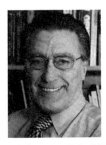

Aaron I. Vinik, MD, PhD, FCP, MACP
Guest Editor

Once the Cinderella of cancer, neuroendocrine tumors (NETS) have found their place in the world of cancer. Indeed, while small gut cancers have not increased in incidence, there has been a fivefold rise in the incidence of neuroendocrine carcinomas over the last 30 years. Once called "carcinoid," the preferred term is now "neuroendocrine carcinoma," and there have emerged European and North American societies focused solely on these tumors. Guidelines have been developed for diagnosis, staging, and the optimum means of localization, using CT, MRI, PET, and radioactive peptide scans. Critical to the evolution of understanding is a pathological grading system based upon cell mitoses and an index (Ki67) of cell division, as well as a staging ranging from G1 localized, G2 local or lymph node spread, and G3 distant spread. It is now clear that the less differentiated and the higher the staging, the worse the prognosis. Recently espoused that "there has been a rapid pace of no progress," it is now apparent that in the era of peptide therapy with somatostatin and its long-acting analogs, 5-year survival of malignant, metastatic NETS has increased from a few months to a greater than 95% 5-year survival. This no doubt has been ably abetted by the introduction of better chemotherapeutic regimens such as temozolamide and capecitabine, monocloncal antibodies to angiogenic agents, chemo- and bland embolization, aggressive surgical debulking and exhaustive search and elimination of the primary tumors, and the introduction of new and effective tyrosine kinase inhibitors and MTOR inhibitors, SIRS therapy, and radiopeptide ablative therapy. What were lacking in the area were good biomarkers for diagnosis during the long latent period from onset of symptoms to identification of the NET, which is approaching 9 years. This too has received a boost with new and better markers and enhanced awareness. Chromogranin was hailed as "the endocrinologist's sedimentation rate" for the diagnosis of these tumors, but now we can quantify by old-fashioned radioimmunoassay peptides such as pancreastatin (a derivative of chromogranin). The success of an intervention and measurement of neurokinin dictates the major difference in 5-year survival. Of course, mere survival

Endocrinol Metab Clin N Am 40 (2011) xvii–xviii
doi:10.1016/j.ecl.2011.01.001
0889-8529/11/$ – see front matter © 2011 Elsevier Inc. All rights reserved.

falls short of an idealistic goal and quality of life has become the rage, and with two tools, including the Norfolk QOLNET, the ability to quantify the impact of an intervention is feasible and appears to relate to tumor bulk and the amine or peptide produced. Perhaps the most exciting aspect of these tumors is the fostering of close interaction between multiple disciplines in medicine, eg, oncology, radiology, surgery, nuclear medicine, endocrinology, and gastroenterology, among others. This cross-discipline attention to NETS has facilitated the recognition of new and emerging syndromes such as the paraneoplastic myopathies, neuropathies, fatigue, and a variety of clinical syndromes still seeking their hormones, peptides, and cytokines, just as there is a plethora of new chemicals being discovered that have yet to have a hormone identified as being responsible. Perhaps the least exciting is the iatrogenic potential for causing these tumors, as appears to be the case with gastric bypass procedures and even the use of certain drugs in managing diabetes. Trust the erudite discipline of neuroendocrinology to guarantee its future and create job security by whatever means possible.

Aaron I. Vinik, MD, PhD, FCP, MACP
Eastern Virginia Medical School
Strelitz Diabetes Center
855 West Brambleton Avenue
Norfolk, VA 23510-1001, USA

E-mail address:
vinikai@evms.edu

The Epidemiology of Gastroenteropancreatic Neuroendocrine Tumors

Ben Lawrence, MBChB, MSc[a], Bjorn I. Gustafsson, MD, PhD[b,c],
Anthony Chan, MD[a], Bernhard Svejda, MD[a], Mark Kidd, PhD[a],
Irvin M. Modlin, MD, PhD, DSc, FRCS(Eng & Ed)[a,*]

KEYWORDS

- Carcinoid • Epidemiology • Incidence • Neuroendocrine tumor
- SEER • Survival

Gastroenteropancreatic neuroendocrine tumors (GEP-NETs) are caused by malignant transformation of cells in the diffuse neuroendocrine system that regulates secretion and motility in the gut.[1] In some instances, this transformation is based on genetic alterations (in 2%–40% of foregut neuroendocrine tumors (NETs), there is a mutation in the multiple endocrine neoplasia 1 gene); however, for most tumors, no identifiable causation is evident.[2] The exception is Type 1 gastric carcinoids, which are directly related to low acid states and pernicious anemia.[3] The traditional assumptions that these cancers are rare and benign are incorrect. NETs have the same incidence as that of testicular cancer, cervical cancer, multiple myeloma, Hodgkin lymphoma, and cancers of the central nervous system.[4] Furthermore, the prevalence of GEP-NETs is higher than that of most gastrointestinal cancers, including pancreatic, gastric, esophageal, and hepatobiliary carcinomas, and is only exceeded by that of colorectal neoplasia.[5] GEP-NETs are not benign, although in many instances, a more indolent course than that of adenocarcinoma is evident. Poorly differentiated GEP-NETs behave very aggressively, and survival may be measured in months. There is thus a substantial clinical imperative to amplify the knowledge of GEP-NETs.

B.L. was supported in part by the Murray Jackson Clinical Fellowship, Genesis Oncology Trust, Auckland, New Zealand.

The authors have nothing to disclose.

[a] Gastrointestinal Pathobiology Research Group, Department of Surgery, Yale University School of Medicine, 310 Cedar Street, PO Box 208602, New Haven, CT 06520-8062, USA

[b] Department of Gastroenterology, St Olavs Hospital, Prinsesse Kristinas Gate 1, 7006 Trondheim, Norway

[c] Department of Cancer Research and Molecular Medicine, Norwegian University of Science and Technology, Prinsesse Kristinas Gate 1, 7006 Trondheim, Norway

* Corresponding author.

E-mail address: imodlin@optonline.net

Endocrinol Metab Clin N Am 40 (2011) 1–18
doi:10.1016/j.ecl.2010.12.005
0889-8529/11/$ – see front matter © 2011 Elsevier Inc. All rights reserved.

GEP-NETs are a heterogeneous group of cancers that have proved to be difficult to assimilate within a globally acceptable classification for more than a century. A diverse array of classification systems has been proposed over the past 5 decades, based on embryologic origin,[6] morphologic differences,[7] or biochemical profile.[8] To date, the most widely accepted system is the World Health Organization classification based on the extent and grade modified by a variety of further subdivisions.[9] Despite attempts at more precise histomorphologic classifications, numerous clinicians have resisted acceptance of this unstable taxonomic landscape and clung to Oberndorfer's original term carcinoid, modified by identification of the primary site/organ in which the tumor occurred. Although this approach is pragmatic and quasi-effective, a more precise and well-defined global classification is required to ensure a clear epidemiologic perspective for each of the GEP-NET primary sites.

Recent studies on NET epidemiology based on the National Cancer Institute Surveillance, Epidemiology and End Results (SEER) cancer registry in the United States as well as the European studies demonstrate an increasing GEP-NET incidence.[5,10–13] It has been hypothesized that at least part of this increase might reflect an increased awareness among physicians, more frequent use of topographic testing (eg, screening endoscopy), and the sensitivity of immunohistochemical (eg, chromogranin A) and radiological (eg, multislice computer tomography [CT] and octreotide scintiscan) diagnostic testing.[14] However, there is little evidence that overall survival has improved for patients with GEP-NETs.[1,12] In some instances, the presence of special interest groups and sophisticated medical centers has resulted in a better outcome,[15] but this may not be adequately reflected in the broader context of an extensive national database.[12] Such findings are contrary to expectation, given the probable survival advantages provided by improved therapeutic options[16] and the increase in relative downstaging of new cases identified by incidental diagnosis based on the increased availability of endoscopic screening. On the other hand, in many countries, including the United States, patients are still seen at general oncology practices where treatment approaches have been anecdotally based and somewhat haphazard. This reflects that few clinicians in general oncology can gain enough experience with each subtype to develop a consistent (let alone evidence-based) approach.

Three years of data have accumulated since the last SEER-based review of GEP-NET epidemiology.[5] In this article, we review the current iteration of the SEER registry to investigate the following questions. First, has the incidence of GEP-NETs continued to increase. Second, has the epidemiologic profile of GEP-NETs altered in each different primary sites. And third, has there been any improvement in survival. This article therefore provides the basis for defining the parameters of the disease problem and its outcome.

METHODS

The SEER program was used to provide comprehensive epidemiology data on GEP-NETs. Data were also identified from the End Results Group (ERG) and the Third National Cancer Survey (TNCS) programs of the National Cancer Institute (NCI) between 1950 and 1971. The SEER program (**Fig. 1**) was established in 1973 by the NCI to provide representative cancer incidence and survival rates in the United States and has collected information on all cancer cases diagnosed in 9 areas or registries (SEER 9 registries) in the United States, including 5 states (Connecticut, Iowa, New Mexico, Utah, and Hawaii) and 4 metropolitan areas (Detroit, San Francisco/Oakland, Seattle, and Atlanta). Over the past 37 years, the NCI has added several other states and population centers into the SEER program to expand the registry. Los Angeles

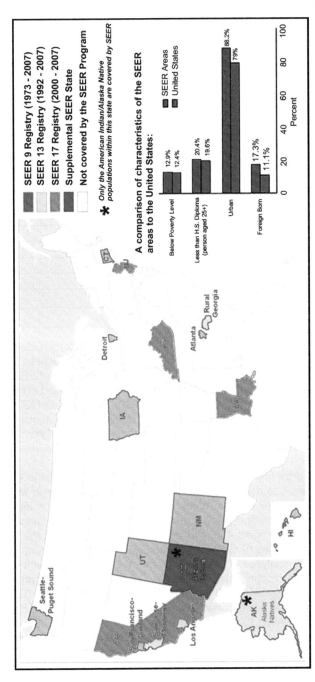

Fig. 1. Geographic distribution of the SEER registries. The blue shaded areas represent the original SEER 9 regions, whereas the regions shaded blue, green, orange, and red are those defined by the SEER 17 registry. (*Adapted from* SEER information brochure. Pub no. 05-4772. Available at: seer.cancer. gov/about/SEER_brochure.pdf.)

Table 1
The NET International Classification of Diseases codes used to interrogate the SEER registry. This table provides information in respect of the NET terminology alterations since 1973 and exhibits the inherent difficulties in uniformity of tumor coding/classification

NET Histology	ICD Code
Carcinoid tumor	8240/3
Enterochromaffin cell carcinoid	8241/3
Goblet cell carcinoid	8243/3
Composite carcinoid	8244/3
Adenocarcinoid	8245/3
Neuroendocrine carcinoma	8246/3
Apudoma	8248/3
Atypical carcinoid tumor	8249/3
Stromal carcinoid	9091/3
Islet cell carcinoma	8150/3
Insulinoma	8151/3
Glucagonoma	8152/3
Gastrinoma	8153/3
Mixed islet cell/exocrine adenocarcinoma	8154/3
VIPoma	8155/3
Somatostatinoma	8156/3

and San-Jose-Monterey, the Alaska Native Tumor Registry, and rural Georgia were added in 1992 (collectively called the SEER 13 registry) and New Jersey, Louisiana, Kentucky, and California in 2000 (SEER 17 registry). At present, the SEER program covers approximately 15% of the population of the United States and provides data on 5,553,822 cancer cases diagnosed from 1973 to 2007. Longitudinal NET incidence was calculated using data from the SEER 9 registry to reflect true changes in disease rates rather than changes attributable to changes in the sample demographic. Figures and tables requiring the most recent dataset for cross-sectional comparison used the SEER 17 registry.

Software provided by the SEER, SEER*Stat 6.6.2, was used to retrieve raw data from the SEER public-use database.[4] The SEER Collaborative Staging Manual and Coding instructions[17] were used to identify areas of interest, which included the primary site, histologic type and grading (the North American Association of Central Cancer Registries item numbers 400, 440, and 522), and the stage of the tumor. We extracted data on all cases of GEP-NETs recorded between 1973 and 2007. The histology of the NETs analyzed in this study (**Table 1**) includes malignant carcinoids (the International Classification of Diseases for Oncology, Third Edition [ICD-O-3] morphology codes: 8240–8249, 9091) and endocrinomas (8150–8156). The primary sites used in our analysis were coded according to the topography section of the ICD-O-3. Information linked to the patient's age and the observed 5-year survival (actuarial method) were also extracted. We also classified NETs based on their embryologic site of origin[6] into foregut (respiratory tract, stomach, duodenum, biliary system, and pancreas), midgut (small bowel, appendix, cecum, and proximal colon), and hindgut (distal colon and rectum) carcinoids. Disease incidence is age-adjusted and presented per 100,000 of the population. Trends in incidence (adjusted for age) and survival between 1973 and 2007 were evaluated using annual percentage change (APC) calculated using a weighted least squares method by SEER*Stat. APC is the relative increase in incidence (or survival) compared with the previous year and is calculated by fitting a least squares regression line to the natural logarithm of the rates, using the calendar year as a regressor variable. Percentage change (PC) in survival was also calculated and represents the relative change between the average survival of the first 2 years and the last 2 years of the period of observation. Alterations in over-all survival (1973–2002) were calculated using the SEER statistical analysis program and GraphPad Prism 4. Survival for each group was modeled using a 1-phase expo-nential decay, and the elapsed time to demise for 50% of patients was calculated from the slope (k value). Statistical significance was accepted at $P<.05$.

The degree of differentiation for a tumor (grade) is reported to the SEER using the system defined by the "Morphology" section of the ICD-O-3. Grade 1 tumors are classed as well differentiated, grade 2 as moderately differentiated, grade 3 as poorly differentiated, and grade 4 as undifferentiated (anaplastic). The grading of tumors is from the primary site and not from the metastatic site or recurrence. If more than one grade is recorded for a single tumor, the highest grade is recorded. Tumor staging is recorded by the SEER using the expanded extent of disease coding.[18] Localized spread is classed as tumors confined within the organ with no obstruction or invasion of regional structures. Regional extension includes spread into surrounding structures, blood vessels, or local lymph nodes. Distant spread includes extension or metastases into other organs or lymph nodes.

RESULTS

A total of 49,012 NETs were included in the SEER epidemiology analysis, including 29,664 patients with GEP-NETs. The distribution of NETs by GEP primary site as accrued in successive national registries is detailed in **Table 2**. In the most recent SEER registry (SEER 17), more than half of all NETs (61.0%) were GEP-NETs, with highest frequency in the rectum (17.7% of NETs), small intestine (17.3% of NETs) and colon (10.1% of NETs). Pancreatic, gastric, and appendiceal sites accounted for 7.0%, 6.0%, and 3.1% of NETs, respectively. Data derived from the earlier ERG and TNCS collations attributed a higher incidence of NETs to appendiceal primaries (43% and 35%, respectively), and nearly 90% of all NETs came from the gastroenter-opancreatic system at the time of the ERG database (1950–1969).

The NET incidence was calculated using data from the SEER 9 registry to allow pro-longed longitudinal comparison. A comprehensive breakdown of GEP-NET incidence by all primary sites per 5-year interval is presented in **Table 3**. The overall incidence of GEP-NETs in the period 1973 to 1977 was 1.00 case per 100,000, and this figure increased to 3.65 cases per 100,000 in the period 2003 to 2007.

The changing incidence of GEP-NETs is demonstrated in **Fig. 2**. The GEP-NET inci-dence persistently increased over the period analyzed (see **Fig. 2**A), and this change was broadly reflected across all GEP-NET embryologic subgroups (see **Fig. 2**B) and primary sites (see **Fig. 2**C). These increases are all statistically significant ($P<.05$). The highest APC was seen in rectal and gastric NETs, the incidence at both sites rising on average by more than 7% per year throughout the 34 years analyzed in the SEER 9 database.

The median age at diagnosis was 63 years, and the incidence of GEP-NETs increased with age (**Fig. 3**A) and indicates a unimodal distribution with a peak at age 80 years. This finding belies some variation between different anatomic sites of GEP-NETs because the incidence of small intestinal NETs peaks at age 80 years, whereas the incidence of rectal NETs peaked at age 50 years, before reducing

Table 2

Frequency of GEP-NETs recorded in successive registries as a percentage of all recorded SEER database NETs (1973–2007). The SEER, ERG, and TNCS databases include 51,849 cases of NETs, including 31,844 cases of GEP-NETs. The most common GEP-NET primary sites in the SEER 17 database in descending incidence are rectum, small intestine, colon, pancreas, stomach, and appendix. NETs also occur with low frequency (<1%) in the esophagus, anal complex, hepatobiliary system, gallbladder, retroperitoneum, peritoneum, omentum, and mesentery

NET Site	ERG (1950–1969)[a]		TNCS (1969–1971)[a]		SEER 9 (1973–1991)		SEER 13 (1992–1999)		SEER 17 (2000–2007)		Pan-SEER (1973–2007)		Total (1950–2007)	
	Number of Patients	Percentage of NETs (%)	Number of Patients	Percentage of NETs (%)	Number of Patients	Percentage of NETs (%)	Number of Patients	Percentage of NETs (%)	Number of Patients	Percentage of NETs (%)	Number of Patients	Percentage of NETs (%)	Number of Patients	Percentage of NETs (%)
All Sites	1867	—	970	—	7278	—	10,575	—	31,159	—	49,012	—	51,849	—
Gastroenteropancreatic Sites	1635	87.57	545	56.19	4636	63.70	6015	56.88	19,013	61.02	29,664	60.52	31,644	61.42
Esophagus	—	—	—	—	6	0.08	18	0.17	75	0.24	99	0.20	99	0.19
Stomach	42	2.25	19	1.96	247	3.39	509	4.81	1876	6.02	2632	5.37	2693	5.19
Small Intestine	353	18.91	—	—	1801	24.75	1933	18.28	5398	17.32	9132	18.63	9485	18.29
Duodenum	33	1.77	22	2.27	136	1.87	305	2.88	1246	4.00	1687	3.44	1742	3.36
Jejunum	19	1.02	19	1.96	134	1.84	111	1.05	300	0.96	545	1.11	583	1.12
Ileum	202	10.82	134	13.81	999	13.73	897	8.48	2204	7.07	4100	8.37	4436	8.56
Meckel diverticulum	—	—	—	—	25	0.34	32	0.30	76	0.24	133	0.27	133	0.26
Overlapping Lesion of Small Intestine	14	0.75	—	—	16	0.22	19	0.18	58	0.19	93	0.19	107	0.21
Small Intestine, NOS	99	5.30	70	7.22	491	6.75	569	5.38	1514	4.86	2574	5.25	2743	5.29
Colon and Rectum	1238	66.31	526	54.23	1766	24.26	2604	24.62	8659	27.79	13,029	26.58	14,793	28.53
Colon Excluding Rectum	—	—	—	—	1052	14.45	1017	9.62	3149	10.11	5218	10.65	5218	10.06
Cecum	50	2.68	29	2.99	286	3.93	315	2.98	956	3.07	1557	3.18	1636	3.16
Appendix	820	43.92	340	35.05	449	6.17	272	2.57	967	3.10	1688	3.44	2848	5.49
Ascending Colon	22	1.18	10	1.03	65	0.89	72	0.68	235	0.75	372	0.76	404	0.78
Hepatic Flexure	—	—	—	—	14	0.19	24	0.23	73	0.23	111	0.23	111	0.21
Transverse Colon	14	0.75	3	0.31	32	0.44	38	0.36	80	0.26	150	0.31	167	0.32

Splenic Flexure	—	—	—	—	9	0.12	10	0.09	28	0.09	47	0.10	47	0.09
Descending Colon	4	0.21	1	0.10	27	0.37	21	0.20	62	0.20	110	0.22	115	0.22
Sigmoid Colon	23	1.23	13	1.34	109	1.50	201	1.90	532	1.71	842	1.72	878	1.69
Large Intestine, NOS	9	0.48	9	0.93	61	0.84	64	0.61	216	0.69	341	0.70	359	0.69
Rectum and Rectosigmoid Junction	—	—	—	—	714	9.81	1587	15.01	5510	17.68	7811	15.94	7811	15.06
Rectosigmoid Junction	15	0.80	2	0.21	84	1.15	187	1.77	384	1.23	655	1.34	672	1.30
Rectum	281	15.05	119	12.27	630	8.66	1400	13.24	5126	16.45	7156	14.60	7556	14.57
Anus, Anal Canal, & Anorectum	—	—	—	—	13	0.18	24	0.23	70	0.22	107	0.22	107	0.21
Liver and Intrahepatic Bile Duct	—	—	—	—	21	0.29	71	0.67	215	0.69	307	0.63	307	0.59
Liver	—	—	—	—	21	0.29	70	0.66	213	0.68	304	0.62	304	0.59
Intrahepatic Bile Duct	—	—	—	—	0	0.00	1	0.01	2	0.01	3	0.01	3	0.01
Gallbladder	1	0.05	—	—	9	0.12	41	0.39	100	0.32	150	0.31	151	0.29
Other Biliary	1	0.05	—	—	18	0.25	43	0.41	128	0.41	189	0.39	190	0.37
Pancreas	—	—	—	—	706	9.70	704	6.66	2188	7.02	3598	7.34	3598	6.94
Retroperitoneum	—	—	—	—	5	0.07	9	0.09	43	0.14	57	0.12	57	0.11
Peritoneum, Omentum, & Mesentery	—	—	—	—	5	0.07	14	0.13	86	0.28	105	0.21	105	0.20
Other Digestive Organs	27	1.45	8	0.82	39	0.54	45	0.43	175	0.56	259	0.53	294	0.57

Abbreviation: NOS, not otherwise specified.

Tumors of the skin are excluded in the figures mentioned.

[a] ERG and TNCS data include carcinoid histology only, whereas SEER data include both carcinoid and endocrinoma histology.

Table 3
Age-adjusted incidence of GEP-NETs at 5-year intervals across the SEER 9 registry from 1973–2007. The GEP-NET incidence over the past 5 years is 3.65 per 100,000. The incidence of GEP-NETs is increasing, and this increase is evident at all GEP-NET primary sites

NET Site	1973–1977	1978–1982	1983–1987	1988–1992	1993–1997	1998–2002	2003–2007	1973–2007
All Sites	1.43	1.48	2.10	3.03	3.80	4.74	5.76	3.46
Gastroenteropancreatic Sites	1.00	1.01	1.30	1.88	2.19	2.94	3.65	2.16
Esophagus	0.00	0.00	0.00	0.00	0.01	0.01	0.01	0.01
Stomach	0.03	0.05	0.08	0.13	0.16	0.29	0.33	0.17
Small Intestine	0.38	0.43	0.54	0.68	0.80	0.89	1.08	0.72
Duodenum	0.02	0.02	0.04	0.08	0.12	0.14	0.25	0.11
Jejunum	0.03	0.03	0.04	0.05	0.05	0.04	0.05	0.04
Ileum	0.26	0.26	0.27	0.33	0.37	0.39	0.45	0.34
Meckel diverticulum	0.00	0.00	0.01	0.01	0.02	0.02	0.01	0.01
Overlapping Lesion of Small Intestine	0.00	0.00	0.00	0.01	0.01	0.01	0.01	0.01
Small Intestine, NOS	0.07	0.12	0.17	0.20	0.24	0.28	0.30	0.21
Colon and Rectum	0.40	0.34	0.48	0.75	0.89	1.32	1.65	0.91
Colon Excluding Rectum	0.30	0.26	0.27	0.33	0.38	0.49	0.60	0.40
Cecum	0.07	0.07	0.09	0.11	0.13	0.16	0.19	0.12
Appendix	0.15	0.12	0.10	0.10	0.10	0.14	0.20	0.13
Ascending Colon	0.02	0.01	0.02	0.02	0.03	0.04	0.04	0.03
Hepatic Flexure	0.00	0.01	0.00	0.01	0.01	0.01	0.01	0.01
Transverse Colon	0.01	0.01	0.01	0.01	0.01	0.01	0.01	0.01
Splenic Flexure	0.00	0.00	0.00	0.01	0.00	0.00	0.01	0.00

Descending Colon	0.01	0.01	0.01	0.01	0.01	0.01	0.01	0.01
Sigmoid Colon	0.01	0.02	0.03	0.05	0.07	0.08	0.09	0.06
Large Intestine, NOS	0.02	0.01	0.02	0.02	0.03	0.04	0.04	0.03
Rectum and Rectosigmoid Junction	0.10	0.08	0.21	0.42	0.51	0.82	1.05	0.52
Rectosigmoid Junction	0.01	0.01	0.02	0.05	0.05	0.07	0.08	0.05
Rectum	0.09	0.08	0.19	0.36	0.46	0.75	0.97	0.47
Anus, Anal Canal, & Anorectum	0.00	0.00	0.00	0.01	0.01	0.01	0.01	0.01
Liver and Intrahepatic Bile Duct	0.00	0.00	0.00	0.02	0.03	0.03	0.04	0.02
Liver	0.00	0.00	0.00	0.02	0.03	0.03	0.04	0.02
Intrahepatic Bile Duct	0.00	0.00	0.00	0.00	0.00	0.00	0.00	0.00
Gall bladder	0.00	0.00	0.00	0.01	0.02	0.01	0.01	0.01
Other Biliary	0.00	0.00	0.01	0.01	0.02	0.02	0.03	0.01
Pancreas	0.17	0.17	0.18	0.26	0.24	0.32	0.43	0.27
Retroperitoneum	0.00	0.00	0.00	0.00	0.00	0.01	0.01	0.00
Peritoneum, Omentum, & Mesentery	0.00	0.00	0.00	0.00	0.01	0.01	0.01	0.01
Other Digestive Organs	0.01	0.01	0.01	0.01	0.02	0.03	0.05	0.02

Abbreviation: NOS, not otherwise specified.

Rates are per 100,000 and age adjusted to the 2000 US standard population (19 age groups, census P25–1130) standard.

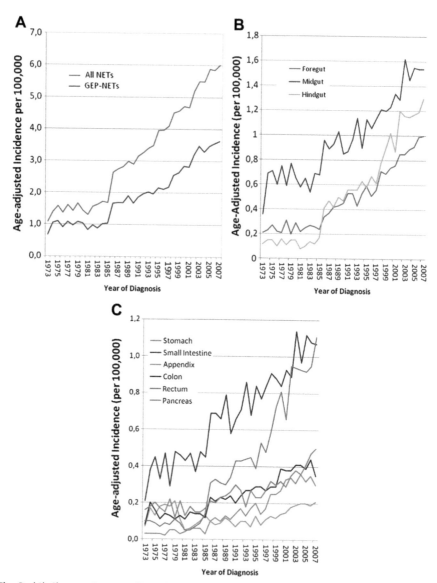

Fig. 2. (*A*) Changes in age-adjusted incidence of GEP-NETs (SEER 9 registry, 1973–2007). (*B*) Age-adjusted incidence based on embryologic site of origin. (*C*) Age-adjusted incidence by GEP-NET primary site (both SEER 9 registry). Total GEP-NETs (*A*) and GEP-NETs of all embryologic classifications (*B*) have increased between 1973 and 2007. The most substantial change in incidence over time occurred in small intestinal and rectal NETs, and these are now the most common GEP-NETs. However, the highest APC (not shown) occurred for rectal primaries (+8.2%), followed by gastric (+7.6%), colonic (+4.4%), small intestinal (+3.5%), pancreatic (+3.4%), and appendiceal primaries (+1.1%). All increases were statistically significant (least weighted squares method, *P*<.05).

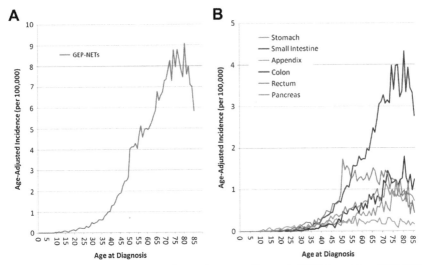

Fig. 3. Mean age-adjusted incidence for each age at diagnosis (SEER 9 registry, 1973–2007). (*A*) All GEP-NETs. (*B*) Individual GEP-NET primary sites. The incidence of GEP-NETs peaks between approximately 70 and 80 years of age, with the median age being 63 years. Small intestinal, gastric, and colonic NET incidences follow a pattern similar to the total GEP-NET group. Rectal NET incidence increases sharply to a peak at age 50 years and decreases gradually as age increases. Pancreatic NET incidence also increases relatively early, with little change beyond age 65 years. Appendiceal NET incidence shows little relationship to age.

over the subsequent 4 decades (see **Fig. 3**B). Appendiceal tumors reveal little change with age.

The changes in incidence for the common GEP-NET primary sites are identified by stage at diagnosis in **Fig. 4**. There has been a substantial increase in the incidence of localized rectal primary sites (see **Fig. 4**A) but only a minimal increase at regional (see **Fig 4**B) and distant (see **Fig 4**C) disease stages. Small intestinal NETs were increasingly diagnosed with local and regional spread, and pancreatic NETs were increasingly likely to show distant disease at the time of diagnosis. However, recent developments in NET identification (^{68}Ga-DOTA-Tyr3-octreotide positron emission tomography) suggest that metastatic lesions are underdetected using less specific imaging modalities, and many tumors are therefore understaged. In addition, it is likely that grade is as important (or more important) than stage in determining survival. Because nearly half of tumors in the SEER 17 database were not assigned a grade; this aspect of the analysis cannot be considered adequately rigorous (**Fig. 5**).

The common primary GEP-NET sites exhibited somewhat different epidemiologic characteristics. For example, rectal NETs occurred in younger patients (peak at age 50 years), were diagnosed while still localized, and demonstrated a high 5-year survival (around 88% between 1973 and 2002 [SEER 17]). Appendiceal NETs occured at all ages but also tend to be localized and demonstrated a high 5-year survival (more than 80%). Pancreatic NETs tended to occur in patients in their 60s and 70s, were diagnosed at a higher stage, and exhibited poor 5-year survival (<40%). The incidence, age at diagnosis, stage at diagnosis, and 5-year survival of each primary GEP-NET can be compared in **Figs. 2–4** and **6**.

The overall observed 5-year survival rate of GEP NETs was 68.1%. Pancreatic NETs showed the lowest 5-year survival rates (37.6%), whereas rectal NETs exhibited the highest 5-year survival rates (88.5%) (see **Fig. 6**). For individual NET primaries, curve

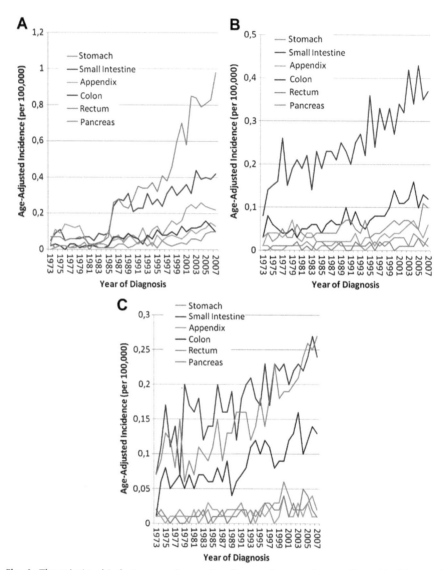

Fig. 4. The relationship between primary site, disease stage, and age-adjusted incidence of GEP-NETs of localized (*A*), regional (*B*), or distant (*C*) stage (SEER 9 registry, 1973–2007). Most rectal primaries were localized at diagnosis, and the incidence of localized rectal NETs increased significantly since 1986 (*A*). Small intestinal NETs were diagnosed with localized disease or regional spread more often than distant disease (*A–C*), but incidence is increasing at all stages. Pancreatic NETs were more likely to be diagnosed with distant spread, and this trend is also increasing (*C*).

modeling demonstrated a linear decline for rectal, appendiceal, and small intestinal primaries, whereas the survival curve for gastric, colonic, and pancreatic primaries best fitted an exponential decay curve. Decay curve analysis enabled calculation of half-lives for these 3 primary sites, with elapsed time to 50% of expected patient deaths being 10.3 months for colonic NETs, 16.7 months for gastric NETs, and 18.9 for pancreatic NETs.

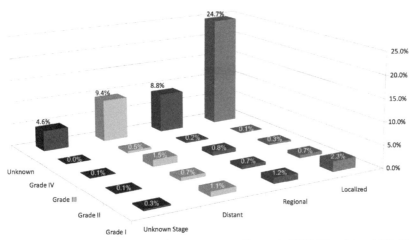

25.0%
20.0%
15.0%
10.0%
5.0%
0.0%

Fig. 5. Stage and grade at diagnosis for GEP-NETs at diagnosis (SEER 17 registry, 1973–2007). Nearly half of the tumors were not graded (47.5%). If data are available, localized tumors tend to have lower grades.

The APC in survival for GEP NETs increased by an average of 0.98% per year across the 34 years of the SEER registry (**Fig. 7**). The PC in survival for GEP-NETs increased by 23.6% during the period of the SEER database (relative change from 1973–1974 to 2001–2002). This change did not occur at a steady rate, and previous analyses had described a change in survival after 1987 in some patients with NET.[5] We compared the mean APC before and after 1988, 1990, and 1992 for patients with GEP-NETs. The mean APC before and after 1988 was +0.62 and +0.92, respectively and before and after 1990 was +0.79 and +1.13, respectively. However, the mean APC before and after 1992 was +0.77 and +0.65, respectively. We interpret this to indicate that the APC seemed to improve after 1988 and 1990 but decline after 1992.

DISCUSSION

The overall incidence of GEP-NETs continues to exhibit a persistent increase, maintaining the trend noted in earlier epidemiologic studies.[5,10–13] Although the incidence increased at all primary sites, the change is mostly accounted for by the escalation in rectal and small intestinal NETs, with the highest proportional change occurring in rectal and gastric NETs. Because the anatomic location exhibiting the most change is luminal, it is appealing to attribute observations of increase to the increasing availability of routine and surveillance endoscopy. The usage of diagnostic modalities, including gastroscopy (gastric and proximal small intestinal NETs), colonoscopy (colonic, rectal, and distal small intestinal NETs), and capsule endoscopy (small intestinal NETs), has escalated in everyday medical and gastroenterological practice. Certainly, the substantial increase in rectal NETs at age 50 years corresponds to the recommended onset of colonoscopic screening programs in the United States.[19] It might also be argued that other opportunities for detection are increasing, such as gynecologic laparoscopy in women.[20] Conversely, because the most common method of appendiceal NET diagnosis is an incidental finding during surgical treatment of acute appendicitis,[21] the relative stability of appendiceal NET incidence mirrors the stable or diminished frequency of appendectomy worldwide[22] and loss of opportunity for tumor detection. Overall, it seems likely that much of the registered

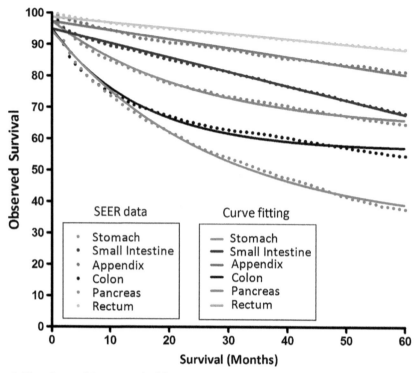

Fig. 6. The observed 5-year survival for GEP-NET primary sites (SEER 17 registry, 1973–2007). Pancreatic NETs exhibited the lowest 5-year survival (37.6%), whereas rectal NETs showed the highest (88.5%). The 5-year survival for colonic, gastric, small intestinal, and appendiceal NETs were 54.6%, 64.1%, 68.1%, and 81.3%, respectively. The slope of the survival curve for each group was modeled using either linear or 1-phase exponential decay. The best fit was achieved with a linear model for rectal, appendiceal, and small intestinal NETs and an exponential decay curve for gastric, colonic, and pancreatic NETs (R^2 for the fitted curves ranged from 0.97–0.99, $P<.001$). Where a decay curve was used, the calculated half-life estimates the time to 50% of expected deaths; colonic NETs (10.3 months), gastric NETs (16.7 months), and pancreatic NETs (18.9 months).

increased incidence of GEP-NETs could be, at least partially, explained by alteration in diagnostic surveillance. Whether or not a real increase in incidence is taking place remains to be elucidated, and more likely than not, it is a combination of both an increasing incidence and amplified diagnostic recognition.

The PC in survival for GEP-NETs increased by 23% from 1973 to 2002; expressed as APC, survival improved by an average of 0.98% relative to each preceding year. It has been previously proposed that overall survival in metastatic NETs improved after 1987[5] and that this reflected the introduction of novel pharmaceutical agents. In the current study of GEP-NETs, survival seemed to improve using a cutoff of 1988 or 1990 but was reduced using a cutoff of 1992. Caution should therefore be exercised in using arbitrary cut-points. Indeed, it is difficult to rigorously separate the effect of novel therapy from a panorama of changes in disease management, which include the introduction of novel diagnostic strategies, alterations in nomenclature, classification, grading, and staging, when attempting to explain perturbations in survival rates. Nevertheless, overall improvement in APC likely reflects the effect of more effective therapy and earlier and more accurate diagnosis with relative downstaging.

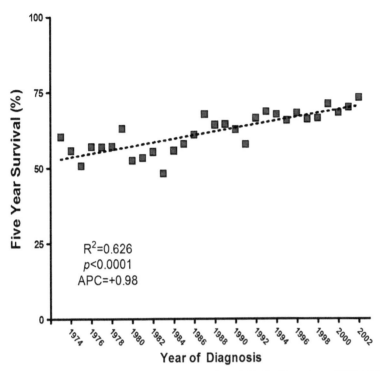

Fig. 7. Annual GEP-NET survival between 1973 and 2002 (SEER 17 registry, 1973–2007). The average survival (1973–2002) for GEP-NETs was 68.1%. Calculation of the APC by regression analysis indicates a linear relationship between survival and year of diagnosis ($R^2 = 0.63$, $P<.001$). The APC has increased by 0.98% per year for the duration of the registry. The overall PC from the beginning to the end of the registry period was 23.1%, and this alteration is significant ($P<.05$).

The 5-year survival rates of GEP-NETs differ depending on the primary site of the tumor. Further, the survival curves showed a different profile of change over time, and curve fitting suggests that gastric, colonic, and pancreatic primaries exhibit an exponential decay in survival over time. A decay curve has 2 implications: (1) survival for these cancers plateau at some point in the future and (2) the curve allows calculation of half life or the time at which half of expected deaths occurs. Despite the poorer 5-year survival rate for pancreatic cancer (37.6%), the time to 50% of expected deaths was longer (18.9 months) than for colonic (10.3 months) primaries, which have a better overall survival rate (54.6%). This steep initial decline may represent a small subset with an aggressive type of tumor who unfortunately meet an early demise, amid a long flat tail corresponding to the bulk of lesions that are less aggressive. These data should be interpreted cautiously but suggest that there must be primary site heterogeneity of NETs and that organ typing of NETs alone is an inadequate prognostic tool. Further molecular descriptors of individual tumors are necessary to identify specific lesions with an aggressive phenotype.

The poor outcome for gastric lesions reflects the heterogeneous nature of NETs at this location, but also suggests some skewing of data based on patient sampling, and limitations in the SEER classification/grading system. It is well recognized that most (70%–80%) gastric NETs are of type I with a survival the same as the general population[3]; therefore the SEER data presumably reflect a disproportionate number of type III lesions; in fact the SEER criteria do not require mandatory reporting of benign lesions[23] and it is likely that type I gastric NETs are regarded as benign by most pathologists and therefore underreported.

International comparison of NET distribution suggests some differences in primary tumor localization. In the SEER 17 registry (2000–2007), the rectum (17.7%) and small intestine (17.3%) are the most common NET primary sites, and the total number of NETs at both these sites has increased markedly; the rectum has now replaced the small intestine as the most common primary site for GEP-NETs. Although European countries show a similar incidence and distribution of tumors,[11] smaller studies from Asian countries exhibit a different pattern. A retrospective series[24] in a single hospital in Taiwan revealed 228 cases of carcinoid tumors diagnosed between 1970 and 2005, of which 60.5% presented in the rectum, and only 4.8% in the small intestine. Similar results were evident in a recent Japanese study of 1027 NETs; 28.2% were of foregut origin, 5.2% of midgut origin, and 66.0% of hindgut origin.[25] Although this finding raises the possibility of genetic/racial variation in NET incidence and tumor localization, an alternative explanation is that this may simply reflect differences in diagnostic practices and the widespread use of endoscopy.

Different geographic localities may also be associated with rates of GEP-NET survival. Among 12 European countries, 5-year survival was considerably better for the Western European countries (64.2%) compared with the United Kingdom and Eastern European countries (55.1%).[26] Similar results were demonstrated in another large European multicenter study that included 7693 patients with GEP-NETs in which the 5-year survival for small intestinal NETs was 64.7%, 54.8% and 39.9%, respectively for Northern, Western, and Eastern Europe.[27] These findings probably reflect the effect of environmental and socioeconomic factors as well as the level of sophistication, structure, and health care delivery systems in influencing long-term outcome. Similarly, it is likely that the level of availability of multidisciplinary clinics and novel targeted pharmacotherapy varies widely in different geographic locations; lack of tertiary or quaternary care and a paucity of diagnostic and therapeutic intervention have a negative effect on the optimization of disease outcome.

SUMMARY

GEP-NET disease is increasing in incidence, and there is evidence that in specific areas such as rectum, small intestine, and stomach, this incidence is escalating at a greater rate. There is a distinct epidemiologic profile for each primary site. For example, rectal NETs are diagnosed at a younger age and a lower stage and demonstrate good survival, whereas colonic NETs are diagnosed at an older age and a higher stage and have poor survival. As might be expected, based on advances in diagnosis and therapy, it is evident that there is an overall improvement in outcome. However, the relatively modest increments reflect limited medical education regarding NETs, inadequate disease awareness, late diagnosis, absence of predictably effective targeted therapy, paucity of research funding, and limitations in the knowledge of the molecular and biologic basis of the diverse spectrum of GEP-NETs.

REFERENCES

1. Modlin IM, Oberg K, Chung DC, et al. Gastroenteropancreatic neuroendocrine tumours. Lancet Oncol 2008;9(1):61–72.
2. Zikusoka MN, Kidd M, Eick G, et al. The molecular genetics of gastroenteropancreatic neuroendocrine tumors. Cancer 2005;104(11):2292–309.

3. Scherubl H, Cadiot G, Jensen RT, et al. Neuroendocrine tumors of the stomach (gastric carcinoids) are on the rise: small tumors, small problems? Endoscopy 2010;42(8):664–71.
4. Surveillance, Epidemiology, and End Results (SEER) Program. SEER*Stat Database: Incidence - SEER 17 Regs Research Data + Hurricane Katrina Impacted Louisiana Cases, Nov 2009 Sub (1973-2007 varying) - Linked To County Attributes - Total U.S., 1969-2007 Counties, National Cancer Institute, DCCPS, Surveillance Research Program, Cancer Statistics Branch, released April 2010, based on the November 2009 submission. Available at: www.seer.cancer.gov. Accessed May 12, 2009.
5. Yao JC, Hassan M, Phan A, et al. One hundred years after "carcinoid": epidemiology of and prognostic factors for neuroendocrine tumors in 35,825 cases in the United States. J Clin Oncol 2008;26(18):3063–72.
6. Williams ED, Sandler M. The classification of carcinoid tumours. Lancet 1963; 1(7275):238–9.
7. Soga J, Tazawa K. Pathologic analysis of carcinoids. Histologic reevaluation of 62 cases. Cancer 1971;28(4):990–8.
8. Pearse AG. The diffuse neuroendocrine system and the apud concept: related "endocrine" peptides in brain, intestine, pituitary, placenta, and anuran cutaneous glands. Med Biol 1977;55(3):115–25.
9. Solcia E, Kloppel G, Sobin L. Histological typing of endocrine tumours: WHO International Histological Classification of Tumours. Berlin: Springer; 2000.
10. Perez EA, Koniaris LG, Snell SE, et al. 7201 carcinoids: increasing incidence overall and disproportionate mortality in the elderly. World J Surg 2007;31(5): 1022–30.
11. Hauso O, Gustafsson BI, Kidd M, et al. Neuroendocrine tumor epidemiology: contrasting Norway and North America. Cancer 2008;113(10):2655–64.
12. Modlin IM, Lye KD, Kidd M. A 5-decade analysis of 13,715 carcinoid tumors. Cancer 2003;97(4):934–59.
13. Gustafsson BI, Siddique L, Chan A, et al. Uncommon cancers of the small intestine, appendix and colon: an analysis of SEER 1973-2004, and current diagnosis and therapy. Int J Oncol 2008;33(6):1121–31.
14. Klimstra DS, Modlin IR, Adsay NV, et al. Pathology reporting of neuroendocrine tumors: application of the Delphic consensus process to the development of a minimum pathology data set. Am J Surg Pathol 2010;34(3):300–13.
15. Modlin IM, Moss SF, Chung DC, et al. Priorities for improving the management of gastroenteropancreatic neuroendocrine tumors. J Natl Cancer Inst 2008;100(18): 1282–9.
16. Rinke A, Muller HH, Schade-Brittinger C, et al. Placebo-controlled, double-blind, prospective, randomized study on the effect of octreotide LAR in the control of tumor growth in patients with metastatic neuroendocrine midgut tumors: a report from the PROMID Study Group. J Clin Oncol 2009;27(28): 4656–63.
17. Shambaugh EM, Weiss MA, Axtell MM, editors. Surveillance Epidemiology and End Results Reporting. Summary staging guide cancer. Bethesda (MD): National Institute of Health; 1977.
18. American Joint Committee on Cancer. Manual for staging of cancer. Chicago: Illinois; 1977.
19. US Preventative Health Services Task Force. Screening for colorectal cancer: U.S. preventive services task force recommendation statement. Rockville (MD): Agency for Health Research and Quality; 2008.

20. Modlin IM. A brief history of endoscopy. Milano (Italy): NextHealth; 1999.
21. Tchana-Sato V, Detry O, Polus M, et al. Carcinoid tumor of the appendix: a consecutive series from 1237 appendectomies. World J Gastroenterol 2006; 12(41):6699–701.
22. Donnelly NJ, Semmens JB, Fletcher DR, et al. Appendicectomy in Western Australia: profile and trends, 1981–1997. Med J Aust 2001;175(1):15–8.
23. SEER Program. Cancer characteristics and selection of cases. Self instructional manual for cancer registrars: book 2 1992. Available at: www.seer.gov/training/manuals/. Accessed July 15, 2009.
24. Li AF, Hsu CY, Li A, et al. A 35-year retrospective study of carcinoid tumors in Taiwan: differences in distribution with a high probability of associated second primary malignancies. Cancer 2008;112(2):274–83.
25. Onozato Y, Kakizaki S, Ishihara H, et al. Endoscopic submucosal dissection for rectal tumors. Endoscopy 2007;39(5):423–7.
26. Lepage C, Ciccolallo L, De Angelis R, et al. European disparities in malignant digestive endocrine tumours survival. Int J Cancer 2009;126(12):2928–34.
27. Gatta G, Ciccolallo L, Kunkler I, et al. Survival from rare cancer in adults: a population-based study. Lancet Oncol 2006;7(2):132–40.

New and Emerging Syndromes due to Neuroendocrine Tumors

Aaron I. Vinik, MD, PhD, FCP, MACP[a],*,
Michael Raymund C. Gonzales, MD[b]

KEYWORDS

- Neuroendocrine tumors ● Biochemical markers
- Differential diagnosis ● Pancreatic neuroendocrine tumors

Neuroendocrine tumors (NETs) are rare, slow-growing neoplasms characterized by their ability to store and secrete different peptides and neuroamines.[1] Some of these substances cause specific clinical syndromes[2] whereas others are not associated with specific syndromes or symptom complexes. There is no "ideal neuroendocrine tumor marker,[3]" but according to the presentation, the sensitivity and specificity of each marker varies, and it is possible to choose those of greatest value for each clinical syndrome.

The biochemical markers are hormones or amines secreted by the neuroendocrine cells from which these tumors are derived. Some are not specific to any tumor, but are secreted by most NETs; other biochemical markers are more specific to a type of tumor whereby their quantification can lead to the diagnosis. **Table 1** summarizes a suggested approach to diagnose a NET based on the clinical presentation, the tumor type, their sites of origin, the possible means of diagnosis, and the biochemical markers that should be measured.

The annual incidence of neuroendocrine tumors (NETs) has risen to 40 to 50 cases per million, due to better diagnosis, the availability of highly specific and sensitive ways to measure these tumors' characteristics, and improved immunohistochemistry techniques for tumor detection (**Fig. 1**). The perceived increase in incidence may be a false-positive one. In a review of the SEER (Surveillance Epidemiology and End Results) database it has now been shown that the prevalence of NETs in the United States is about 100,000 cases, which is twice the prevalence of gastric and pancreatic

[a] Eastern Virginia Medical School, Strelitz Diabetes Center, 855 West Brambleton Avenue, Norfolk, VA 23510, USA
[b] Division of Endocrinology and Metabolism, Department of Internal Medicine, Eastern Virginia Medical School, Norfolk, VA 23501-1980, USA
* Corresponding author.
E-mail address: vinikai@evms.edu

Endocrinol Metab Clin N Am 40 (2011) 19–63
doi:10.1016/j.ecl.2010.12.010
0889-8529/11/$ – see front matter © 2011 Elsevier Inc. All rights reserved.

Table 1
Clinical presentations, syndromes, tumor types, sites, and hormones[4]

Clinical Presentation	Syndrome	Tumor Type	Sites	Hormones
Flushing	Carcinoid Medullary carcinoma of thyroid Pheochromocytoma	Carcinoid C-cell tumor Tumor of chromaffin cells	Mid/foregut adrenal medulla gastric Thyroid C cells Adrenal and sympathetic nervous system	Serotonin, CGRP, calcitonin Metanephrine and normetanephrine
Diarrhea, abdominal pain, and dyspepsia	Carcinoid, WDHHA, ZE, PP, MCT	Carcinoid, VIPoma, gastrinoma, PPoma, medullary carcinoma thyroid, mastocytoma	As above, pancreas, mast cells, thyroid	As above, VIP, gastrin, PP, calcitonin
Diarrhea/steatorrhea	Somatostatin Bleeding GI tract	Somatostatinoma, neurofibromatosis	Pancreas Duodenum	Somatostatin
Wheezing	Carcinoid	Carcinoid	Gut/pancreas/lung	SP, CGRP, serotonin
Ulcer/dyspepsia	Zollinger-Ellison	Gastrinoma	Pancreas/duodenum	Gastrin
Hypoglycemia	Whipple's triad	Insulinoma, sarcoma, hepatoma	Pancreas, retroperitoneal liver	Insulin, IGF-1, IGF-11
Dermatitis	Sweet syndrome Pellagra	Glucagonoma Carcinoid	Pancreas Midgut	Glucagon Serotonin
Dementia	Sweet syndrome	Glucagonoma	Pancreas	Glucagon
Diabetes	Glucagonoma Somatostatin	Glucagonoma Somatostatinoma	Pancreas Pancreas	Glucagon Somatostatin
DVT, steatorrhea, cholelithiasis, neurofibromatosis	Somatostatin	Somatostatinoma	Pancreas Duodenum	Somatostatin
Silent, liver metastases	Silent	PPOMA	Pancreas	PP

Abbreviations: CGRP, calcitonin gene-related peptide; PP, pancreatic polypeptide; IGF, insulin-like growth factor; VIP, vasoactive intestinal peptide; MCT, medullary carcinoma of thyroid; SP, substance P.

Data from Vinik A, O'Dorisio T, Woltering E, et al. Neuroendocrine tumors: a comprehensive guide to diagnosis and management. 1st edition. Inglewood (CA): Interscience Institute; 2006.

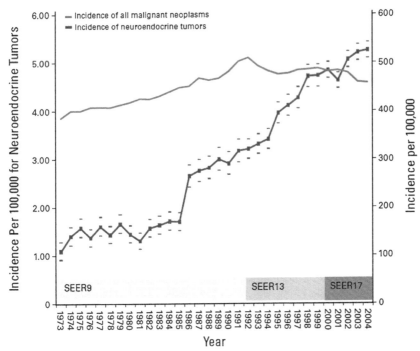

Fig. 1. Incidence of neuroendocrine tumors (NETs) over time. Annual age-adjusted incidence of NETs by year (1973–2004). The incidence is presented as the number of tumors per 100,000 (with 95% confidence intervals) age-adjusted for the 2000 United States standard population. Cases were selected from the Surveillance, Epidemiology, and End Results database (1973–2004). (*Data from* Yao JC, Hassan M, Phan A, et al. One hundred years after "carcinoid": epidemiology of and prognostic factors for neuroendocrine tumors in 35,825 cases in the United States. J Clin Oncol 2008;26:3063–73.)

cancer combined. The great majority (56%) of these tumors are carcinoid and the remainder are pancreatic neuroendocrine (PNETs).

There are impediments to the diagnosis of these tumors. First, they comprise less than 2% of gastrointestinal malignancies and are therefore not the first diagnosis considered. Symptoms are often nonspecific and do not lend themselves to identifying the specific underlying tumor. The manifestations are protean and mimic a variety of disorders. For example, midgut carcinoids may be confused with irritable bowel syndrome (IBS). The natural history of this disease is invariably attended by a long history of vague abdominal symptoms, visits to a primary care practitioner, and referral to a gastroenterologist, with a misdiagnosis of IBS. In terms of natural history, the median latency to correct diagnosis of carcinoid tumors is 9.2 years by which time the tumor has metastasized, causing symptoms like flushing and diarrhea, and progressing slowly until the patient dies (**Fig. 2**). Thus, a greater index of suspicion and a carcinoid tumor profile screen is warranted for all patients presenting with "traditional IBS symptoms." Midgut carcinoids are associated with mesenteric fibrosis, which can compress mesenteric vessels and cause bowel ischemia and malabsorption, which may be found in the absence of an abdominal mass. The diagnosis of metastases to the liver often takes place after a delay of many years. Even then an incorrect diagnosis is not uncommon; unless biopsy material is examined for the secretory peptides chromogranin, synaptophysin, or neuron-specific enolase (NSE),

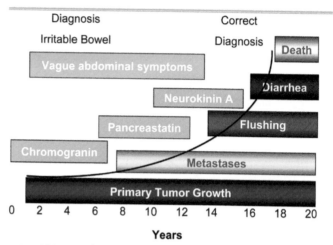

Fig. 2. The natural history of carcinoid tumors. Vague symptoms such as abdominal pain precede the diagnosis by a median of 9.2 years, and flushing and diarrhea, the major manifestations of carcinoid NETs, occur after the tumor has metastasized. Also shown is the relationship between tumor extent and when the biochemical markers are positive when measured in blood. Pancreastatin and neurokinin are both important, as they correlate with mortality, metastases, and survival, respectively. (*Data from* Vinik A. Biochemical testing for neuroendocrine tumors. Pancreas 2009;38:876–89.)

tumors may be labeled erroneously as adenocarcinoma, affecting management and underestimating prospects for survival.[4] This holds true for all NETs, as a delay in diagnosis with resulting tumor progression directly affects survival (**Fig. 3**).

FLUSHING

Cutaneous flushing, a common presenting complaint to dermatologists, internists, and family practitioners, results from changes in cutaneous blood flow triggered by

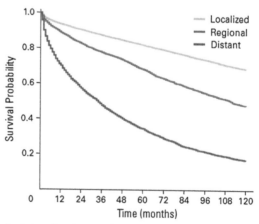

Fig. 3. Median Survival duration in months based on extent of tumor. (*Data from* Yao JC, Hassan M, Phan A, et al. One hundred years after "carcinoid": epidemiology of and prognostic factors for neuroendocrine tumors in 35,825 cases in the United States. J Clin Oncol 2008;26:3063–73.)

multiple conditions. Most cases are caused by very common, benign diseases, such as rosacea or climacterum, which are readily apparent after a thorough taking of history and physical examination. However, in some cases accurate diagnosis requires studies to differentiate important entities such as carcinoid syndrome and pheochromocytoma (**Table 2**). Obtaining a good history of the nature of the flushing is vital to ascertain whether this can be ascribed to a NET. Is the flushing wet or dry? If dry it is almost always caused by a NET. If it is wet it may still be due to a NET with diaphoresis caused by coexistent anxiety. Intermittent flushing suggests menopause or a NET, for example, systemic mastocytosis or pheochromocytoma. Constant flushing is found with alcoholism, polycythemia, and mitral valve stenosis or prolapse. If there is a facial rash it may be rosacea and, if more diffuse, mastocytosis with the attendant dermatographia or dermatomyositis should be considered. Associated symptoms or signs such as diarrhea suggest a NET, either carcinoid or medullary carcinoma of the thyroid. Headache occurs with mastocytosis or pheochromocytoma and syncope suggests autonomic neuropathy, pheochromocytoma, or epilepsy. Flushing in NETs varies depending on the location of the tumor.

In foregut, carcinoid tumor flushing is dry, long lasting, intense, and has a purplish or violet hue in contrast to the common red/pink hue seen in other NE-related flushing. Telangiectasia and skin hypertrophy occurs in the face and upper neck but can also involve the limbs, and can lead to a leonine appearance after repeated episodes.

In midgut tumors, flushing is a faint pink to red color involving the face and upper trunk as far as the nipple line. The flush is provoked by exercise, alcohol, and food containing tyramines (eg, blue cheese, chocolate, red sausage, and red wine). With time, it may occur spontaneously and without provocation. It becomes ephemeral, lasting only a few minutes, and may occur many times per day; however, after years patients may develop a persistent flush with a purpuric malar and nasal complexion. As mentioned, the differential diagnosis for flushing is numerous and in order to

Table 2	
Differential diagnosis of flushing and recommended tests	
Clinical Condition	**Tests**
Carcinoid	Serotonin, 5-HIAA, NKA, TCP, PP, CGRP, VIP, SP, PGD2, PGE1, PGF2
Medullary carcinoma of the thyroid	Calcitonin, Ca^{2+} infusion, RET proto-oncogene
Pheocromocytoma	CgA, Plasma free metanephrines, urine metanephrines, VMA, Epi, Norepi, glucagon stimulation, MIBG
Diabetic autonomic neuropathy	HRV, 2hs PP glucose
Menopause	FSH
Epilepsy	EEG
Panic attack	Pentagastrin, ACTH
Mastocytosis	Plasma histamine, urine tryptase
Hypomastia and mitral valve prolapse	Cardiac echo

Abbreviations: ACTH, adrenocorticotropic hormone; CgA, chromogranin A; EEG, electroencephalography; Epi, epinephrine; FSH, follicle-stimulating hormone; 5-HIAA, 5-hydroxyindoleacetic acid; HRV, heart rate variability; 2hs PP, 2-hour postprandial blood sugar; MIBG, metaiodobenzylguanidine; NKA, neurokinin A; Norepi, norepinephrine; PGD2, prostaglandin D2; PGE1, prostaglandin E1; PGE2, prostaglandin E2; PP, pancreatic polypeptide; TCP, tricalcium phosphate; VMA, vanillylmandelic acid.

differentiate all those causes from a carcinoid tumor, besides knowing the characteristics of the flushing it is also necessary to know what is producing the flushing.

Flushing in carcinoid syndrome has been ascribed to prostaglandins, kinins, and serotonin (5-HT). The advent of sophisticated radioimmunoassay methods and region-specific antisera has resulted in several neurohumors thought to be secreted by carcinoid tumors, including serotonin, dopamine, histamine, 5-hydroxyindole acetic acid (5-HIAA), kallikrein, substance P (SP), neurotensin, motilin, somatostatin, vasoactive intestinal polypeptide (VIP), prostaglandins, neuropeptide K, and gastrin-releasing peptide (GRP).

Several provocative tests have been developed to identify the cause of flushing in carcinoid syndrome. These tests are based on the need to distinguish the flushing from that in other conditions such as panic syndrome, where the associated anxiety and phobias establishes the cause but frequently there is a need to rule out an underlying malignancy.

Feldman and O'Dorisio[5] have previously reported the incidence of elevated levels of plasma neuropeptide concentrations in patients with flushing. Despite the elevated basal concentrations of SP and neurotensin, these investigators documented further increases in these neuropeptides during ethanol-induced facial flushing.

Ahlman and colleagues[6] reported the results of pentagastrin (PG) provocation in 16 patients with midgut carcinoid tumors and hepatic metastases. All patients had elevated urinary 5-HIAA levels, and 12 had profuse diarrhea requiring medication. PG uniformly induced facial flushing and gastrointestinal (GI) symptoms in patients with liver metastases, but had no effect in healthy control patients. All patients with PG-induced GI symptoms demonstrated elevated serotonin levels in peripheral blood. Administration of a serotonin-receptor antagonist had no effect on serotonin release but completely aborted the GI symptoms. The investigators emphasized the improved reliability of PG compared with calcium infusion—another provocative test popularized by Kaplan and colleagues[7]—and pointed out that PG provocation occasionally can be falsely negative in patients with subclinical disease. Vinik and colleagues[8] reported that PG uniformly induced flushing in patients with gastric carcinoid tumors that was associated with an increase in circulating levels of SP in 80%. Thus, SP is one neurohumor that may be involved in the flushing of carcinoid syndrome.

SP has also been found in tumor extracts and plasma from patients with carcinoid tumors and, in one reported case, was useful for tumor localization. Neurokinin A, its amino-terminally extended form, neuropeptide K, and SP are a group of peptides (ie, tachykinins) with common biologic properties. Norheim and colleagues[9] measured peptide responses to PG or ingestion of food or alcohol in 16 patients with metastatic carcinoid tumors, and demonstrated twofold or greater increases in neurokinin A and neuropeptide K in 75% of patients, as well as variable increases in SP in approximately 20% of patients.

Conlon and colleagues[10] used region-specific antisera to SP and neurokinin A to measure circulating tachykinins during a meal-induced flush in 10 patients with metastatic carcinoid tumors. Five patients had undetectable levels of neurokinin A and SP after stimulation, thus suggesting that elevated tachykinin concentrations are not a constant feature of such patients. The investigators also studied the effect of a somatostatin-analogue administration on meal-induced tachykinin responses in 3 patients with carcinoid tumors. Flushing was aborted in 2 patients, but tachykinin levels were only partially suppressed, indicating that these peptides cannot be solely responsible for the carcinoid flush. When the diagnosis of the underlying cause of flushing has been established, pathogenesis-oriented treatment can be very helpful.

Cunningham and colleagues[11] also performed a study in which they used patients with metastasizing ileocecal serotonin-producing carcinoid tumors (MISPCs) and looked for the relationship of flushing to tachykinin production. These investigators concluded that MISPCs produce many biologically active substances with partially overlapping biologic functions. The biologic processes underlying the specific symptoms of the carcinoid syndrome are probably multifactorial. This study confirmed results from earlier studies showing that tachykinins and 5-HIAA levels are elevated in patients with daily episodes of flushing. The hormone effects were not mutually independent. It is possible that the development of flushing is the result of multihormonal stimulation. Other biologically active substances, such as kallikrein and prostaglandins, may also contribute.

DIARRHEA, ABDOMINAL PAIN, DYSPEPSIA

The key question to ask is whether the diarrhea persists with fasting. Diarrhea of NETs is always secretory whereas diarrhea from other gastrointestinal causes is usually malabsorptive. The most vexing question is to differentiate the diarrhea and abdominal pain and dsyspepsia from IBS. IBS affects a large proportion of the American population (6%–12%) and in Pakistan, Mexico, and Brazil may be as high as 40%. IBS occurs more frequently in young white females, begins before the age of 35 years in 50% of cases, and the symptoms do not disturb sleep, quite unlike those of NETs. Bleeding, fever, weight loss, and persistent severe pain are not features of IBS. Most sufferers (7.4%) report alternating constipation and diarrhea, distinguishing them from NETs, and the diarrhea does not persist with fasting. Secretory diarrhea is characteristic of NETs, causing large-volume stools, persists with fasting, and there is no osmotic gap between serum and stool. Other causes of secretory diarrhea included in the differential diagnosis are: watery diarrhea, hypokalemia, hyperchlorhydria and acidosis (WDHHA) syndrome, the Zollinger-Ellison syndrome (ZES), carcinoid tumors, medullary carcinoma of the thyroid (MCT), secreting villous adenoma of the rectum, surreptitious laxative abuse, and idiopathic cause. Diarrhea that disappears with the use of a proton pump inhibitor (PPI) is very suspicious of a gastrinoma. The use of somatostatin analogues can change the character of diarrhea from secretory to malabsorptive. Somatostatin analogues cause inhibition of pancreatic enzyme secretion and the intestinal absorption of fluid and nutrients, resulting in steatorrhea.

NETs can produce diarrhea by different mechanisms depending on their secretory products. Gastrin increases the acid secretion by the stomach, which in turn inactivates lipase, amylase, and trypsin, and damages the mucosa of the small bowel, leading to decreased absorption and impaired digestion in the small bowel, giving an increased fecal volume as in malabsorptive syndromes and sometimes steatorrhea. Carcinoid or other NETs can produce other substances such as VIP, pancreatic polypeptide (PP), SP, calcitonin gene related peptide (CGRP), and/or thyrocalcitonin, which act on the small bowel, increasing the secretion of fluids and ions, exceeding the colonic absorptive capacity, and producing an increased fecal volume and loss of electrolytes.

Laxative abuse is difficult to detect and, in all circumstances, a potassium hydroxide stool preparation to detect laxatives is mandatory. Measurement of intestinal secretion by passing a multilumen tube and quantifying electrolytes and water transport, in addition to the measurement of stool electrolytes, which should account for the total osmolarity, helps to exclude laxative abuse but is rarely performed.

It is important to mention that Cunningham and colleagues[11] found, in their study of tachykinins and neuroendocrine tumors, that there is an association between the elevation of tachykinins and the severity of the diarrhea. It was concluded that all biochemical marker concentrations were elevated in patients with daily episodes of diarrhea, although the association between increased plasma tachykinins and the severity of diarrhea was independent of both chromogranin A (CgA) and 5-HIAA concentrations.

Bronchoconstriction

Wheezing due to bronchospasm occurs in up to one-third of patients with carcinoid syndrome. Lung function tests show a prolonged forced expiratory volume in the first second (FEV$_1$). Differential diagnoses are asthma and chronic obstructive pulmonary disease. In the carcinoid syndrome the cause of bronchoconstriction is usually SP, histamine, or serotonin.[4]

Dyspepsia or Peptic Ulcer

The ZES is characterized by peptic ulcers and diarrhea that responds to therapy with PPIs, in the setting of hypergastrinemia and low gastric pH. Gastrinomas are localized 90% of the time in the "gastrinoma triangle." As discussed in the previous section, the measurements that should be drawn for these tumors are fasting serum gastrin and gastric acid output, to differentiate gastrinoma from other causes of hypergastrinemia.

Hypoglycemia

The Whipple Triad (symptoms of hypoglycemia, low blood glucose levels <40 mg/dl, and relief of symptoms with glucose) is the clinical presentation of insulinomas, but other causes should be ruled out. Patients with noninsulinoma pancreatogenous hypoglycemia (NIPHS) present with postprandial neuroglycopenia symptoms (within 4 hours of meal ingestion) have negative 72-hour fasting test and tumor localization studies, and on histologic diagnosis, hypertrophy or nesidioblastosis are found.[12,13] Other possible causes include insulin antibodies, counter-regulatory hormone deficiency, and drug-induced and factitious hypoglycemia. To exclude all other causes, clinical suspicion together with measurement of hormones or peptides should be used.

In the case of hypoglycemia the recommended biochemical markers are insulin, insulin-like growth factor (IGF)-2, C-peptide, glucagon-like peptide type 1 (GLP-1), gastrointestinal peptide (GIP), sulfonylurea, adrenocorticotropic hormone (ACTH), growth hormone (GH), insulin antibodies, and liver enzymes.[4]

Dumping Syndrome

This manifestation occurs after surgery when the pylorus has been resected or inactivated. The early syndrome resembles shock, whereas the late presents as hypoglycemia. Provocative testing for diagnosis is done giving the patient a high-calorie, carbohydrate-rich breakfast with 750 kcal (21 g protein, 30 g fat, and 99 g carbohydrate) that should be ingested in 10 minutes to produce the maximum response. After the meal a blood sample is collected at 10, 15, 30, 45, 60, 120, and 180 minutes to measure glucose, insulin, C-peptide, motilin, PP, and GLP-1 levels.[4] An exaggerated insulin and GLP-1 response to the meal is found in gastric bypass patients with the syndrome, although the case and relationship between the hormonal overproduction and the clinical syndrome remain controversial.

Pellagra

Pellagra is caused by the deficiency of niacin, whereby the precursor tryptophan is shunted toward the production of increased amounts of serotonin.

DIAGNOSIS OF GASTRIC CARCINOID TUMORS

Fasting serum gastrin levels are important to differentiate types I and II gastric carcinoids from type III. Gastrin levels are elevated in both type I and type II gastric carcinoids but not in type III. It is important to note that patients with type I gastric carcinoid are hypochlorhydric or achlorhydric whereas patients with type II gastric carcinoids have high acid levels. 5-HIAA levels are generally not high because development of the carcinoid syndrome is uncommon.[14] Plasma chromogranin A (CgA) levels are recommended because CgA is frequently elevated in patients with types I and II as well as type III gastric carcinoid tumors,[15] and changes in CgA levels may be helpful in follow-up.[15] In patients treated with somatostatin analogues, CgA levels should be interpreted cautiously, because these agents significantly reduce plasma CgA levels.[15,16] In patients on stable doses of somatostatin analogues, consistent increases in plasma CgA levels over time may reflect loss of secretory control and/or tumor growth. Plasma CgA levels also have prognostic value in patients with metastatic disease.[15,17]

PATHOLOGY

Neuroendocrine tumors (NETs) arise throughout the body sharing basic characteristics. NETs are classified according to site, differentiation (well vs poorly differentiated), a marker of cell proliferation, for example, Ki-67, grade and stage, the hormones or amines produced, and markers of behavior such as CgA and synaptophysin. Tumor differentiation refers to the extent of resemblance to the normal cellular counterpart or loss of this resemblance. Tumor grade refers to the degree of biologic aggressiveness. Tumor stage refers to the extent of spread of the tumor. The extent of invasion into the organ of origin and involvement of nodes or distant sites are critical factors. There are several different systems to classify, grade, and stage neuroendocrine tumors and, although the criteria differ among systems, the underlying basic data are similar. The World Health Organization classification for NET uses a combination of gross and histologic features to place all NETs into 1 of 4 categories: (1) well-differentiated endocrine tumor of probable benign behavior, (2) well-differentiated endocrine tumor of uncertain behavior, (3) well-differentiated endocrine carcinoma, and (4) poorly differentiated endocrine carcinoma. A quick glance shows that it can be summarized as a 3-tiered classification (**Fig. 4**). A review of nomenclature, grading,

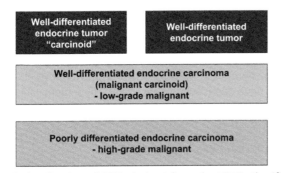

Fig. 4. Three-tiered Classification of NETs derived from the WHO Classification. Elements required to allow proper classification include gross description, microscopic profile including Immunohistochemistry, and finally level of invasion for gastrointestinal tumors. (*Data from* Ramage JK, Davies AH, Ardill J, et al. Guidelines for the management of gastroenteropancreatic neuroendocrine tumors. Gut 2005;54:1–16.)

and staging system has been summarized in previous articles on the pathologic classification of NETs adapted by the development of the North American Neuroendocrine Tumor Society Consensus Guidelines.

IMMUNOHISTOCHEMISTRY

While most agree that a mitotic rate or Ki-67 is necessary in specific cases, whether Ki-67 staining is needed in all cases remains hotly debated. An experienced pathologist familiar with NETs will likely be able to determine the tumor's grade in the majority of resected specimens, and a Ki-67 can be obtained as needed in difficult cases. In small biopsy specimens, there may not be sufficient material to differentiate between grade 1 versus 2 neuroendocrine carcinomas with or without Ki-67.

SPECIAL PATHOLOGIC CONSIDERATION AMONG NETs of the midgut

In addition to classic NETs, mixed histology tumors having neuroendocrine as well as glandular features, such as goblet cell carcinoids and adenocarcinoids, can be observed. Midgut tumors are more frequent in the appendix and cecum. For example, mixed histology tumors account for 1% of jejunal/ileal NETs and 7.3% of cecal NETs (P<.001).[18] While the numerical fraction of appendiceal NETs of mixed histology in the SEER registry is even higher, the exact percentage is difficult to ascertain. The reason for this is that small appendiceal carcinoids are often considered benign and are not reported to the registries, and mixed histology tumors such as goblet cell carcinoids are generally considered malignant and are more like to be reported.

Similarly, the distribution of poorly differentiated NETs among midgut tumors is different. Poorly differentiated NETs account for only 0.9% and 1.1% of appendiceal and jejunal/ileal NETs, respectively. However, they account for 14.2% of NETs arising from the cecum.[18]

These pathologic descriptors provide important information for patient management, as mixed histology tumors such as goblet cell carcinoids can be more aggressive and prone to peritoneal dissemination. Poorly differentiated NETs are often rapidly progressive and require cytotoxic chemotherapy.

MOLECULAR GENETICS

The genetics of neuroendocrine tumorigenesis have yet to be elucidated. Although small familial clusters of midgut carcinoids have been described, there are no known genetic cancer syndromes associated with them. Tumors have clustered in several small families without multiple endocrine neoplasia type 1 (MEN-1), and multiplicity of tumors is a feature in one-quarter of isolated cases. Among sporadic midgut carcinoids, several studies using comparative genomic hybridization or microsatellite markers have shown frequent allelic deletion of chromosome 18.[19,20] On an epigenetic level, midgut NETs have been found to have global hypomethylation.[21] There are few data about genetic aspects in NETs of the appendix or cecum. Tumor multiplicity is much less frequent in the appendix and cecum than the ileum.

BLOOD AND URINE BIOMARKERS IN MIDGUT NETs

Several circulating tumor markers have been evaluated for the follow-up management of NETs. However, isolated elevation of marker levels is generally not sufficient for diagnosis without tissue confirmation. The most important of these markers, CgA, is a 49-kDa acidic polypeptide that is present in the secretory granules of neuroendocrine cells. Plasma CgA is elevated in 60% to 100% of patients with either functioning or nonfunctioning NETs. The sensitivities and specificities of CgA for the detection of NETs range between 70% and 100%.[22–25] CgA level may correlate with tumor volume, but this should be interpreted carefully. For example, because somatostatin analogues affect blood levels of CgA, serial CgA levels should be measured at approximately the same interval from injection of long-acting somatostatin analogues. Spuriously elevated levels of CgA have also been reported in patients using PPIs, in patients with renal or liver failure, and in those patients with chronic gastritis.

Urinary 5-HIAA (24-hour collection) is a useful laboratory marker for carcinoid tumors. It is a surrogate measure of serotonin metabolism and is perhaps more useful than the direct measurement of serotonin, as serum values vary considerably during the day according to activity and stress level. The specificity of this test has been reported to be 88%.[26] However, certain foods and medications can increase urinary 5-HIAA levels and should be avoided during specimen collection.[27] High serotonin concentrations occur with the ingestion of bananas, kiwis, pineapple, plantains, plums, and tomatoes. Moderate elevations are found with avocado, black olives, spinach, broccoli, cauliflower, eggplant, cantaloupe, dates, figs, grapefruit, and honeydew melon. Drugs that can increase 5-HIAA are acetanilide, phenacetin, reserpine, glyceryl guaiacolate (found in many cough syrups), and methocarbamol. Drugs that can decrease 5-HIAA levels include chlorpromazine, heparin, imipramine, isoniazid, levodopa, monoamine oxidase inhibitors, methenamine, methyldopa, phenothiazines, promethazine, and tricyclic antidepressants. In addition, foregut carcinoids do not produce 5-HIAA but rather only 5-hydroxytryptophan (5-HTP), limiting the usefulness of these measures as a diagnostic or screening tool.

Another useful blood marker, NSE, is a dimer of the glycolytic enzyme enolase. NSE is present in the cytoplasmic compartment of the cell, and its serum level is thought to be unrelated to the secretory activity of the tumor.[25] Although it is less specific than CgA, it may be a useful marker for follow-up of patients with known diagnosis of NETs.

A variety of other secreted molecules can be measured among patients with midgut NETs. These include other chromogranins such as chromogranins B and C, pancreastatin, and substance B. The general principle of biomarker measurement is to identify a few biomarkers that are elevated in the particular patient in question and to follow these over time.

PANCREATIC NEUROENDOCRINE TUMORS

PNETs have an estimated incidence of less than 1 per 100,000 individuals.[28–30] PNETs are divided into 2 groups: those associated with a functional syndrome due to ectopic secretion of a biologically active substance and those that are not associated with a functional syndrome (generally called nonfunctional PNETs [NF-PNETs]).[28–31] Functional PNETs include insulinomas, gastrinomas, VIPomas, somatostatinomas, glucagonomas, growth hormone releasing factor secreting (GRFomas), and a group of less common PNETs including PNETs secreting ACTH (ACTHomas) and causing Cushing syndrome, PNETs causing the carcinoid syndrome, PNETs causing hypercalcemia, and very rarely PNETs ectopically secreting luteinizing hormone, renin, or erythropoietin (Table 3).[28] Functional PNETs and NF-PNETs also frequently secrete several other substances: chromogranins, NSE, subunits of human chorionic gonadotropin, neurotensin, and ghrelin.[28–31] In terms of relative frequency, NF-PNETs are at present the most frequently found PET, occurring approximately twice as frequently as insulinomas, which are generally more frequent than gastrinomas, followed by glucagonomas, VIPomas, somatostatinomas, and others.[28,29,31,32]

Table 3
Clinical presentation, syndrome, tumor type, sites, and the hormones produced

Clinical Presentation	Syndrome	Tumor Type	Sites	Hormones
Acromegaly	Acromegaly, gigantism	NET, PNET, Pheo	Pancreas islet	GHRH
Cushing	Cushing	NET, PNET, Pheo	Pancreas islet, Lung, Pheo, MTC	CRH, ACTH
Pigmentation	Pigmentation	NET	Pancreas islet	MSH
Anorexia, nausea, vomiting, abdominal pain	Hypercalcemia	NET, PNET, Pheo	Pancreas islet, Pheo	PTH-rp, PTH, TGFβ, IL, 25 OHD, 1,25 OHD – bone Alk phos, NTx
Hypoglycemia	Autonomic and CNS symptoms of hypoglycemia	NET, PNET	Pancreas, carcinoid	IGF, IGF2 and proIGF, GLP-1, GLP-2
Weakness, lethargy, apathy	Hyponatremia, SIADH	NET, PNET, Pheo	Lung, pancreas, Pheo	ADH, ANP
Hyperandrogenism, gynecomastia, hyperthyroidism	—	PET	Pancreas	LH, FSH, prolactin, TSH
Hypertension	Malignant hypertension	PET, Pheo, paraganglioma	Paraganglioma, NET	Renin, prorenin, aldosterone

Abbreviations: ACTH, adrenocorticotropic hormone; ADH, antidiuretic hormone; Alk phos, alkaline phosphatase; ANP, atrial natriuretic peptide; CNS, central nervous system; CRH, corticotropin-releasing hormone; FSH, follicle-stimulating hormone; GHRH, growth hormone releasing hormone; IGF, insulin-like growth factor; LH, leuteinizing hormone; MTC, medullary thyroid carcinoma; NET, neuroendocrine tumor; NTx, N-telopeptide; 25 OHD, 25-hydroxyvitamin D; PNET, pancreatic NET; Pheo, pheochromocytoma; PTH, parathyroid hormone; PTH-rp, parathyroid hormone related peptide; SIADH, syndrome of inappropriate secretion of antidiuretic hormone; TGF, transforming growth factor; TSH, thyrotropin-stimulating hormone.

PNETs can occur both sporadically and in patients with various inherited disorders.[28,33] PNETs occur in 80% to 100% of patients with MEN-1; 10% to 17% of patients with von Hippel-Lindau syndrome (VHL); up to 10% of patients with von Recklinghausen disease (neurofibromatostis-1 [NF-1]); and occasionally in patients with tuberous sclerosis.[33] Of these autosomal dominant disorders, MEN-1 is the most frequent in patients with PNETs.[33,34] MEN-1 is caused by mutations in the chromosome 11q13 region resulting in alterations in the MEN1 gene, which has important effects on transcriptional regulation, genomic stability, cell division, and cell cycle control.[33] Patients with MEN-1 develop hyperplasia or tumors of multiple endocrine and nonendocrine tissues, including parathyroid adenomas (95%–100%) resulting in hyperparathyroidism; pituitary adenomas (54%–65%); adrenal adenomas (27%–36%); various carcinoid tumors (gastric, lung, thymic) (0%–10%); thyroid adenomas (up to 10%); various skin tumors (80%–95%); central nervous system tumors (up to 8%); and smooth muscle tumors (up to 10%).[33] In MEN-1 patients 80% to 100% develop pancreatic NF-PNETs, but in most patients they are small and microscopic, causing symptoms in only 0% to 13%.[33] Gastrinomas (>80% duodenal) develop in 54% of MEN-1 patients, insulinomas in 18%, and glucagonomas, VIPomas, GRFomas, and somatostatinomas in less than 5%.[33] In VHL, 98% of all the PNETs that develop in 10% to 17% of the patients are NF-PNETs; in the 0% to 10% of NF-1 patients developing a PET they are characteristically duodenal somatostatinomas that do not cause the somatostatinoma syndrome; and in tuberous sclerosis, rare functional and NF-PNETs are reported.[33]

Insulinoma

Insulinoma patients characteristically present with symptoms of hypoglycemia, neuroglycopenic symptoms (confusion, altered consciousness), and symptoms of sympathetic overdrive weakness and sweating.[28,35,36] The diagnosis of insulinoma can be established by determining plasma proinsulin, insulin, C-peptide, and glucose levels, which are usually performed during a 72-hour fast.[28,35,36]

There are 6 criteria for the diagnosis of insulinomas: documented blood glucose levels $\leq$2.2 mmol/L ($\leq$40 mg/dL); concomitant insulin levels $\geq$6 μU/mL ($\geq$36 pmol/L; $\geq$3 μU/mL by immunochemiluminometic assay); C-peptide levels $\geq$200 pmol/L; proinsulin levels $\geq$5 pmol/L; β-hydroxybutyrate levels $\leq$2.7 mmol/L; and absence of sulfonylurea (metabolites) in the plasma and/or urine. The 72-hour fast is the gold standard for establishing the diagnosis of insulinoma.[36] In fact 98% of patients with insulinomas will develop symptomatic hypoglycemia within 72 hours.[1] When the patient develops symptoms and the blood glucose levels are 2.2 mmol/L or less ($\leq$40 mg/dL), C-peptide, proinsulin, and insulin are drawn and the fast should be stopped. Failure of appropriate insulin suppression in the presence of hypoglycemia substantiates an autonomously secreting insulinoma.[36] It has been proposed that the sensitivity of the 48-hour fasting test is between 94.5% and 95.7% and that this should be enough for the diagnosis of insulinoma instead of the 72-hour fast test.[37,38] In the case of suspected insulinoma it is important to keep in mind the possible differential diagnosis: nesidioblastosis, noninsulinoma pancreatogenous hypoglycemia syndrome (NIPHS) (see discussion later), and multiple adenomas.

Insulinomas have an estimated annual incidence of 1 to 4 per million persons. Approximately 4% to 5% of patients with insulinoma have MEN-1.[33] Insulinomas are usually single tumors (except in patients with MEN-1), generally small (ie, <1 cm), almost always (>99%) intrapancreatic in location and, in contrast to all other PNETs, are benign in upward of 85% to 90% of patients.[33,35,36,39]

Gastrinoma

Patients typically present with abdominal pain due to peptic ulcer disease [PUD], diarrhea, and reflux esophagitis.[40] ZES should be suspected in patients with PUD with diarrhea; with ulcers in unusual locations; with severe PUD or with complications of PUD; with PUD without *Helicobacter pylori* present; with PUD with a family history of PUD or endocrinopathies or with PUD with prominent gastric folds; in the presence of an endocrinopathy; or with hypergastrinemia.[28,40–43] The diagnosis requires the demonstration of inappropriate hypergastrinemia.[28,40–43] The initial determination in most centers is a fasting gastrin level, because it will be elevated in 99% to 100% of ZES patients.[28,42,43] The diagnosis can be complicated by other conditions that can cause hypergastrinemia in a range seen with ZES patients.[28,40–45] These conditions either cause hypochlorhydria/achlorhydria (atrophic gastritis, PPI treatment) or can be associated with increased acid secretion similar to ZES.[28,40,42,43,46] Recent studies[46,47] show the widespread use of PPIs can particularly complicate and delay the diagnosis of ZES by controlling the symptoms in most ZES patients with conventional doses, thus masking the diagnosis.[28,43,46] Furthermore, PPIs cause hypergastrinemia in patients without ZES, in the range that is normal in ZES patients.[41,43,46–48] Fasting serum gastrin (FSG) level of 1000 ng/L (pg/mL) or more, gastric pH less than 2.5, and if the patient is normocalcemic, free of pyloric obstruction, and has normal renal function establish the diagnosis of gastrinoma.[13] The 2006 European Neuroendocrine Tumor Society (ENETS) guidelines had cutoff values of greater than 10-fold elevation for FSG and gastric pH of 2 or greater.[41] Because of the presence of other conditions that can also cause hypergastrinemia and an acidic pH, the diagnosis of ZES may require the assessment of basal acid output as well as a secretin provocative gastrin test.[28,41,43,44] In the case that the FSG values are not high enough to make a definitive diagnosis, a provocative test should be done. Secretin is administered after an overnight fast, and serum for estimation of gastrin levels is collected fasting and 2, 5, 10, 15, and 30 minutes after the secretin bolus. In healthy people the increase in gastrin is not higher than 50% above the baseline level; in the presence of a gastrinoma the increase is greater than 100 ng/L above the baseline levels, which will also distinguish patients with hypergastrinemia from achlorhydric states (ie, type 1 gastric carcinoids, use of PPIs, pernicious anemia, atrophic gastritis).[4]

With some patients suspected of having ZES, there can be risk of stopping PPIs to assess fasting gastrin levels or perform acid secretory studies, or secretin provocative testing, therefore it is best that these patients be referred to a clinical unit experienced in making the diagnosis of ZES.

At present gastrinomas, in contrast to older studies, are found in the duodenum in more than 60% of patients with sporadic ZES (>85% with MEN-1/ZES); are usually single in sporadic ZES and invariably multiple in MEN-1/ZES; are usually small in size the duodenum (<1 cm); and are malignant in 60% to 90% of cases.[33,49–53] Recent studies show that pancreatic tumors are more aggressive than duodenal tumors, are much more likely to metastasize to liver and/or bone, and are more likely to be present in the 25% of ZES patients with aggressive gastrinomas.[28,54–56]

The diagnosis of ZES in patients with MEN-1 can be complicated by the fact that the presence or absence of hyperparathyroidism with the resultant hypercalcemia can have a marked effect on fasting gastrin levels, basal acid output, and the secretin test results.[33,34,57–59] Each of these parameters can markedly decrease after correction of the hyperparathyroidism, by an effective parathyroidectomy ($\geq$3.5 glands removed), and thus can mask the diagnosis of ZES in a MEN-1 patient.[33,34,57–59]

Glucagonoma

Glucagonoma or the "Sweet" syndrome

Diabetes accompanied by the 4D syndrome (Dermatosis and necrolytic migratory erythema; Depression; Deep venous thrombosis; Diarrhea), is the clinical presentation of glucagonomas. Glucagonomas cause glucose intolerance (40%–90%), weight loss (80%), and a pathognomonic rash characterized by a migratory necrolytic erythema (70%–90%).[28,32,60–62] Fasting plasma glucagon levels tend to be higher in patients with large hepatic metastases than in those without hepatic metastases,[63] and all patients with large hepatic metastases have glucose intolerance. Massive hepatic metastases may decrease the ability of the liver to metabolize splanchnic glucagon, thus increasing peripheral levels. Another factor may be variation in the molecular species of glucagon that is present in each case, and its biologic potency.[64]

Glucagonomas are generally single, large tumors (mean 6 cm) associated with liver metastases in more than 60% of cases at diagnosis, and are almost entirely intrapancreatic in location.[28,32,60–62] Clinically significant hyperglycemia occurs in only half of such patients. Patients are frequently initially diagnosed by a dermatologist, after presenting with necrolytic migratory erythema. This rash, characterized by raised erythematous patches beginning in the perineum and subsequently involving the trunk and extremities, is found in more than two-thirds of all patients.[28,32,60–62] However, it is not specific for glucagonomas because it can also occur in cirrhosis, pancreatitis, and celiac disease.[28] The diagnosis requires the demonstration of increased plasma glucagon levels (usually 500–1000 pg/mL, normal <50) in the presence of the appropriate symptoms.[28,32,60–62] In previously reported cases using radioimmunoassays, fasting plasma glucagon concentrations were 2100 ± 334 pg/mL. These levels are markedly higher than in normal, fasting subjects (ie, 150 pg/mL) or in those with other disorders where fasting plasma glucagon concentrations often are elevated but less than 500 pg/mL, including diabetes mellitus, burn injury, acute trauma, bacteremia, cirrhosis, renal failure, or Cushing syndrome. As with other islet cell neoplasms, glucagonomas may overproduce multiple hormones such as insulin, ACTH, PP, parathyroid hormone (PTH) or substances with PTH-like activity, gastrin, serotonin, VIP, and melanocyte stimulating hormone (MSH), in that order of frequency.[65]

VIPomas

VIPomas (also called Verner-Morrison syndrome, pancreatic cholera, WDHA syndrome for Watery Diarrhea, Hypokalemia, and Achlorhydria) are PNETs ectopically secreting VIP, which leads to profound, large-volume diarrhea (100% >700 mL/d), hypokalemia, and achlorhydria.[28,30,32,60,66] VIPomas are single tumors, metastatic at presentation in 70% to 80% of cases and in adults are intrapancreatic in location in more than 95% of cases, whereas in children they often are ganglioneuromas/ganglioblastomas.[28,30,32,60,66] Elevated plasma VIP levels in a patient with large-volume secretory diarrhea establishes the diagnosis.[28,30,32,60,66]

Somatostatinoma

Somatostatin (SRIF) is a tetradecapeptide that inhibits numerous endocrine and exocrine secretory functions. Almost all gut hormones that have been studied are inhibited by SRIF, including insulin, PP, glucagon, gastrin, secretin, GIP, and motilin.[67] SRIF also has direct effects on several target organs.[68] For example, it inhibits basal and PG-stimulated gastric acid secretion. It also affects GI transit time, intestinal motility, and absorption of nutrients from the small intestine. The major effect in the small intestine appears to be a delay in the absorption of fat and reduced absorption of calcium.

The salient features of the somatostatinoma syndrome are diabetes, diarrhea or steatorrhea, gallbladder disease, hypochlorhydria, and weight loss.[69–71] The first cases of the somatostatinoma syndrome were reported in 1977 by Ganda and colleagues.[69] The authors have examined the cases reported since 1977 and describe here the features now recognized to be a part of the syndrome. Different syndromes manifest among tumors arising from the pancreas and the intestine or extrapancreatic sites, and these are considered separately.

Clinical features
Most patients were between 40 and 60 years of age. There is a 2:1 ratio of female to male patients, which contrasts with the equal sex incidence for other islet cell tumors.[72]

Plasma somatostatin-like immunoreactivity
The mean plasma somatostatin-like immunoreactivity (SLI) concentration in patients with pancreatic somatostatinoma was 50 times higher than normal (range, 1–250 times). Intestinal somatostatinomas, however, had only slightly elevated or normal SLI concentrations.

Diabetes mellitus and hypoglycemia
Seventy-five percent of patients with pancreatic tumors had diabetes mellitus. By contrast, diabetes occurred only in 11% of patients with intestinal tumors. In all instances, the diabetes was mild and could be controlled with diet and/or oral hypoglycemic agents or with small doses of insulin. The differential inhibition of insulin and diabetogenic hormones may explain the usually mild degree of diabetes and the rarity of ketoacidosis in these cases. Replacement of functional islet cell tissue by pancreatic tumor may be another cause for diabetes in most patients with pancreatic somatostatinoma, contrasting with the low incidence in patients with intestinal tumors.

Gallbladder disease
Fifty-nine percent of patients with pancreatic tumors and 27% of patients with intestinal tumors had gallbladder disease. Somatostatin has been shown to inhibit gallbladder emptying,[68,73] and may be the cause the observed high rate of gallbladder disease in patients with somatostatinoma. This thesis is supported by the observation of massively dilated gallbladders without stones or other pathology[74,75] in patients with these tumors.

Diarrhea and steatorrhea
Diarrhea consisting of 3 to 10 frequently foul-smelling stools per day and/or steatorrhea from 20 to 76 g of fat per 24 hours is common in patients with pancreatic somatostatinoma. The high levels of somatostatin within the pancreas, serving as a paracrine mediator to inhibit exocrine secretion or, alternatively, from the somatostatinoma's causing duct obstruction, are possible causes. The severity of diarrhea and steatorrhea parallels the course of the disease, worsening as the tumor advances and metastatic disease spreads, and improving after tumor resection. Somatostatin has been shown to inhibit the pancreatic secretion of proteolytic enzymes, water, bicarbonate,[76] and gallbladder motility.[77] In addition, it inhibits the absorption of lipids.[78] All but one patient with diarrhea and steatorrhea had high plasma somatostatin concentrations. The rarity of diarrhea and/or steatorrhea in patients with intestinal somatostatinomas may result from the lower SLI levels.

Hypochlorhydria

Infusion of somatostatin has been shown to inhibit gastric acid secretion in human subjects.[79] Thus, hypochlorhydria in patients with somatostatinoma in the absence of gastric mucosal abnormalities likely results from elevated somatostatin concentrations. Basal and stimulated acid secretion was inhibited in 87% of patients with pancreatic tumors tested but in only 12% of patients with intestinal tumors.

Weight loss

Weight loss ranging from 9 to 21 kg over several months occurred in one-third of patients with pancreatic tumors and one-fifth of patients with intestinal tumors. The weight loss may relate to malabsorption and diarrhea, but in small intestinal tumors anorexia, abdominal pain, and as yet unexplained reasons may be relevant.

Associated endocrine disorders

Of great interest is the presence of café-au-lait spots, neurofibromatosis, and paroxysmal hypertension in patients with intestinal tumors. Approximately 50% of all patients have other endocrinopathies in addition to their somatostatinoma. Occurrence of MEN-1 has been recognized in patients with islet cell tumors, and MEN-2A or MEN-2B syndromes are present in association with pheochromocytomas and neurofibromatosis, respectively. These possibilities should be considered during endocrine workups of patients with islet cell tumors and their relatives.

Tumor location

Somatostatinomas are PNETs that can occur in the duodenum or pancreas.[28,32,60,80,81] Of the reported primary tumors, 60% were found in the pancreas and 40% in the duodenum or jejunum. Of the pancreatic tumors, 50% were located in the head and 25% in the tail, and the remaining tumors either infiltrated the whole pancreas or were found in the body. Regarding extrapancreatic locations, approximately 50% originate in the duodenum, approximately 50% originate in the ampulla and, rarely, one is found in the jejunum. Thus, approximately 60% of somatostatinomas originate in the upper intestinal tract, which probably is a consequence of the relatively large number of normal D cells in this region.

Tumor size

Somatostatinomas tend to be large, similar to glucagonomas,[82] but unlike insulinomas and gastrinomas which, as a rule, are small.[83–85] Within the intestine, tumors have tended to be smaller. Symptoms associated with somatostatinomas and glucagonomas are less pronounced and probably do not develop until very high blood levels of the respective hormones have been attained, resulting in a later diagnosis.

Incidence of malignancy

Eighty percent of pancreatic patients with pancreatic somatostatinomas were metastatic at diagnosis, and 50% with intestinal tumors had evidence of metastatic disease. Metastasis to the liver is most frequent, and regional lymph node involvement and metastases to bone are less so. In approximately 70% of cases, metastatic disease is present at diagnosis. This is similar to the high incidence of malignancy in glucagonoma[83] and in gastrinoma,[84] but it is different from the low incidence in insulinoma.[85] The high prevalence of metastatic disease may be a consequence of late diagnosis but apparently is not dependent on the tissue of origin.

Microscopic appearance

On light microscopy, most tumors appear to be well-differentiated islet cell or carcinoid-type tumors. Some show a mixed picture, consisting of separate zones of differentiated and anaplastic cells. In the differentiated areas, cells are arranged in lobular or acinar patterns that are separated by fibrovascular stroma. Less well-differentiated areas consist of sheets of cells interrupted by fibrous septa.

Diffuse positive immunoreactivity for somatostatin usually is found, which contrasts with the rarity of somatostatin-positive cells in gastrinomas and other tumors. There is a unique occurrence of psammoma bodies in somatostatinomas localized within the duodenum. In addition, there is abundant immunologic evidence for the presence of cells containing insulin, calcitonin, gastrin and VIP, ACTH, prostaglandin E2, and SP. In tumors with multiple hormones, however, SLI-containing cells represent the large majority of all cells containing hormones detected by immunopathology.

Somatostatin-containing tumors outside the GI tract

Somatostatin has been found in many tissues outside the GI tract including the hypothalamic and extrahypothalamic regions of the brain, the peripheral nervous system (including the sympathetic adrenergic ganglia), and the C cells of the thyroid gland. Not surprisingly, high concentrations of somatostatin have been found in tumors originating from these tissues. Sano and colleagues[86] and Saito and colleagues[87] reported 7 patients with MCT who had high basal plasma SLI concentrations and high tumor SLI concentrations. Roos and colleagues[88] reported elevated plasma SLI concentrations in 3 of 7 patients with MTC and high tissue SLI concentrations in 3 of 5 MTC tumors. Some, but not all, of these patients exhibited the clinical somatostatinoma syndrome.

Elevated plasma SLI concentrations also have been reported in patients with small cell lung cancer.[88] One case of metastatic bronchial oat cell carcinoma caused Cushing syndrome, diabetes, diarrhea, steatorrhea, anemia, and weight loss, and had a plasma SLI concentration 20 times greater than normal.[89] A patient with a bronchogenic carcinoma presenting with diabetic ketoacidosis and high levels of SLI (>5000 pg/mL) has been reported.[90] Pheochromocytomas[91,92] and catecholamine-producing extra-adrenal paragangliomas[88] are other examples of endocrine tumors producing and secreting somatostatin in addition to other hormonally active substances. One-quarter of 37 patients with pheochromocytomas had elevated SLI levels.[88]

Diagnosis

In the reported series cited, somatostatinomas were found accidentally. The tumors were found either during exploratory laparotomy or upper GI radiographic studies, computed tomography (CT), or ultrasonography (US), or endoscopy performed because of various symptoms, like abdominal pain, melena, hematemesis, persistent diarrhea, or in search of insulinomas or ACTH-secreting tumors. Once found, the tumors were identified as somatostatinoma by the demonstration of elevated tissue concentrations of SLI and/or prevalence of D cells by immunocytochemistry, or demonstration of elevated plasma SLI concentrations. In other islet cell tumors, the clinical symptoms and signs usually suggest the diagnosis, followed by elevated blood hormone levels, then tumor localization. It can be expected that the same sequence of diagnostic procedures will be followed in the future for the diagnosis of somatostatinoma, mainly for 2 reasons: (a) the increasing familiarity of physicians with the clinical somatostatinoma syndrome and (b) the greater availability of reliable radioimmunoassays for the determination of SLI in blood that has increased the yield. At present, these assays are complicated by the need for cumbersome extraction procedures and are not readily available. (Assay available at Inter Science Institute, Inglewood, CA, USA, Tel. 800-255-2873.) It should be recognized, however, that the syndrome is rare. Of 1199 cases screened for somatostatinoma at the University of Michigan between 1982 and 1986, only 8 had diagnostic serum levels.

The diagnosis of somatostatinoma at a time when blood SLI concentrations are normal or only marginally elevated requires reliable provocative tests. Increased plasma SLI concentrations have been reported after intravenous infusion of tolbutamide and arginine, and decreased SLI concentrations have been observed after intravenous infusion of diazoxide. Arginine is a well-established stimulant for normal D cells and thus is unlikely to differentiate between normal and supranormal somatostatin secretion. The same may be true for diazoxide, which has been shown to decrease SLI secretion from normal dog pancreas as well as in patients with somatostatinoma.[93] Tolbutamide stimulates SLI release from normal dog and rat pancreas,[76,77,93] but no change was found in the circulating SLI concentrations of 3 normal human subjects after intravenous injection of 1 g of tolbutamide.[94] Therefore, at present tolbutamide appears to be a candidate for a provocative agent in the diagnosis of somatostatinoma, but its reliability must be established in a greater number of patients and controls. Until then, it may be necessary to measure plasma SLI concentrations during routine workups for postprandial dyspepsia and gallbladder disorders,[70] for diabetes in patients without a family history, and for unexplained steatorrhea, as these findings can be early signs of somatostatinomas.

Other Rare Functional PNETs

GRFomas ectopically secrete growth hormone-releasing factor, which results in acromegaly that is clinically indistinguishable from that caused by pituitary adenomas.[28,60,95] GRFomas in the pancreas are generally single, large tumors at diagnosis; one-third have liver metastases and they are found in the pancreas in 30% of cases, 54% in the lung, and the remainder primarily in other abdominal locations.[28,60,95] PNETs causing hypercalcemia usually secrete PTH-related peptide (PTH-rp) as well as other biologically active peptides, and are usually large tumors at diagnosis, with 80% to 90% associated with liver metastases.[28,60,96,97]

Nonfunctioning Pancreatic Endocrine Tumors

NF-PNETs are intrapancreatic in location, characteristically large (70% >5 cm), and at an advanced stage when first diagnosed, with 60% to 85% having liver metastases in most series.[28,30,31,60,98] NF-PNETs are not associated with a clinical hormonal syndrome presenting with symptoms due to the tumor per se, which include abdominal pain (40%–60%), weight loss, or jaundice.[28,30,31,60,98] In recent years, they are increasingly being discovered by chance on imaging studies performed for nonspecific abdominal symptoms.[28,99] Although NF-PNETs do not secrete peptides causing a clinical syndrome, they characteristically secrete several other peptides, which are helpful in their diagnosis. These include chromogranins, especially CgA (70%–100%) and PP (50%–100%).[28,30,31,60,98] The presence of an NF-PET is suggested by the presence of a pancreatic mass in a patient without hormonal symptoms, with an elevated serum PP or CgA level or a positive octreoscan (somatostatin receptor scintigraphy) (discussed in the next section). However, an elevated PP level or CgA level is not specific for NF-PNETs.[28,30,31,60,98]

Miscellaneous Pancreatic NETs

For VIPomas, glucagonomas, somatostatinomas, and PPomas the biochemical markers are VIP, glucagon, somatostatin, and PP, respectively.[1] For every pancreatic NET always screen for MEN type 1 syndrome by measuring ionized calcium, serum PTH, and prolactin.[100] For the biochemical screening for pancreatic NETs, in the presence of suspected MEN-1 syndrome gastrin, insulin/proinsulin, PP, glucagon, and CgA together have a sensitivity of approximately 70%, which can be increased if α- and β-human chorionic gonadotropin subunits, VIP, and postprandial gastrin and PP measurements are added.[13]

Acromegaly and gigantism

Acromegaly or gigantism can present when any NET secretes GH or GH-releasing hormone. Basal levels of GH and IGF-1 are usually enough to make a diagnosis; but in 15% to 20% of the patients further investigation is needed to show nonsuppressibility of GH to an oral glucose tolerance test (OGTT), a somatostatin inhibition test, or a bromocriptine suppression test. In the case of the OGTT, lipids, and insulin, these should also be suppressed. Other pituitary and hypothalamic hormones should also be measured, such as prolactin, the α- and β-subunits of gonadotropins, and thyroid-stimulating hormone (TSH).[4]

Cushing syndrome

A pituitary tumor, small cell carcinoma of the lung (known to produce ACTH), or an ACTH-secreting NET will present clinically as the Cushing syndrome from oversecretion of cortisol, adrenal androgens, and 11-deoxycorticosterone. To reach the diagnosis several steps should be followed. New guidelines for the diagnosis of Cushing syndrome have been published, though some of the recommendations are based on low-quality evidence. Their proposed approach is as follows.

After excluding exogenous glucocorticoid use (iatrogenic Cushing syndrome), patients with age-unusual features such as osteoporosis or hypertension, other features predictive of Cushing syndrome (easy bruising, facial plethora, proximal myopathy or muscle weakness, reddish/purple striae, weight gain in children with decreasing growth velocity), and those with adrenal incidentaloma compatible with adenoma should undergo testing for Cushing syndrome starting with one test with high diagnostic accuracy: urine free cortisol (at least 2 measurements), late night salivary cortisol (2 measurements), 1 mg overnight dexamethasone suppression test (DST), or longer low-dose DST (2 mg/d for 48 hours). If the test is negative and the pretest probability is low then follow-up in 6 months is recommended if progression of symptoms; in case of a negative test but with a high pretest probability then more than one test should be performed. In some cases a serum midnight cortisol or dexamethasone–corticotropin-releasing hormone test should be done.[101]

Biochemical assessment and monitoring for PNETs

Specific hormonal assays are needed to establish the diagnosis of each functional PET as outlined in the discussion of each tumor type in the aforementioned. Armed with knowledge about the characteristics and associated biomarkers with NETs, a simple but effective algorithm can be used (**Fig. 5**). Specifically, for insulinomas an assessment of plasma insulin, proinsulin, and C-peptide are needed at the time of glucose determinations, usually during a fast.[28,36,102] For ZES, serum gastrin is needed either alone or during a secretin provocation test.[28,36,42,44,102] For VIPomas a plasma VIP level is needed; for glucagonoma plasma glucagon levels; for GRFomas plasma GH and GRF levels; for Cushing syndrome urinary cortical, plasma ACTH, and appropriate ACTH suppression studies; for hypercalcemia with PET both serum PTH levels and PTH-rp levels are indicated; and for a PET with carcinoid syndrome, urinary 5-H1AA should be measured.[28,32,60,102,103] Plasma chromogranin A (CgA) can be used as a marker in patients with both functional and nonfunctional pancreatic endocrine tumors.[28,102–104] CgA should be used cautiously in patients treated with somatostatin

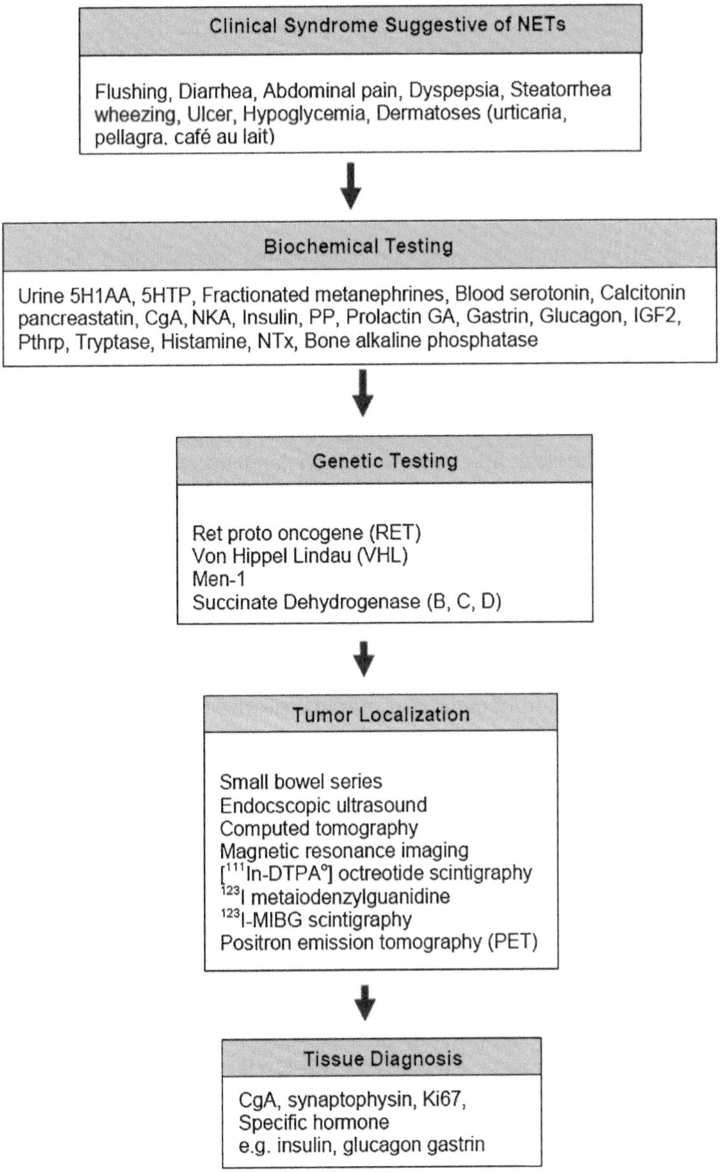

Clinical Syndrome Suggestive of NETs
Flushing, Diarrhea, Abdominal pain, Dyspepsia, Steatorrhea wheezing, Ulcer, Hypoglycemia, Dermatoses (urticaria, pellagra. café au lait)

↓

Biochemical Testing
Urine 5H1AA, 5HTP, Fractionated metanephrines, Blood serotonin, Calcitonin pancreastatin, CgA, NKA, Insulin, PP, Prolactin GA, Gastrin, Glucagon, IGF2, Pthrp, Tryptase, Histamine, NTx, Bone alkaline phosphatase

↓

Genetic Testing
Ret proto oncogene (RET) Von Hippel Lindau (VHL) Men-1 Succinate Dehydrogenase (B, C, D)

↓

Tumor Localization
Small bowel series Endocscopic ultrasound Computed tomography Magnetic resonance imaging [^{111}In-DTPA°] octreotide scintigraphy ^{123}I metaiodenzylguanidine ^{123}I-MIBG scintigraphy Positron emission tomography (PET)

↓

Tissue Diagnosis
CgA, synaptophysin, Ki67, Specific hormone e.g. insulin, glucagon gastrin

Fig. 5. Algorithm for diagnosis of NETs.[74–76] Based on the clinical presentations, specific measures are selected for evaluation of each patient. 5H1AA, 5-hydroxyindolacetic acid; 5HTP, 5-hydroxytryptophan; CgA, chromogranin A; GH, growth hormone; IGF2, insulin-like growth factor 2; NKA, neurokinin A; NTx, N-telopeptide; PP, pancreatic polypeptide; Pthrp, parathyroid hormone-related peptide. (*Data from* Vinik A. Diffuse hormonal systems and endocrine tumor syndromes. Available at: www.endotext.org.)

analogues, because these agents significantly reduce plasma CgA levels.[16,103] In patients on stable doses of somatostatin analogues, consistent increases in plasma CgA levels over time may reflect loss of secretory control and/or tumor growth.[17,39,102–104]

Pheochromocytomas

The main signs and symptoms of catecholamine excess include hypertension, palpitations, headache, sweating, and pallor. Less common signs and symptoms are fatigue, nausea, weight loss, constipation, flushing, and fever. Patients may present with myocardial infarction, arrhythmia, stroke, or other vascular manifestations (eg, any organ ischemia). Similar signs and symptoms are produced by numerous other clinical conditions and therefore pheochromocytoma is often referred to as the "great mimic."

In general, about 80% of pheochromocytomas are located in the adrenal medulla.[105] Extra-adrenal sympathetic paragangliomas in the abdomen most commonly arise from chromaffin tissue around the inferior mesenteric artery (the organ of Zuckerkandl) and aortic bifurcation, AND less commonly from any other chromaffin tissue in the abdomen, pelvis, and thorax.[106] Extra-adrenal parasympathetic paragangliomas are most commonly found in the neck and head.

Pheochromocytomas and sympathetic extra-adrenal paragangliomas almost all produce, store, metabolize, and secrete catecholamines or their metabolites. Head and neck paragangliomas, however, rarely produce significant amounts of catecholamines (<5%).

Epidemiology

Pheochromocytomas and paragangliomas are rare and occur in about 0.05% to 0.1% of patients with sustained hypertension. However, this probably accounts for only 50% of people harboring pheochromocytoma or paraganglioma because about half the patients with pheochromocytoma or paraganglioma have paroxysmal hypertension or normotension. The prevalence of pheochromocytoma and paraganglioma can be estimated to lie between 1:6500 and 1:2500, with the annual incidence in the United States being 500 to 1600 cases per year.

Pathology and molecular genetics

At present it is estimated that at least 24% to 27% of pheochromocytomas or paragangliomas are associated with known genetic mutations, and in children this prevalence may be as high as 40%.[107–112]

Pheochromocytomas may occur sporadically or as part of hereditary syndrome. According to the latest studies, among patients with nonsyndromic pheochromocytoma, up to about 24% of tumors may be hereditary.[107,112,113] Hereditary pheochromocytoma is associated with MEN-2A or MEN-2B, NF-1, VHL syndrome, and familial paragangliomas and pheochromocytomas due to germ-line mutations of genes encoding succinate dehydrogenase subunits B, C, and D (SDHB, SDHC, SDHD). In general, the traits are inherited in an autosomal dominant pattern.[113]

Specifically, pheochromocytomas related to MEN-1 and NF-1 secrete epinephrine, VHL-related pheochromocytomas secrete norepinephrine, and elevation of dopamine with norepinephrine is seen in some SDHB-related paragangliomas. In contrast to MEN-2, VHL, and NF-1 tumors that are almost always found in the adrenal gland, SDHB-related tumors are found in extra-adrenal localizations. In those patients with malignant disease secondary to an extra-adrenal paraganglioma, almost 50% had SDHB mutations.[114] Some studies suggested that more than two-thirds of patients with SDHB-related pheochromocytoma or paraganglioma will develop metastatic disease.[115,116] Family history is often helpful in MEN-2, VHL, and NF-1 tumors, but only 10% of the currently investigated patients with SDHB mutations have a positive family history for pheochromocytoma or paraganglioma.[115]

Biochemical markers for pheochromocytomas and paragangliomas
Independent studies have now confirmed that measurements of fractionated meta-nephrines (ie, normetanephrine and metanephrine measured separately) in urine or plasma provide superior diagnostic sensitivity over measurement of the parent cate-cholamines (see **Table 3**).[117–119] It is strongly recommended to obtain blood samples in the supine position to preserve diagnostic sensitvity.[120]

Current recommendations are that initial testing for pheochromocytoma or paragan-glioma must include measurements of fractionated metanephrines in plasma, urine, or both, as available.[121] Blood sampling should be performed at a supine position after about 15 to 20 minutes of intravenous catheter insertion. Food, caffeinated beverages, strenuous physical activity, or smoking are not permitted for at least about 8 to 12 hours before the testing. The elevation of plasma metanephrines of more than fourfold above the upper reference limit is associated with close to 100% probability of the tumor.[122]

Should additional biochemical testing be necessary, the possibility of false-positive results due to medications, clinical conditions (as described earlier), or inadequate sampling conditions (eg, blood sampling while seated) should first be considered and eliminated.[122] In patients with plasma metanephrine values above the upper refer-ence limit and less than fourfold above that limit, the clonidine suppression test combined with measurements of plasma catecholamines and normetanephrine may prove useful.[122] Guller and colleagues[123] published in 2006 that the tests of choice to establish the diagnosis of pheochromocytomas are urinary normetanephrine and platelet norepinephrine with sensitivities of 96.9% and 93.8%, respectively. In a study conducted in Switzerland by Giovanella and colleagues[124] in 2006, plasma meta-nephrine and CgA showed 95% sensitivity with comparable high specificity and diagnostic accuracy (96% and 96% for CgA, 94% and 95% for metanephrine, respec-tively). If both were used then sensitivity increased to 100%. The difference found between these 2 markers is that only CgA was correlated with tumor mass. In 2008 Bilek and colleagues[125] also studied the use of CgA for pheochromocytoma and found that it is a useful marker for following response to treatment, and that the levels of CgA were correlated with the size and the malignancy of the tumor.

Paragangliomas Paragangliomas are NETs that arise from the paravertebral axis. Sympathetic paragangliomas usually hypersecrete catecholamines and are localized in the thorax, abdomen, or pelvis. Parasympathetic paragangliomas are nonsecretory tumors usually localized in the head and neck area.[126]

Diagnosis of paragangliomas is similar to that of pheochromocytomas because these 2 entities only differ in their place of origin, extra-adrenal versus adrenal respec-tively. Algeciras-Schimnich and colleagues[127] suggested that when plasma fraction-ated metanephrines are measured and values are not fourfold above upper normal limit, serum or plasma CgA and urine fractionated metanephrines should be measured to confirm the diagnosis. After surgery the biochemical follow-up should be done 1 to 2 weeks later with 24-hour urine fractionated catecholamines and metanephrines; if these are normal complete resection is claimed, but if elevated levels persist a second primary or occult metastasis should be suspected and investigated. Young and colleagues[128] also proposed an annual biochemical testing follow-up for life, with 24-hour urinary excretion of fractionated catecholamines and metanephrines or plasma fractionated metanephrines, with imaging follow-up being considered only in the case of elevated levels.

All patients with paragangliomas should be considered for genetic testing with VHL, RET, NF1, SDHD, SDHB, and SDHC genes.[126] If positive then first-degree relatives genetic testing should be suggested and genetic counseling should be offered.

First-degree relatives should always undergo biochemical testing with 24-hour urine fractionated metanephrines and catecholamines.[128]

Medullary carcinoma of the thyroid MCTs originate from the parafollicular cells of the thyroid, which secrete calcitonin. They represent 4% to 10% of all thyroid neoplasms.[129] MCT can present as 2 different forms, sporadic (75%) or inherited (25%), and the latter can be either isolated or part of the MEN-2 syndrome.[130] A germ-line autosomal dominant mutation in the RET proto-oncogene, which encodes for a transmembrane tyrosine kinase receptor, predisposes individuals to develop MCT. Screening for RET germline mutations has allowed for early and accurate diagnosis of patients at risk of developing MCT.[131,132]

The most common clinical presentation of MCT is a thyroid nodule, either single or as multinodular goiter. Usually no other manifestations are present unless the tumor is already in stage IV (metastatic disease), when diarrhea and/or flushing can present.[133]

The fact that calcitonin is almost exclusively secreted by C cells explains why this hormone is the preferred biochemical marker for the diagnosis and follow-up of this disease; besides which calcitonin measurement is more sensitive than fine-needle aspiration for the diagnosis of MCT.[133] A 10-year survival of only 50% for MTC patients is reported in several series. The only possible means to improve the cure and survival rate of these patients consists in early diagnosis and early surgical treatment while the MTC is still intrathyroid.[133] Costante and colleagues[129] reported on 2007 that the positive predictive value (PPV) of basal calcitonin levels above 100 pg/mL is 100% for MCT and if the pentagastrin stimulation test is used calcitonin levels above 100 pg/mL had a PPV of 40%, but below this cutoff value the false-positive results increase until the PPV of basal calcitonin levels above 20 pg/mL is less than 25%. Cohen and colleagues[130] found that calcitonin levels are not only useful as diagnostic marker but are also correlated with tumor size and metastasis, giving prognostic value. When levels are less than 50 pg/mL preoperatively, the normalization of calcitonin levels postoperatively is found in 97.8% of the patients. Scheuba and colleagues[134] recently published that values of basal calcitonin greater than 64 pg/mL or stimulated calcitonin levels greater than 560 pg/mL had a sensitivity of 100% for MCT. Calcitonin increase can be observed also in parafollicular c-cell hyperplasia (CCH) and other extrathyroidal conditions. The cutoff value of calcitonin response between patients with MTC and CCH remains to be established.[135] The pentagastrin stimulation test is no longer available in the United States; it consisted of the intravenous injection of 0.5 μg/kg body weight of pentagastrin and measurements of calcitonin at 0, 1, 2, 5, and 10 minutes after the injection; healthy people do not experience an increase in calcitonin above 200 pg/mL after the administration of pentagastrin.[4] Calcitonin provocation can also be accomplished with an intravenous calcium infusion, with a risk of cardiac arrhythmias.

C-cell hyperplasia This entity has been proposed to be a precancerous lesion that eventually transforms into MCT. Schley and colleagues[136] submitted 3 cases in which patients presented with flushing, abdominal pain, diarrhea, and facial telangiectasia, resembling carcinoid syndrome, and the only biochemical abnormalities were elevated calcitonin levels and positive pentagastrin and calcium infusion tests. Venous sampling localized the overproduction of calcitonin to the thyroid and histology showed C-cell hyperplasia. After thyroidectomy symptoms resolved and calcitonin levels normalized. They proposed that the condition might be a gene mutation, but this has not been identified. The RET proto-oncogene was negative in the 3 patients. These findings suggest that every case of flushing and diarrhea should have a calcitonin measurement, with CCH or MCT in the differential diagnosis.[136]

Multiple endocrine neoplasia syndromes This entity is classified as either MEN type 1 or type 2, which are both inherited in an autosomal dominant pattern. Mutations on the MEN-1 tumor suppressor gene (inactivated) or the RET proto-oncogene (activated) are found in MEN type 1 and type 2, respectively.[137]

MEN type 1 MEN-1 is characterized by hyperplasia and/or neoplasm of the parathyroid glands, enteropancreatic NETs, and pituitary adenomas. Some patients do not present with all these tumors, so it has been agreed that diagnosis is made when a patient presents with 2 of these concomitantly. To diagnose familial MEN-1 syndrome, a first-degree relative has to present at least one of the tumors mentioned.[138] Hyperparathyroidism occurs in about 90% of patients; endocrine pancreatic tumors in 60% of patients; usually they are small and nonfunctional, the most common hormonally active ones being insulinomas or gastrinomas. Pituitary adenomas are present in 40% of patients and in 60% of the patients, skin manifestations can also be present.[138,139] Genetic studies are available for MEN type 1 syndrome; MEN-1 germline mutations are found in these patients, but its presence does not prompt any immediate intervention.[140] Piecha and colleagues[138] proposed a recommendation for carriers of MEN-1 mutation to be screened biochemically every 1 to 3 years for hyperparathyroidism, prolactinoma, gastrinoma, insulinoma, and other enteropancreatic tumors.

MEN type 2 This syndrome is subclassified into types 2A, 2B, and familial medullary carcinoma of the thyroid, all sharing the presence of MCT; and they are all characterized by an activating germline mutation in the RET proto-oncogene, specific for each type, and which can be identified in almost 100% of the patients by genetic testing. Once the genetic test demonstrates the mutation, a total thyroidectomy is mandatory either prophylactically in carriers or as treatment in patients who already present with manifestations of the syndrome.[141] MEN type 2A presents with MCT, bilateral pheochromocytomas, and primary hyperparathyroidism; it has been published recently that Hirschsprung disease could also be a manifestation of this syndrome, and genetic screening for RET proto-oncogene mutation is recommended for these patients[142]; MEN type 2B is an association of MCT, pheochromocytomas, and mucosal neuromas[143]; these patients usually present with a marfanoid phenotype.

The biochemical studies recommended for these syndromes are the same as previously proposed for each tumor type, depending on the clinical syndrome; and in the case of MEN syndrome being suspected, genetic testing should also be performed in the patient, and if positive, first-degree relatives should also be tested.

CLASSIFICATION OF THE BIOCHEMICAL MARKERS ACCORDING TO THEIR USE

The measurement of general and specific biochemical markers in patients with neuroendocrine tumors assists with diagnosis and gives an indication of the effectiveness of treatment, and they may be used as prognostic indicators. A review of tumor type and associated markers as well as the specificity of each marker shows not only great diversity but the close overlap of markers (**Table 4**).

Diagnostic

Chromogranin A and chromogranin B
Both CgA and CgB are part of the granin family. CgA and CgB are stored and secreted from vesicles present in the neuroendocrine cells, together with other peptides, amines, and neurotransmitters.[144] CgA is the best studied[145] and most used, but is not perfect. Stridsberg and colleagues[146] reported common conditions that can

Table 4
Specific biochemical markers for each tumor type[212]

Site	Tumor Type	Marker	Specificity
All	—	CgA and B	High
		PP, NSE, neurokinin,	Intermediate
		neurotensin	Low
		HCG α and β	
Thymus	Foregut carcinoid	ACTH	Intermediate
Bronchus	Foregut carcinoid,	ACTH, ADH,	Intermediate
	small cell lung	serotonin, 5-HIAA,	Low
	carcinoma	histamine, GRP,	
		GHRH, VIP, PTH-rp	
Stomach	Foregut carcinoid,	Histamine, gastrin	Intermediate
	gastrinoma,	Ghrelin	Low
	ghrelinoma		
Pancreas	Gastrinoma,	Gastrin, insulin,	High
	insulinoma,	proinsulin,	Low
	glucagonoma,	glucagon,	
	somatostatinoma,	somatostatin	
	PPoma, VIPoma	C-peptide,	
		neurotensin, VIP,	
		PTH-rp, calcitonin	
Duodenum	Gastrinoma,	Somatostatin,	High
	somatostatinoma	gastrin	
Ileum	Midgut carcinoid	Serotonin, 5-HIAA	High
		Neurokinin A,	Intermediate
		neuropeptide K,	
		substance P	
Colon and rectum	Hindgut carcinoid	Peptide YY,	Intermediate
		somatostatin	
Bone	Metastasis	Bone alkaline	High (blastic lesions),
		phosphatase,	modest (lytic
		N-telopeptide	lesions)
		PTH-rp	Intermediate
Cardiac involvement	Carcinoid	BNP	Intermediate

Abbreviations: 5-HIAA, 5-hydroxyindoleacetic acid; ACTH, adrenocorticotropic hormone; ADH, antidiuretic hormone; BNP, brain natriuretic peptide; CgA and B, chromogranin A and B; GHRH, growth hormone releasing hormone; GRP, gastrin-releasing peptide; HCG, human chorionic gonadotropin; NSE, neuron-specific enolase; PP, pancreatic polypeptide; PTH-rp, parathyroid hormone related peptide; VIP, vasointestinal peptide.
Data from Modlin IM, Oberg K, Chung DC, et al. Gastroenteropancreatic neuroendocrine tumours. Lancet Oncol 2008;9:61–72.

increase the levels of this marker and give false-positive measurements, including decreased renal function and treatment with PPIs and even essential hypertension[147]; these problems are not seen with CgB, with complementary measurement therefore being proposed.[146]

The most important characteristic of these markers is that they are not only secreted by the functional tumors but also by those less well-differentiated NETs that do not secrete known hormones.[2]

High CgA has been shown to be increased in 50% to 100% of patients with NETs.[148] CgA levels may be associated with the primary tumor (gastrinomas 100%, pheochromocytomas 89%, carcinoid tumors 80%, nonfunctioning tumors of the endocrine pancreas 69%, and medullary thyroid carcinomas 50%). In addition, blood levels depend on tumor mass, burden, or progression, and malignant nature of the tumor.[125,149] Small tumors may be associated with normal CgA levels.

Sensitivity and specificity of CgA depend on many factors. For example, sensitivity varies from 77.8% to 84% and specificity from 71.3% to 85.3% depending on the assay used, and of great importance is to establish the cutoff value that gives the highest sensitivity without compromising the specificity.[150] Another use of CgA is to discriminate between patients with or without metastasis, which also depends on the assay and the cutoff values used, with a sensitivity of 57% to 63.3% and specificity 55.6% to 71.4%.[150]

Pancreatic polypeptide

PP is considered another nonspecific biochemical marker. In a study conducted by Panzuto and colleagues[151] in Rome, Italy in 2004, PP sensitivity was 54% in functioning tumors, 57% in nonfunctioning tumors, 63% in pancreatic tumors, and 53% in gastrointestinal tumors. Specificity was 81% compared with disease-free patients, and 67% compared with patients with nonendocrine tumors; but when combined with CgA the sensitivity increased compared with either of the markers alone. When used in combination, the sensitivity of these markers is: for gastro-entero-pancreatic neuroendocrine tumors (GEP NETs) 96%; for nonfunctioning tumors 95%; and for pancreatic tumors 94%.

Neuron-specific enolase

NSE enzymes occur mainly in cells of neuronal and neuroectodermal origin. NSE has been found in thyroid and prostatic carcinomas, neuroblastomas, small-cell lung carcinoma, carcinoids, GEP NETs, and pheochromocytomas. Despite its high sensitivity (100%), its use is limited as a blood biochemical marker for neuroendocrine tumors due to its very low specificity (32.9%).[25]

DETERMINING PROGNOSIS
Chromogranin A

Other than the applications of CgA previously discussed, this marker can be used for prognosis and follow-up. Jensen and colleagues[152] found that a reduction on CgA levels of 80% or more after cytoreductive surgery for carcinoid tumors predicts symptom relief and disease control; it is associated with improved patient outcomes, even after incomplete cytoreduction.

Pancreastatin

One of the post-translational processing products of CgA, pancreastatin has found to be an indicator of poor outcome in patients with NETs when its concentration in plasma is elevated before treatment. A level greater than 500 pmol/L is an independent indicator of poor outcome. This marker is also known to correlate with the number of liver metastases, so it would be appropriate to use it in the follow-up of NET patients. Furthermore, Stronge and colleagues[153] found that an increase in pancreastatin levels following somatostatin analogue therapy is associated with a poor survival. Other studies have shown that pancreastatin should be measured before treatment and monitored during and after it. Plasma levels of this marker above 5000 pg/mL pretreatment were associated with increased periprocedure mortality in patients with NETs who underwent hepatic artery chemoembolization.[154]

These observations suggest that pancreastatin is potentially a very useful marker not only for diagnosis but more importantly for monitoring treatment response.

Neurokinin A

Neurokinin A (NKA) has been shown to have strong prognostic value. Turner and colleagues[155] showed in 2006 that in patients with midgut carcinoid who have raised plasma NKA, a reduction of the this biochemical marker after somatostatin analogue (SSA) therapy was associated with an 87% survival at 1 year compared with 40% if it increased. These investigators also concluded that any alteration in NKA predicts improved or worsening survival.

DIAGNOSIS OF BONE METASTASIS

Metastases from NETs can be either lytic and/or osteoblastic.

There may be an increased osteoclast activity contributing to lytic lesions and or an increase osteoblastic activity responsible for blastic metastases. Bone markers in lytic and osteoblastic metastases therapy include bone alkaline phosphatase (bAP), an indicator of osteoblast function, and urinary N-telopeptide, which reflects osteoclast activity or bone resorption. Somewhat paradoxically, only blastic metastases show an increase in both markers.[156]

Increased osteoclast activity predicts a poor outcome, with a relative risk (RR) for high N-telopeptide (>100 nmol BCE/mM creatinine) of: skeletal related events RR: 3.3 ($P<.001$); disease progression RR: 2.0 ($P<.001$); death RR: 4.6 ($P<.001$).[157]

BIOCHEMICAL DIAGNOSIS OF CARDIAC INVOLVEMENT

Carcinoid heart disease is a unique cardiac disease associated with NETs, and may be seen in up to 60% of patients with metastatic carcinoid. Valvular disease is the most common pathologic feature, and tricuspid damage is found in 97% and pulmonary valve disease in 88% with 88% displaying insufficiency and 49% stenosis. The distinctive carcinoid lesion consists of deposits of fibrous tissue devoid of elastic fibers, known as carcinoid plaque. The deposits are found on the endocardial surface on the ventricular aspect of the tricuspid leaflet and on the arterial aspect of the pulmonary valve cusps.[158]

The cause for the plaque formation is unclear, but the direct actions of serotonin and bradykinin have been implicated in animal studies. This finding is corroborated by the observation that the appetite suppressant drug fenfluramine, which releases serotonin, has been noted to cause valvular distortion similar to that seen in carcinoid heart disease.[159] Values of serotonin greater than 1000 ng/mL seem to consort with the development of carcinoid heart disease.

Pro-brain natriuretic peptide (NT-pro-BNP) can be used as a biomarker for the detection of carcinoid heart disease with high specificity and sensitivity, and is used as an adjunct to deciding who might require echocardiography.[160]

IMAGING OF THE PATIENT WITH A SUSPECTED NET
Imaging of Gastric Carcinoid Tumors

Most gastric carcinoid tumors are directly imaged and diagnosed during endoscopy. For larger lesions, endoscopic ultrasonography (EUS) may be performed to assess whether the gastric carcinoid is invasive. This technique, when used with tattooing of the gastric lesion, offers the endoscopist the opportunity to observe the lesion in a serial fashion. This method is highly valuable in the case of type I gastric carcinoids, which rarely need a formal gastric resection. In patients with more aggressive gastric carcinoids such as type II gastric carcinoids, EUS offers the endoscopist the opportunity to access nearby nodes as well as the depth of tumor invasion. Cross-sectional imaging with CT or magnetic resonance imaging (MRI) is recommended to assess for metastases in patients with type I or type II gastric carcinoids of more than 2 cm in diameter, or for patients with type III gastric carcinoids in whom metastatic risk is a concern.[15] The predominant site of distant metastatic spread in patients with gastric carcinoid tumors is the liver. Carcinoid liver metastases are often hypervascular, and may become isodense relative to the liver with the administration of intravenous contrast. CT scans should thus be performed both before and after the administration of intravenous contrast agents.[161] Somatostatin receptor scintigraphy provides a second useful imaging modality for the detection of metastatic disease in patients with malignant gastric carcinoids.[15,161,162]

Imaging of Midgut NETs

Imaging studies for NETs are generally done for initial staging and subsequent follow-up. Goals for initial staging include identification of primary tumor, assessment of extent of disease, and treatment planning. Subsequent follow-up imaging studies are done for surveillance following complete resection or during periods of stability, and evaluation of response following treatment. Imaging modalities commonly employed include:

- Small bowel series
- Computed tomography
- Magnetic resonance imaging
- [^{111}In-DTPA]octreotide scintigraphy
- [^{123}I]metaiodobenzylguanidine ([^{123}I]MIBG) scintigraphy
- Positron emission tomography (PET).

Initial Staging of Midgut NETs

Imaging studies generally recommended at time of initial staging include plain film of the chest, cross-sectional imaging of (CT or MRI) the abdomen and pelvis, and [^{111}In-DTPA]octreotide scintigraphy. In cases where a midgut primary is suspected but not directly identified (eg, a mesenteric mass in the ileal mesentery), often small bowel series or multiphasic CT of abdomen and pelvis with thin section and negative bowel contrast can be used to locate the primary tumor.

Techniques for Cross-Sectional Imaging

NETs are generally vascular tumors that enhance intensely with intravenous contrast during early arterial phases of imaging with washout during the delayed portal venous phase. The key to detecting small NETs on CT is to maximize the contrast between the tumor and the adjacent normal parenchyma. For abdominal and pelvic imaging the authors recommend multiphasic CT that includes the arterial phase (beginning 25–30 seconds after the start of contrast injection) and the portal venous phase (beginning approximately 60 seconds after the start of contrast injection). Rapid intravenous bolus of contrast at 4 to 5 mL per second is also recommended. Thin sectioning and the use of a negative oral contrast agent also may be helpful in detecting a small primary tumor in the small bowel that may not otherwise be seen.

MRI is preferred over CT for patients with a history of allergy to iodine contrast material or for those with renal insufficiency. NETs can have variable appearances on non-contrast MRI. They can be hypo- or isointense on T1-weighted images. Metastases to the liver typically are usually high signal on T2-weighted images.[163] Because T2-weighted images are obtained without intravenous contrast, they do not have the problems of variations in the timing of phases of contrast enhancement. T2-weighted imaging can be especially useful for patients unable to receive contrast. However, these metastases, especially when cystic or necrotic, can mimic the appearance of other T2 high signal intensity lesions, such as hemangiomas and occasionally cysts.[164] Dynamic contrast-enhanced imaging can provide additional information about the nature of the lesions, and helps to detect smaller lesions. The authors recommend T1- and T2-weighted imaging, and multiphasic (arterial, portal venous, and delayed) dynamic MRI for NETs.[163,165]

Some have reported that MRI may be more sensitive than CT for the detection of small liver metastases.[166,167] However, the CT may be better for the evaluation of peritoneal and mesenteric disease. Whether CT or MRI is better overall for NETs will continue to be debated, and may vary depending on the expertise of the local center.

Nuclear Imaging of NETs

The ^{111}In-labeled somatostatin analogue [^{111}In-DTPA]octreotide was developed for scintigraphy of NETs. It shares the receptor-binding profile of octreotide, which makes it a good radiopharmaceutical for imaging of tumors positive for somatostatin receptors 2 and 5.[168] The overall sensitivity of [^{111}In-DTPA]octreotide scintigraphy appears to be about 80% to 90%.[168] Unlike cross-sectional imaging, which are generally site directed, [^{111}In-DTPA]octreotide scintigraphy is generally done as whole body imaging and thus can detect disease at unsuspected sites.

Imaging is generally performed at 4 to 6 hours and again at 24 hours. Imaging at 24 hours provides better contrast due to lower background activity. However, there is often physiologic bowel activity that may produce false-positive results. At 4 to 6 hours, some lesions may be obscured by relatively high background activity; however, bowel activity is limited. Single-photon emission CT (SPECT) imaging with Ct coregistration may be helpful in resolving the nature of indeterminate lesions found on CT, and enhance the sensitivity and specificity study.

[^{111}In-DTPA]Octreotide scintigraphy can be performed for patients on long-acting octreotide, but is best performed at the end of the dosing interval (3–6 weeks after the last dose). While [^{111}In-DTPA]octreotide scintigraphy can provide useful information about the site of disease, it does not give information about size. Some agents such as interferon may upregulate somatostatin receptors and thus can lead to increased uptake without disease progression.

PET [^{18}F]fluoro-2-deoxy-D-deoxyglucose (FDG) imaging, though successful for many solid tumors, has not been helpful for NETs because of their generally lower proliferative activity. Prior studies have shown [^{11}C]5-HTP PET to be a promising imaging modality for the detection of NETs.[169] The serotonin precursor 5-HTP labeled with ^{11}C showed an increased uptake and irreversible trapping of this tracer in NETs.[169] [^{11}C]5-HTP PET proved better results than somatostatin receptor scintigraphy for tumor visualization. However, the short half-life of [11]C ($t_{1/2}$ = 20 minutes) makes it difficult to apply in clinical practice, and is not available in the United States.

Imaging of Pancreatic Neuroendocrine Tumors

General

Imaging of the primary tumor location and the extent of the disease is needed for all phases of management of patients with PNETs. It is necessary to determine whether surgical resection for possible cure or possible cytoreductive surgery is needed and whether treatment for advanced metastatic disease is appropriate, and during follow-up to assess the effects of any antitumor treatment as well as the need for deciding whether additional treatments directed at the PNETs are indicated.[28,60,170,171] Functional PNETs (especially insulinomas and duodenal gastrinomas) are often small in size, and localization may be difficult.[28,60,170,171] Several different imaging modalities have been widely used including conventional imaging studies (CT, MRI, US, angiography),[161,172–174] EUS,[28,175,176] functional localizations studies measuring hormonal gradients[28,177–179]; intraoperative methods, particularly intraoperative ultrasonography[28,180,181]; and recently, the use of PET preoperatively.[169,174,182,183] A few important points with regard to each are made here.

Conventional imaging studies for PNET studies (CT, MRI, US, angiography)

Even though PNETs are highly vascular tumors and most of these studies are now performed with contrast agents, the results with conventional imaging studies are dependent to a large degree on the tumor size.[28,161,170,184,185] Although conventional imaging studies detect more than 70% of PNETs larger than 3 cm, they detect less than 50% of most PNETs smaller than 1 cm, therefore frequently miss small primary PNETs (especially insulinomas and duodenal gastrinomas) and small liver metastases.[28,161,170,184,185] At least one of these modalities is generally available in most centers, with CT scanning with contrast being most frequently used as the first imaging modality.

Somatostatin receptor scintigraphy

PNETs, similar to carcinoid tumors, frequently (>80%, except insulinomas) overexpress somatostatin receptors (particularly subtypes sst 2, 5), which bind various synthetic analogues of somatostatin (octreotide, lanreotide) with high affinity.[28,172–174,186] Several radiolabeled somatostatin analogues have been developed to take advantage of this finding to image PNETs, with the most widely used worldwide and the only one available in the United States being [^{111}In-DTPA]octreotide (octreoscan).[28,172–174,186] Somatostatin receptor scintigraphy (SRS) combined with SPECT imaging is more sensitive than conventional imaging for detection of both the primary (except insulinomas) PET and metastatic PNETs to liver, bone, or other distant sites.[56,172–174,186,187] This sensitivity allows SRS to detect 50% to 70% of primary PNETs (less frequent with insulinomas or duodenal gastrinomas) and more than 90% of patients with metastatic disease.[28,172–174,188,189] SRS has the advantage of allowing total body scanning quickly at one time, and its use has resulted in a change in management of 24% to 47% of patients with PNETs.[28,172–174,188,189] False-positive localizations can occur in up to 12% of patients, so it is important to interpret the result within the clinical context of the patient and by doing this, the false-positive rate can be reduced to 3%.[28,173,189,190]

Endoscopic ultrasonography

EUS combined with fine-needle aspiration can be useful in distinguishing an NF-PET from adenocarcinoma or some other cause of a pancreatic mass.[28,175,176] Fine-needle aspiration is rarely used to diagnose functional PNETs, because they are suggested by symptoms and the diagnosis is established by hormonal assays.[28,60] EUS is much more effective for localizing intrapancreatic PNETs than extrapancreatic PNETs such as duodenal gastrinomas or somatostatinomas.[28,60,175] EUS is particularly helpful in localizing insulinomas, which are small, almost always intrapancreatic, and frequently missed by conventional imaging studies and SRS.[28,60,175] EUS can identify an intrapancreatic PET in about 90% of cases.[28,175] EUS can also play an important role in the management of patients with MEN-1 who harbor NF-PNETs in 80% to 100% of cases or in patients with NF-PNETs with VHL syndrome, occurring in 10%

to 17%, which are often small and whose management is controversial.[28,33,39,191–193] EUS can detect many of these small NF-PNETs, and it has been proposed that serial evaluations with EUS be used to select which MEN-1 or VHL patients should have surgery.[28,33,39,192–194]

Functional localization (assessing hormonal gradients) and PET scanning for PNETs

Assessment of hormonal gradients is now rarely used except in occasional patients with insulinomas or gastrinomas not localized by other imaging methods.[28,177–179,184,195] When used it is now usually performed at the time of angiography, and combined with selective intra-arterial injections of calcium for primary insulinomas or secretin for a primary gastrinoma or possible metastatic gastrinoma in the liver with hepatic venous hormonal sampling.[28,177–179,184,195] PET scanning is receiving increasing attention because of its increased sensitivity.[28,169,182–184] With PNETs, [^{11}C]5-HTP or ^{68}Ga-labeled somatostatin analogues have been shown to have greater sensitivity than SRS or conventional imaging studies, and therefore may be clinically useful in the future. Neither of these methods is approved for use in the United States and are not available in the United States at the current time.[28,169,174,182,183]

Intraoperative localization of PNETs

During surgery the routine use of intraoperative US is recommended, especially for pancreatic PNETs,[28,180,181] and for small duodenal tumors (especially duodenal gastrinomas) endoscopic transillumination[28,196,197] in addition to routine duodenotomy are recommended.[28,53,175,197–199]

Imaging for Pheochromocytomas and Paragangliomas

Either CT or MRI is recommended for initial tumor localization, with MRI preferred in children and pregnant or lactating women because of concerns regarding radiation exposure. Recent data suggest that adrenergic blockade in pheochromocytoma or paraganglioma patients as a specific precautionary measure before intravenous nonionic contrast enhanced CT imaging is not necessary (Brahm Shapiro, unpublished observations). Although CT and MRI have excellent sensitivity for detecting most catecholamine-producing tumors, these anatomic imaging approaches lack the specificity required to unequivocally identify a mass as a pheochromocytoma or paraganglioma.[200] The specificity of functional imaging using ^{123}I-labeled meta-iodobenzylguanidine scintigraphy ([^{123}I]-MIBG) offers an approach that overcomes the specificity limitations of anatomic imaging. Reduced sensitivity of MIBG scans in familial paraganglioma syndromes, malignant disease, and extra-adrenal paragangliomas has been described.[201–204] Newer compounds such as [^{18}F]fluorodopamine ([^{18}F]-FDA), [^{18}F]-fluoro-dihydroxyphenylalanine ([^{18}F]-FDOPA), and [^{18}F]-FDG have emerged for use in PET. The superiority of [^{18}F]-FDA PET imaging over [^{131}I]-MIBG scintigraphy, especially in malignant tumors, has been reported.[205] [^{18}F]-FDOPA PET imaging has been described to outperform [^{123}I]-MIBG scintigraphy in the detection of pheochromocytoma.[206] However, the sensitivity of [^{18}F]-FDOPA for metastatic paragangliomas is limited.[207] Studies have revealed that most pheochromocytomas show uptake of [^{18}F]-FDG in PET imaging.[208,209] Recently, [^{18}F]-FDG was demonstrated to be a superior tool in the evaluation of metastatic SDHB-associated adult pheochromocytoma and paraganglioma.[210] It is recommended that functional imaging be used on all pheochromocytomas and paragangliomas, except adrenal pheochromocytomas, that are less than 5 cm in size and associated with elevations of plasma or urine metanephrine (practically all epinephrine-producing pheochromocytomas are found in the adrenal gland or are recurrences of previously resected adrenal tumors).

Summary of Imaging for NETs

The preliminary workup of a neuroendocrine tumor often starts in the emergency department with plain abdominal radiographs done to work up an abdominal pain syndrome. Any abnormal finding leads to CT scanning, and the discovery of liver metastasis inevitably leads to CT-guided liver biopsy. These tests are often used nonspecifically because of the presence of vague symptom complexes. Once the NET diagnosis is suspected, more specific means of imaging are typically employed. For detecting the primary NET tumor, a multimodality approach is best and may include CT, MRI, SRS, EUS, endoscopy, and less commonly digital selective angiography or venous sampling. CT is probably superior for localizing the primary tumor, mesenteric invasion, and thoracic lesions, whereas gadolinium-enhanced MRI is superior in characterizing liver lesions. Technique is critical and meticulous attention to detail is necessary, and multidetector-row CT and MRI gradients have enhanced diagnostic performance. While some investigators in Europe advocate the use of enteroclysis with CT imaging, this technique is not readily available in most United States hospitals and thus is rarely done in this country.

The most sensitive imaging modality for detecting widespread metastatic disease in NETs is SRS (Octreoscan). However, SRS is less sensitive for metastatic insulinomas because only 40% to 50% express type 2 somatostatin receptors (sst 2) needed for SRS. Recent findings using glucagon receptor[211,212] imaging suggest that this may replace Octreoscans when insulinomas have not been identified, but this has not been done in the United States. Octreoscans are extremely useful in confirming the diagnosis and in evaluating tumor distribution and burden. The use of PET scanning in undifferentiated tumors or small cell-like lesions of the bronchus or thymus is highly effective. The role of PET scanning for well-differentiated NETs is less delineated. Only tumors with high proliferative activity and dedifferentiation show FDG-PET uptake. PET with tracers based on metabolic features (5-HTP) and receptor characteristics (DOTATOC) have shown promising results in a limited number of studies.

Once a gut-based NET is suspected, barium studies or endoscopy may rarely be helpful in localizing the primary tumor. The use of capsule endoscopy and double-balloon push-pull enteroscopy has been useful in cases of midgut-based NETs. EUS combined with biopsy is the most sensitive method to detect pancreatic NETs.

Recently [123I]MIBG scanning has been added to the diagnostic tools of US for the physician working up NETs. This scan offers information that is additive to the information gained by SRS imaging. In some patients SRS scanning is negative and other lesions light up on MIBG scanning. In other patients SRS imaging and MIBG scans both are positive or negative. In the case where both scans are positive, patients may be candidates for future therapy with [131I]MIBG or peptide receptor radionuclide therapy with radiolabeled somatostatin analogues.

SUMMARY

To conclude, an algorithm proposes a summary of the steps for diagnosis of NETs starting at the presentation of a suggestive clinical scenario (**Fig. 6**).[100]

NETs are small, slow-growing neoplasms, usually with episodic expression that makes diagnosis difficult, erroneous, and often late; for these reasons a high index of suspicion is needed, and it is important to understand the pathophysiology of

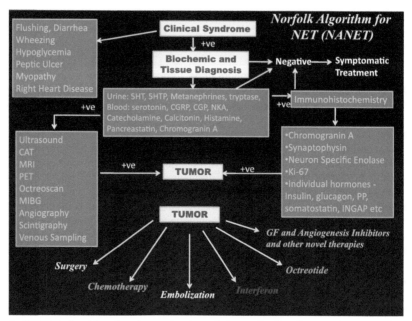

Fig. 6. NANETS algorithm for the evaluation of the patient with a suspected neuroendocrine tumor. (*Data from* Vinik A. Diffuse hormonal systems and endocrine tumor syndromes. Available at: www.endotext.org.)

each tumor to decide which biochemical markers are more useful and when they should be used.

It is the purpose of this guideline to show the importance of recognizing, as early as possible, the clinical syndromes that suggest a NET as one of the differential diagnoses, and once suspected, to look for the appropriate biochemical markers and radiological or other means that will confirm the diagnosis or confidently discard it. Ultimately all 3 modalities are important in creating a platform for monitoring response to therapy, determining prognosis, and choosing the right therapeutic intervention.

REFERENCES

1. Massironi S, Sciola V, Peracchi M, et al. Neuroendocrine tumors of the gastro-entero-pancreatic system. World J Gastroenterol 2008;14:5377–84.
2. Eriksson B, Oberg K, Stridsberg M. Tumor markers in neuroendocrine tumors. Digestion 2000;62(Suppl 1):33–8.
3. Lamberts SW, Hofland LJ, Nobels FR. Neuroendocrine tumor markers. Front Neuroendocrinol 2001;22:309–39.
4. Vinik A, O'Dorisio T, Woltering E, et al. Neuroendocrine tumors: a comprehensive guide to diagnosis and management. 1st edition. Inglewood (CA): Interscience Institute; 2006.
5. Feldman JM, O'Doriso TM. Role of neuropeptides and serotonin in the diagnosis of carcinoid tumors. Am J Med 1986;81:41–8.
6. Ahlman H, Dahlstrom A, Gronstad K, et al. The pentagastrin test in the diagnosis of the carcinoid syndrome. Blockade of gastrointestinal symptoms by ketanserin. Ann Surg 1985;201:81–6.

7. Kaplan EL, Jaffe BM, Peskin GW. A new provocative test for the diagnosis of the carcinoid syndrome. Am J Surg 1972;123:173–9.

8. Vinik AI, Gonin J, England BG, et al. Plasma substance-P in neuroendocrine tumors and idiopathic flushing: the value of pentagastrin stimulation tests and the effects of somatostatin analog. J Clin Endocrinol Metab 1990;70:1702–9.

9. Norheim I, Theodorsson-Norheim E, Brodin E, et al. Tachykinins in carcinoid tumors: their use as a tumor marker and possible role in the carcinoid flush. J Clin Endocrinol Metab 1986;63:605–12.

10. Conlon JM, Deacon CF, Richter G, et al. Circulating tachykinins (substance P, neurokinin A, neuropeptide K) and the carcinoid flush. Scand J Gastroenterol 1987;22(1):97–105.

11. Cunningham JL, Janson ET, Agarwal S, et al. Tachykinins in endocrine tumors and the carcinoid syndrome. Eur J Endocrinol 2008;159:275–82.

12. Won JG, Tseng HS, Yang AH, et al. Clinical features and morphological characterization of 10 patients with noninsulinoma pancreatogenous hypoglycaemia syndrome (NIPHS). Clin Endocrinol (Oxf) 2006;65:566–78.

13. Kaltsas GA, Besser GM, Grossman AB. The diagnosis and medical management of advanced neuroendocrine tumors. Endocr Rev 2004;25:458–511.

14. Rindi G, Bordi C, Rappel S, et al. Gastric carcinoids and neuroendocrine carcinomas: pathogenesis, pathology, and behavior. World J Surg 1996;20:168–72.

15. Ruszniewski P, Delle FG, Cadiot G, et al. Well-differentiated gastric tumors/carcinomas. Neuroendocrinology 2006;84:158–64.

16. Oberg K, Kvols L, Caplin M, et al. Consensus report on the use of somatostatin analogs for the management of neuroendocrine tumors of the gastroenteropancreatic system. Ann Oncol 2004;15:966–73.

17. Janson ET, Holmberg L, Stridsberg M, et al. Carcinoid tumors: analysis of prognostic factors and survival in 301 patients from a referral center. Ann Oncol 1997;8:685–90.

18. National Cancer Institute. Surveillance, Epidemiology, and End Results (SEER) Program. Available at: www.seer.cancer.gov. SEER*Stat Database: SEER 17 Regs Nov 2006 sub (1973–2004), ed released April 2006, National Cancer Institute, DCCPS, Surveillance Research Program, Cancer Statistic Branch. National Cancer Institute; 2006. Ref Type: Report.

19. Wang GG, Yao JC, Worah S, et al. Comparison of genetic alterations in neuroendocrine tumors: frequent loss of chromosome 18 in ileal carcinoid tumors. Mod Pathol 2005;18:1079–87.

20. Kytola S, Hoog A, Nord B, et al. Comparative genomic hybridization identifies loss of 18q22-qter as an early and specific event in tumorigenesis of midgut carcinoids. Am J Pathol 2001;158:1803–8.

21. Choi IS, Estecio MR, Nagano Y, et al. Hypomethylation of LINE-1 and Alu in well-differentiated neuroendocrine tumors (pancreatic endocrine tumors and carcinoid tumors). Mod Pathol 2007;20:802–10.

22. Goebel SU, Serrano J, Yu F, et al. Prospective study of the value of serum chromogranin A or serum gastrin levels in the assessment of the presence, extent, or growth of gastrinomas. Cancer 1999;85:1470–83.

23. Bernini GP, Moretti A, Ferdeghini M, et al. A new human chromogranin 'A' immunoradiometric assay for the diagnosis of neuroendocrine tumours. Br J Cancer 2001;84:636–42.

24. Nehar D, Lombard-Bohas C, Olivieri S, et al. Interest of chromogranin A for diagnosis and follow-up of endocrine tumours. Clin Endocrinol (Oxf) 2004;60:644–52.

25. Bajetta E, Ferrari L, Martinetti A, et al. Chromogranin A, neuron specific enolase, carcinoembryonic antigen, and hydroxyindole acetic acid evaluation in patients with neuroendocrine tumors. Cancer 1999;86:858–65.

26. Tormey WP, FitzGerald RJ. The clinical and laboratory correlates of an increased urinary 5-hydroxyindoleacetic acid. Postgrad Med J 1995;71:542–5.

27. Feldman JM, Lee EM. Serotonin content of foods: effect on urinary excretion of 5-hydroxyindoleacetic acid. Am J Clin Nutr 1985;42:639–43.

28. Metz DC, Jensen RT. Gastrointestinal neuroendocrine tumors: pancreatic endocrine tumors. Gastroenterology 2008;135:1469–92.

29. Kloppel G, Anlauf M. Epidemiology, tumour biology and histopathological classification of neuroendocrine tumours of the gastrointestinal tract. Best Pract Res Clin Gastroenterol 2005;19:507–17.

30. Oberg K, Eriksson B. Endocrine tumours of the pancreas. Best Pract Res Clin Gastroenterol 2005;19:753–81.

31. Falconi M, Plockinger U, Kwekkeboom DJ, et al. Well-differentiated pancreatic nonfunctioning tumors/carcinoma. Neuroendocrinology 2006;84:196–211.

32. O'Toole D, Salazar R, Falconi M, et al. Rare functioning pancreatic endocrine tumors. Neuroendocrinology 2006;84:189–95.

33. Jensen RT, Berna MJ, Bingham DB, et al. Inherited pancreatic endocrine tumor syndromes: advances in molecular pathogenesis, diagnosis, management, and controversies. Cancer 2008;113:1807–43.

34. Gibril F, Schumann M, Pace A, et al. Multiple endocrine neoplasia type 1 and Zollinger-Ellison syndrome: a prospective study of 107 cases and comparison with 1009 cases from the literature. Medicine (Baltimore) 2004;83:43–83.

35. Grant CS. Insulinoma. Best Pract Res Clin Gastroenterol 2005;19:783–98.

36. de Herder WW, Niederle B, Scoazec JY, et al. Well-differentiated pancreatic tumor/carcinoma: insulinoma. Neuroendocrinology 2006;84:183–8.

37. Hirshberg B, Livi A, Bartlett DL, et al. Forty-eight-hour fast: the diagnostic test for insulinoma. J Clin Endocrinol Metab 2000;85:3222–6.

38. Quinkler M, Strelow F, Pirlich M, et al. Assessment of suspected insulinoma by 48-hour fasting test: a retrospective monocentric study of 23 cases. Horm Metab Res 2007;39:507–10.

39. Kann PH, Balakina E, Ivan D, et al. Natural course of small, asymptomatic neuroendocrine pancreatic tumours in multiple endocrine neoplasia type 1: an endoscopic ultrasound imaging study. Endocr Relat Cancer 2006;13:1195–202.

40. Roy PK, Venzon DJ, Shojamanesh H, et al. Zollinger-Ellison syndrome. Clinical presentation in 261 patients. Medicine (Baltimore) 2000;79:379–411.

41. Jensen RT, Niederle B, Mitry E, et al. Gastrinoma (duodenal and pancreatic). Neuroendocrinology 2006;84:173–82.

42. Berna MJ, Hoffmann KM, Serrano J, et al. Serum gastrin in Zollinger-Ellison syndrome: I. Prospective study of fasting serum gastrin in 309 patients from the National Institutes of Health and comparison with 2229 cases from the literature. Medicine (Baltimore) 2006;85:295–330.

43. Gibril F, Jensen RT. Zollinger-Ellison syndrome revisited: diagnosis, biologic markers, associated inherited disorders, and acid hypersecretion. Curr Gastroenterol Rep 2004;6:454–63.

44. Berna MJ, Hoffmann KM, Long SH, et al. Serum gastrin in Zollinger-Ellison syndrome: II. Prospective study of gastrin provocative testing in 293 patients from the National Institutes of Health and comparison with 537 cases from the literature. evaluation of diagnostic criteria, proposal of new criteria, and correlations with clinical and tumoral features. Medicine (Baltimore) 2006;85:331–64.

45. Arnold R. Diagnosis and differential diagnosis of hypergastrinemia. Wien Klin Wochenschr 2007;119:564–9.
46. Corleto VD, Annibale B, Gibril F, et al. Does the widespread use of proton pump inhibitors mask, complicate and/or delay the diagnosis of Zollinger-Ellison syndrome? Aliment Pharmacol Ther 2001;15:1555–61.
47. Agreus L, Storskrubb T, Aro P, et al. Clinical use of proton-pump inhibitors but not H2-blockers or antacid/alginates raises the serum levels of amidated gastrin-17, pepsinogen I and pepsinogen II in a random adult population. Scand J Gastroenterol 2009;44:564–70.
48. Jensen RT. Consequences of long-term proton pump blockade: insights from studies of patients with gastrinomas. Basic Clin Pharmacol Toxicol 2006;98:4–19.
49. Thom AK, Norton JA, Axiotis CA, et al. Location, incidence, and malignant potential of duodenal gastrinomas. Surgery 1991;110:1086–91.
50. Jensen R, Gardner J. Gastrinoma. In: Go VL, DiMagno EP, Gardner JD, et al, editors. The pancreas: biology, pathobiology and disease. 2nd edition. New York: Raven Press Publishing Co; 1993. p. 931–78.
51. Thakker RV. Multiple endocrine neoplasia. Horm Res 2001;56(Suppl 1):67–72.
52. Hoffmann KM, Furukawa M, Jensen RT. Duodenal neuroendocrine tumors: classification, functional syndromes, diagnosis and medical treatment. Best Pract Res Clin Gastroenterol 2005;19:675–97.
53. Norton JA, Fraker DL, Alexander HR, et al. Surgery to cure the Zollinger-Ellison syndrome. N Engl J Med 1999;341:635–44.
54. Weber HC, Venzon DJ, Lin JT, et al. Determinants of metastatic rate and survival in patients with Zollinger-Ellison syndrome: a prospective long-term study. Gastroenterology 1995;108:1637–49.
55. Yu F, Venzon DJ, Serrano J, et al. Prospective study of the clinical course, prognostic factors, causes of death, and survival in patients with long-standing Zollinger-Ellison syndrome. J Clin Oncol 1999;17:615–30.
56. Gibril F, Doppman JL, Reynolds JC, et al. Bone metastases in patients with gastrinomas: a prospective study of bone scanning, somatostatin receptor scanning, and magnetic resonance image in their detection, frequency, location, and effect of their detection on management. J Clin Oncol 1998;16:1040–53.
57. Jensen RT. Management of the Zollinger-Ellison syndrome in patients with multiple endocrine neoplasia type 1. J Intern Med 1998;243:477–88.
58. Norton JA, Cornelius MJ, Doppman JL, et al. Effect of parathyroidectomy in patients with hyperparathyroidism, Zollinger-Ellison syndrome, and multiple endocrine neoplasia type I: a prospective study. Surgery 1987;102:958–66.
59. Norton JA, Venzon DJ, Berna MJ, et al. Prospective study of surgery for primary hyperparathyroidism (HPT) in multiple endocrine neoplasia-type 1 and Zollinger-Ellison syndrome: long-term outcome of a more virulent form of HPT. Ann Surg 2008;247:501–10.
60. Jensen RT. Endocrine neoplasms of the pancreas. In: Yamada T, Alpers DH, Kalloo AN, et al, editors. Textbook of gastroenterology. 5th edition. Oxford (England): Wiley-Blackwell; 2009. p. 1875–920.
61. Kindmark H, Sundin A, Granberg D, et al. Endocrine pancreatic tumors with glucagon hypersecretion: a retrospective study of 23 cases during 20 years. Med Oncol 2007;24:330–7.
62. van Beek AP, de Haas ER, van Vloten WA, et al. The glucagonoma syndrome and necrolytic migratory erythema: a clinical review. Eur J Endocrinol 2004;151:531–7.
63. Montenegro F, Lawrence GD, Macon W, et al. Metastatic glucagonoma. improvement after surgical debulking. Am J Surg 1980;139:424–7.

64. Conlon JM. The glucagon-like polypeptides—order out of chaos? Diabetologia 1980;18:85–8.
65. Vinik AI. Glucagonoma syndrome. Diffuse hormonal systems and endocrine tumor syndromes. In: Neuroendocrine tumors: a comprehensive guide to diagnosis and management. Inglewood (CA): Inter Science Institute; 2004.
66. Nikou GC, Toubanakis C, Nikolaou P, et al. VIPomas: an update in diagnosis and management in a series of 11 patients. Hepatogastroenterology 2005;52:1259–65.
67. Vale W, Rivier C, Brown M. Regulatory peptides of the hypothalamus. Annu Rev Physiol 1977;39:473–527.
68. Creutzfeldt W, Arnold R. Somatostatin and the stomach: exocrine and endocrine aspects. Metabolism 1978;27:1309–15.
69. Ganda OP, Weir GC, Soeldner JS, et al. "Somatostatinoma": a somatostatin-containing tumor of the endocrine pancreas. N Engl J Med 1977;296:963–7.
70. Krejs GJ, Orci L, Conlon JM, et al. Somatostatinoma syndrome. Biochemical, morphologic and clinical features. N Engl J Med 1979;301:285–92.
71. Larsson LI, Hirsch MA, Holst JJ, et al. Pancreatic somatostatinoma. Clinical features and physiological implications. Lancet 1977;1:666–8.
72. Crain EL Jr, Thorn GW. Functioning pancreatic islet cell adenomas; a review of the literature and presentation of two new differential tests. Medicine (Baltimore) 1949;28:427–47.
73. Fisher RS, Rock E, Levin G, et al. Effects of somatostatin on gallbladder emptying. Gastroenterology 1987;92:885–90.
74. Axelrod L, Bush MA, Hirsch HJ, et al. Malignant somatostatinoma: clinical features and metabolic studies. J Clin Endocrinol Metab 1981;52:886–96.
75. Penman E, Wass JA, Besser GM, et al. Somatostatin secretion by lung and thymic tumours. Clin Endocrinol (Oxf) 1980;13:613–20.
76. Boden G, Baile CA, McLaughlin CL, et al. Effects of starvation and obesity on somatostatin, insulin, and glucagon release from an isolated perfused organ system. Am J Physiol 1981;241:E215–20.
77. Creutzfeldt W, Lankisch PG, Folsch UR. [Inhibition by somatostatin of pancreatic juice and enzyme secretion and gallbladder contraction in man induced by secretin and cholecystokinin-pancreozymin administration (author's transl)]. Dtsch Med Wochenschr 1975;100:1135–8 [in German].
78. Schwartz TW. Atropine suppression test for pancreatic polypeptide. Lancet 1978; 2:43–4.
79. Bloom SR, Mortimer CH, Thorner MO, et al. Inhibition of gastrin and gastric-acid secretion by growth-hormone release-inhibiting hormone. Lancet 1974;2:1106–9.
80. Moayedoddin B, Booya F, Wermers RA, et al. Spectrum of malignant somatostatin-producing neuroendocrine tumors. Endocr Pract 2006;12:394–400.
81. Tanaka S, Yamasaki S, Matsushita H, et al. Duodenal somatostatinoma: a case report and review of 31 cases with special reference to the relationship between tumor size and metastasis. Pathol Int 2000;50:146–52.
82. Bhathena S, Higgins G, Recant L. Glucagonoma and glucagonoma syndrome. New York: Elsesvier/North Holland; 1981. p. 413.
83. Vinik AI, Delbridge L, Moattari R, et al. Transhepatic portal vein catheterization for localization of insulinomas: a ten-year experience. Surgery 1991;109:1–11.
84. Jensen RT, Gardner JD, Raufman JP, et al. Zollinger-Ellison syndrome: current concepts and management. Ann Intern Med 1983;98:59–75.
85. Vinik AI, Levitt NS, Pimstone BL, et al. Peripheral plasma somatostatin-like immunoreactive responses to insulin hypoglycemia and a mixed meal in healthy

subjects and in noninsulin-dependent maturity-onset diabetics. J Clin Endocrinol Metab 1981;52:330–7.

86. Sano T, Kagawa N, Hizawa K. Demonstration of somatostatin production in medullary carcinoma of the thyroid. Jpn J Cancer Res 1980;10:221.

87. Saito S, Saito H, Matsumura M, et al. Molecular heterogeneity and biological activity of immunoreactive somatostatin in medullary carcinoma of the thyroid. J Clin Endocrinol Metab 1981;53:1117–22.

88. Roos BA, Lindall AW, Ells J, et al. Increased plasma and tumor somatostatin-like immunoreactivity in medullary thyroid carcinoma and small cell lung cancer. J Clin Endocrinol Metab 1981;52:187–94.

89. Ghose RR, Gupta SK. Oat cell carcinoma of bronchus presenting with somatostatinoma syndrome. Thorax 1981;36:550–1.

90. Jackson J, Raju U, Janakivamon N. Metastatic pulmonary somatostatinoma presenting with diabetic ketoacidosis: clinical biochemical and morphologic characterization. Clin Res 1986;34:196A.

91. Vinik AI, Shapiro B, Thompson NW. Plasma gut hormone levels in 37 patients with pheochromocytomas. World J Surg 1986;10:593–604.

92. Berelowitz M, Szabo M, Barowsky HW, et al. Somatostatin-like immunoactivity and biological activity is present in a human pheochromocytoma. J Clin Endocrinol Metab 1983;56:134–8.

93. Samols E, Weir GC, Ramseur R, et al. Modulation of pancreatic somatostatin by adrenergic and cholinergic agonism and by hyper- and hypoglycemic sulfonamides. Metabolism 1978;27:1219–21.

94. Pipeleers D, Couturier E, Gepts W, et al. Five cases of somatostatinoma: clinical heterogeneity and diagnostic usefulness of basal and tolbutamide-induced hypersomatostatinemia. J Clin Endocrinol Metab 1983;56:1236–42.

95. Gola M, Doga M, Bonadonna S, et al. Neuroendocrine tumors secreting growth hormone-releasing hormone: Pathophysiological and clinical aspects. Pituitary 2006;9:221–9.

96. Maton PN, Gardner JD, Jensen RT. Cushing's syndrome in patients with the Zollinger-Ellison syndrome. N Engl J Med 1986;315:1–5.

97. Mao C, Carter P, Schaefer P, et al. Malignant islet cell tumor associated with hypercalcemia. Surgery 1995;117:37–40.

98. Plockinger U, Wiedenmann B. Diagnosis of non-functioning neuro-endocrine gastro-enteropancreatic tumours. Neuroendocrinology 2004;80(Suppl 1):35–8.

99. Gullo L, Migliori M, Falconi M, et al. Nonfunctioning pancreatic endocrine tumors: a multicenter clinical study. Am J Gastroenterol 2003;98:2435–9.

100. Vinik AI, Silva MP, Woltering EA, et al. Biochemical testing for neuroendocrine tumors. Pancreas 2009;38:876–89.

101. Nieman LK, Biller BM, Findling JW, et al. The diagnosis of Cushing's syndrome: an Endocrine Society Clinical Practice Guideline. J Clin Endocrinol Metab 2008; 93:1526–40.

102. de Herder WW. Biochemistry of neuroendocrine tumours. Best Pract Res Clin Endocrinol Metab 2007;21:33–41.

103. Oberg K, Eriksson B. Best practice & research clinical endocrinology metabolism. Oxford (England): Elsevier, Ltd; 2007.

104. Ardill JE. Circulating markers for endocrine tumours of the gastroenteropancreatic tract. Ann Clin Biochem 2008;45:539–59.

105. Lenders JW, Eisenhofer G, Mannelli M, et al. Phaeochromocytoma. Lancet 2005; 366:665–75.

106. Manger WM, Gifford RW. Pheochromocytoma. J Clin Hypertens (Greenwich) 2002;4:62–72.

107. Neumann HP, Bausch B, McWhinney SR, et al. Germ-line mutations in nonsyndromic pheochromocytoma. N Engl J Med 2002;346:1459–66.

108. Barontini M, Levin G, Sanso G. Characteristics of pheochromocytoma in a 4- to 20-year-old population. Ann N Y Acad Sci 2006;1073:30–7.

109. de Krijger RR, Petri BJ, van Nederveen FH, et al. Frequent genetic changes in childhood pheochromocytomas. Ann N Y Acad Sci 2006;1073:166–76.

110. Ludwig AD, Feig DI, Brandt ML, et al. Recent advances in the diagnosis and treatment of pheochromocytoma in children. Am J Surg 2007;194:792–6.

111. Benn DE, Gimenez-Roqueplo AP, Reilly JR, et al. Clinical presentation and penetrance of pheochromocytoma/paraganglioma syndromes. J Clin Endocrinol Metab 2006;91:827–36.

112. Gimenez-Roqueplo AP, Favier J, Rustin P, et al. Mutations in the SDHB gene are associated with extra-adrenal and/or malignant phaeochromocytomas. Cancer Res 2003;63:5615–21.

113. Bryant J, Farmer J, Kessler LJ, et al. Pheochromocytoma: the expanding genetic differential diagnosis. J Natl Cancer Inst 2003;95:1196–204.

114. Brouwers FM, Eisenhofer G, Tao JJ, et al. High frequency of SDHB germline mutations in patients with malignant catecholamine-producing paragangliomas: implications for genetic testing. J Clin Endocrinol Metab 2006;91: 4505–9.

115. Timmers HJ, Kozupa A, Eisenhofer G, et al. Clinical presentations, biochemical phenotypes, and genotype-phenotype correlations in patients with succinate dehydrogenase subunit B-associated pheochromocytomas and paragangliomas. J Clin Endocrinol Metab 2007;92:779–86.

116. Amar L, Bertherat J, Baudin E, et al. Genetic testing in pheochromocytoma or functional paraganglioma. J Clin Oncol 2005;23:8812–8.

117. Lenders JW, Pacak K, Walther MM, et al. Biochemical diagnosis of pheochromocytoma: which test is best? JAMA 2002;287:1427–34.

118. Eisenhofer G, Lenders JW, Linehan WM, et al. Plasma normetanephrine and metanephrine for detecting pheochromocytoma in von Hippel-Lindau disease and multiple endocrine neoplasia type 2. N Engl J Med 1999; 340:1872–9.

119. Sawka AM, Jaeschke R, Singh RJ, et al. A comparison of biochemical tests for pheochromocytoma: measurement of fractionated plasma metanephrines compared with the combination of 24-hour urinary metanephrines and catecholamines. J Clin Endocrinol Metab 2003;88:553–8.

120. Lenders JW, Willemsen JJ, Eisenhofer G, et al. Is supine rest necessary before blood sampling for plasma metanephrines? Clin Chem 2007;53:352–4.

121. Grossman A, Pacak K, Sawka A, et al. Biochemical diagnosis and localization of pheochromocytoma: can we reach a consensus? Ann N Y Acad Sci 2006;1073: 332–47.

122. Eisenhofer G, Goldstein DS, Walther MM, et al. Biochemical diagnosis of pheochromocytoma: how to distinguish true- from false-positive test results. J Clin Endocrinol Metab 2003;88:2656–66.

123. Guller U, Turek J, Eubanks S, et al. Detecting pheochromocytoma: defining the most sensitive test. Ann Surg 2006;243:102–7.

124. Giovanella L, Squin N, Ghelfo A, et al. Chromogranin A immunoradiometric assay in diagnosis of pheochromocytoma: comparison with plasma metanephrines and ^{123}I-MIBG scan. Q J Nucl Med Mol Imaging 2006;50:344–7.

125. Bilek R, Safarik L, Ciprova V, et al. a member of neuroendocrine secretory proteins as a selective marker for laboratory diagnosis of pheochromocytoma. Physiol Res 2008;57(Suppl 1):S171–9.

126. Klein RD, Lloyd RV, Young WF. Hereditary paraganglioma-pheochromocytoma syndromes. Gene Reviews 2008 [online].

127. Algeciras-Schimnich A, Preissner CM, Young WF Jr, et al. Plasma chromogranin A or urine fractionated metanephrines follow-up testing improves the diagnostic accuracy of plasma fractionated metanephrines for pheochromocytoma. J Clin Endocrinol Metab 2008;93:91–5.

128. Young WF Jr. Paragangliomas: clinical overview. Ann N Y Acad Sci 2006;1073: 21–9.

129. Costante G, Meringolo D, Durante C, et al. Predictive value of serum calcitonin levels for preoperative diagnosis of medullary thyroid carcinoma in a cohort of 5817 consecutive patients with thyroid nodules. J Clin Endocrinol Metab 2007;92:450–5.

130. Cohen R, Campos JM, Salaun C, et al. Preoperative calcitonin levels are predictive of tumor size and postoperative calcitonin normalization in medullary thyroid carcinoma. Groupe d'Etudes des Tumeurs a Calcitonine (GETC). J Clin Endocrinol Metab 2000;85:919–22.

131. Kebebew E, Ituarte PH, Siperstein AE, et al. Medullary thyroid carcinoma: clinical characteristics, treatment, prognostic factors, and a comparison of staging systems. Cancer 2000;88:1139–48.

132. Etit D, Faquin WC, Gaz R, et al. Histopathologic and clinical features of medullary microcarcinoma and C-cell hyperplasia in prophylactic thyroidectomies for medullary carcinoma: a study of 42 cases. Arch Pathol Lab Med 2008;132: 1767–73.

133. Elisei R. Routine serum calcitonin measurement in the evaluation of thyroid nodules. Best Pract Res Clin Endocrinol Metab 2008;22:941–53.

134. Scheuba C, Kaserer K, Moritz A, et al. Sporadic hypercalcitoninemia: clinical and therapeutic consequences. Endocr Relat Cancer 2009;16(1):243–53.

135. Colombo P, Locatelli F, Travaglini P. [Useful and limits of the biochemical markers for the diagnosis of thyroid carcinoma]. Ann Ital Chir 2006;77:209–14 [in Italian].

136. Schley E, Shin S, Nakave AA, et al. Symptomatic isolated C-cell hyperplasia: masquerading as carcinoid syndrome. Pancreas 2009.

137. Marx SJ, Agarwal SK, Kester MB, et al. Multiple endocrine neoplasia type 1: clinical and genetic features of the hereditary endocrine neoplasias. Recent Prog Horm Res 1999;54:397–438.

138. Piecha G, Chudek J, Wiecek A. Multiple endocrine neoplasia type 1. Eur J Intern Med 2008;19:99–103.

139. Perry R. Multiple Endocrine Neoplasia Type 1 and MEN II. Diffuse hormonal systems and endocrine tumor syndromes. 2006. Available at: www.Endotext. org. Accessed December 30, 2010.

140. Brandi ML, Gagel RF, Angeli A, et al. Guidelines for diagnosis and therapy of MEN type 1 and type 2. J Clin Endocrinol Metab 2001;86:5658–71.

141. Gertner ME, Kebebew E. Multiple endocrine neoplasia type 2. Curr Treat Options Oncol 2004;5:315–25.

142. Fialkowski EA, DeBenedetti MK, Moley JF, et al. RET proto-oncogene testing in infants presenting with Hirschsprung disease identifies 2 new multiple endocrine neoplasia 2A kindreds. J Pediatr Surg 2008;43:188–90.

143. Raue F, Frank-Raue K. Multiple endocrine neoplasia type 2: 2007 update. Horm Res 2007;68(Suppl 5):101–4.

144. Taupenot L, Harper KL, O'Connor DT. The chromogranin-secretogranin family. N Engl J Med 2003;348:1134–49.
145. Nobels FR, Kwekkeboom DJ, Bouillon R, et al. Chromogranin A: its clinical value as marker of neuroendocrine tumours. Eur J Clin Invest 1998;28:431–40.
146. Stridsberg M, Eriksson B, Fellstrom B, et al. Measurements of chromogranin B can serve as a complement to chromogranin A. Regul Pept 2007;139:80–3.
147. Takiyyuddin MA, Cervenka JH, Hsiao RJ, et al. Chromogranin A. Storage and release in hypertension. Hypertension 1990;15:237–46.
148. Oberg K. Biochemical diagnosis of neuroendocrine GEP tumor. Yale J Biol Med 1997;70:501–8.
149. Nobels FR, Kwekkeboom DJ, Coopmans W, et al. Chromogranin A as serum marker for neuroendocrine neoplasia: comparison with neuron-specific enolase and the alpha-subunit of glycoprotein hormones. J Clin Endocrinol Metab 1997; 82:2622–8.
150. Zatelli MC, Torta M, Leon A, et al. Chromogranin A as a marker of neuroendo-crine neoplasia: an Italian Multicenter Study. Endocr Relat Cancer 2007;14: 473–82.
151. Panzuto F, Severi C, Cannizzaro R, et al. Utility of combined use of plasma levels of chromogranin A and pancreatic polypeptide in the diagnosis of gastroines-tinal and pancreatic endocrine tumors. J Endocrinol Invest 2004;27:6–11.
152. Jensen EH, Kvols L, McLoughlin JM, et al. Biomarkers predict outcomes following cytoreductive surgery for hepatic metastases from functional carcinoid tumors. Ann Surg Oncol 2007;14:780–5.
153. Stronge RL, Turner GB, Johnston BT, et al. A rapid rise in circulating pancreast-atin in response to somatostatin analogue therapy is associated with poor survival in patients with neuroendocrine tumours. Ann Clin Biochem 2008;45: 560–6.
154. Bloomston M, Al-Saif O, Klemanski D, et al. Hepatic artery chemoembolization in 122 patients with metastatic carcinoid tumor: lessons learned. J Gastrointest Surg 2007;11:264–71.
155. Turner GB, Johnston BT, McCance DR, et al. Circulating markers of prognosis and response to treatment in patients with midgut carcinoid tumours. Gut 2006;55:1586–91.
156. Lipton A, Costa L, Ali S, et al. Use of markers of bone turnover for moni-toring bone metastases and the response to therapy. Semin Oncol 2001; 28:54–9.
157. Brown JE, Cook RJ, Major P, et al. Bone turnover markers as predictors of skel-etal complications in prostate cancer, lung cancer, and other solid tumors. J Natl Cancer Inst 2005;97:59–69.
158. Roberts WC. A unique heart disease associated with a unique cancer: carcinoid heart disease. Am J Cardiol 1997;80:251–6.
159. Fox DJ, Khattar RS. Carcinoid heart disease: presentation, diagnosis, and management. Heart 2004;90:1224–8.
160. Bhattacharyya S, Toumpanakis C, Caplin ME, et al. Usefulness of N-terminal pro-brain natriuretic peptide as a biomarker of the presence of carcinoid heart disease. Am J Cardiol 2008;102:938–42.
161. Rockall AG, Reznek RH. Imaging of neuroendocrine tumours (CT/MR/US). Best Pract Res Clin Endocrinol Metab 2007;21:43–68.
162. Gibril F, Reynolds JC, Lubensky IA, et al. Ability of somatostatin receptor scin-tigraphy to identify patients with gastric carcinoids: a prospective study. J Nucl Med 2000;41:1646–56.

163. Semelka RC, Custodio CM, Cem BN, et al. Neuroendocrine tumors of the pancreas: spectrum of appearances on MRI. J Magn Reson Imaging 2000; 11:141–8.
164. Pamuklar E, Semelka RC. MR imaging of the pancreas. Magn Reson Imaging Clin N Am 2005;13:313–30.
165. Kelekis NL, Semelka RC. MRI of pancreatic tumors. Eur Radiol 1997;7:875–86.
166. Dromain C, de BT, Baudin E, et al. MR imaging of hepatic metastases caused by neuroendocrine tumors: comparing four techniques. AJR Am J Roentgenol 2003;180:121–8.
167. Debray MP, Geoffroy O, Laissy JP, et al. Imaging appearances of metastases from neuroendocrine tumours of the pancreas. Br J Radiol 2001;74:1065–70.
168. Krenning EP, Kooij PP, Bakker WH, et al. Radiotherapy with a radiolabeled somatostatin analogue, [^{111}In-DTPA-D-Phe1]-octreotide. A case history. Ann N Y Acad Sci 1994;733:496–506.
169. Orlefors H, Sundin A, Garske U, et al. Whole-body (11)C-5-hydroxytryptophan positron emission tomography as a universal imaging technique for neuroendocrine tumors: comparison with somatostatin receptor scintigraphy and computed tomography. J Clin Endocrinol Metab 2005;90:3392–400.
170. Noone TC, Hosey J, Firat Z, et al. Imaging and localization of islet-cell tumours of the pancreas on CT and MRI. Best Pract Res Clin Endocrinol Metab 2005;19: 195–211.
171. Kloppel G, Couvelard A, Perren A, et al. ENETS guidelines for the standards of care in patients with neuroendocrine tumors: towards a standardized approach to the diagnosis of gastroenteropancreatic neuroendocrine tumors and their prognostic stratification. Neuroendocrinology 2009;90(2):162–6.
172. Virgolini I, Traub-Weidinger T, Decristoforo C. Nuclear medicine in the detection and management of pancreatic islet-cell tumours. Best Pract Res Clin Endocrinol Metab 2005;19:213–27.
173. Gibril F, Jensen RT. Diagnostic uses of radiolabelled somatostatin receptor analogues in gastroenteropancreatic endocrine tumours. Dig Liver Dis 2004; 36(Suppl 1):S106–20.
174. Sundin A, Garske U, Orlefors H. Nuclear imaging of neuroendocrine tumours. Best Pract Res Clin Endocrinol Metab 2007;21:69–85.
175. Norton JA, Jensen RT. Resolved and unresolved controversies in the surgical management of patients with Zollinger-Ellison syndrome. Ann Surg 2004;240: 757–73.
176. McLean AM, Fairclough PD. Endoscopic ultrasound in the localisation of pancreatic islet cell tumours. Best Pract Res Clin Endocrinol Metab 2005;19: 177–93.
177. Doppman JL, Miller DL, Chang R, et al. Gastrinomas: localization by means of selective intraarterial injection of secretin. Radiology 1990;174:25–9.
178. Doppman JL, Chang R, Fraker DL, et al. Localization of insulinomas to regions of the pancreas by intra-arterial stimulation with calcium. Ann Intern Med 1995; 123:269–73.
179. Strader D, Doppman J, Orbuch M, et al. Functional localization of pancreatic endocrine tumors. In: Mignon M, Jensen RT, editors. Endocrine tumors of the pancreas: recent advances in research and management. Series: frontiers of gastrointestinal research. Basel (Switzerland): Karger Publishing Co; 1995. p. 282–97.
180. Norton JA. Surgical treatment of islet cell tumors with special emphasis on operative tumors. In: Mignon M, Jensen RT, editors. Endocrine tumors of the

pancreas: recent advances in research and management. Basel (Switzerland): S. Karger; 1995. p. 309–32.

181. Shin LK, Brant-Zawadzki G, Kamaya A, et al. Intraoperative ultrasound of the pancreas. Ultrasound Q 2009;25:39–48.

182. Gabriel M, Decristoforo C, Kendler D, et al. ^{68}Ga-DOTA-Tyr3-octreotide PET in neuroendocrine tumors: comparison with somatostatin receptor scintigraphy and CT. J Nucl Med 2007;48:508–18.

183. Eriksson B, Orlefors H, Oberg K, et al. Developments in PET for the detection of endocrine tumours. Best Pract Res Clin Endocrinol Metab 2005;19:311–24.

184. Jackson JE. Angiography and arterial stimulation venous sampling in the localization of pancreatic neuroendocrine tumours. Best Pract Res Clin Endocrinol Metab 2005;19:229–39.

185. Sundin A, Vullierme MP, Kaltsas G, et al. ENETS guidelines for the standards of care in patients with neuroendocrine tumours: radiological examinations in patients with neuroendocrine tumours. Neuroendocrinology 2009;90(2):167–83.

186. Krenning EP, Kwekkeboom DJ, Oei HY, et al. Somatostatin-receptor scintigraphy in gastroenteropancreatic tumors. An overview of European results. Ann N Y Acad Sci 1994;733:416–24.

187. Gibril F, Reynolds JC, Doppman JL, et al. Somatostatin receptor scintigraphy: its sensitivity compared with that of other imaging methods in detecting primary and metastatic gastrinomas. A prospective study. Ann Intern Med 1996;125:26–34.

188. Termanini B, Gibril F, Reynolds JC, et al. Value of somatostatin receptor scintigraphy: a prospective study in gastrinoma of its effect on clinical management. Gastroenterology 1997;112:335–47.

189. Berna M, Jensen R. Use of radiolabeled somatostatin receptor analogues in diagnosis of gastrointestinal neuroendocrine tumors. In: Modlin IM, Oberg K, editors. A century of advances in neuroendocrine tumor biology and treatment. Hanover: Felstein C.C.C.P; 2007. p. 328–39.

190. Gibril F, Reynolds JC, Chen CC, et al. Specificity of somatostatin receptor scintigraphy: a prospective study and effects of false-positive localizations on management in patients with gastrinomas. J Nucl Med 1999;40:539–53.

191. Hellman P, Hennings J, Akerstrom G, et al. Endoscopic ultrasonography for evaluation of pancreatic tumours in multiple endocrine neoplasia type 1. Br J Surg 2005;92:1508–12.

192. Libutti SK, Choyke PL, Bartlett DL, et al. Pancreatic neuroendocrine tumors associated with von Hippel Lindau disease: diagnostic and management recommendations. Surgery 1998;124:1153–9.

193. Langer P, Kann PH, Fendrich V, et al. Prospective evaluation of imaging procedures for the detection of pancreaticoduodenal endocrine tumors in patients with multiple endocrine neoplasia type 1. World J Surg 2004;28:1317–22.

194. Manfredi S, Pagenault M, de Lajarte-Thirouard AS, et al. Type 1 and 2 gastric carcinoid tumors: long-term follow-up of the efficacy of treatment with a slow-release somatostatin analogue. Eur J Gastroenterol Hepatol 2007;19:1021–5.

195. Gibril F, Doppman JL, Chang R, et al. Metastatic gastrinomas: localization with selective arterial injection of secretin. Radiology 1996;198:77–84.

196. Frucht H, Norton JA, London JF, et al. Detection of duodenal gastrinomas by operative endoscopic transillumination. A prospective study. Gastroenterology 1990;99:1622–7.

197. Norton JA, Doppman JL, Jensen RT. Curative resection in Zollinger-Ellison syndrome. Results of a 10-year prospective study. Ann Surg 1992;215:8–18.

198. Norton JA, Alexander HR, Fraker DL, et al. Does the use of routine duodenotomy (DUODX) affect rate of cure, development of liver metastases, or survival in patients with Zollinger-Ellison syndrome? Ann Surg 2004;239:617–25.

199. Sugg SL, Norton JA, Fraker DL, et al. A prospective study of intraoperative methods to diagnose and resect duodenal gastrinomas. Ann Surg 1993;218:138–44.

200. Pacak K, Eisenhofer G, Goldstein DS. Functional imaging of endocrine tumors: role of positron emission tomography. Endocr Rev 2004;25:568–80.

201. Lumachi F, Tregnaghi A, Zucchetta P, et al. Sensitivity and positive predictive value of CT, MRI and 123I-MIBG scintigraphy in localizing pheochromocytomas: a prospective study. Nucl Med Commun 2006;27:583–7.

202. van der HE, de Herder WW, Bruining HA, et al. [(123)I]metaiodobenzylguanidine and [(111)In]octreotide uptake in benign and malignant pheochromocytomas. J Clin Endocrinol Metab 2001;86:685–93.

203. Bhatia KS, Ismail MM, Sahdev A, et al. ^{123}I-metaiodobenzylguanidine (MIBG) scintigraphy for the detection of adrenal and extra-adrenal phaeochromocytomas: CT and MRI correlation. Clin Endocrinol (Oxf) 2008;69:181–8.

204. Mackenzie IS, Gurnell M, Balan KK, et al. The use of 18-fluoro-dihydroxyphenylalanine and 18-fluorodeoxyglucose positron emission tomography scanning in the assessment of metaiodobenzylguanidine-negative phaeochromocytoma. Eur J Endocrinol 2007;157:533–7.

205. Ilias I, Yu J, Carrasquillo JA, et al. Superiority of 6-[^{18}F]-fluorodopamine positron emission tomography versus [^{131}I]-metaiodobenzylguanidine scintigraphy in the localization of metastatic pheochromocytoma. J Clin Endocrinol Metab 2003;88:4083–7.

206. Hoegerle S, Nitzsche E, Altehoefer C, et al. Pheochromocytomas: detection with ^{18}F DOPA whole body PET–initial results. Radiology 2002;222:507–12.

207. Timmers HJ, Hadi M, Carrasquillo JA, et al. The effects of carbidopa on uptake of 6-^{18}F-Fluoro-L-DOPA in PET of pheochromocytoma and extraadrenal abdominal paraganglioma. J Nucl Med 2007;48:1599–606.

208. Shulkin BL, Koeppe RA, Francis IR, et al. Pheochromocytomas that do not accumulate metaiodobenzylguanidine: localization with PET and administration of FDG. Radiology 1993;186:711–5.

209. Shulkin BL, Thompson NW, Shapiro B, et al. Pheochromocytomas: imaging with 2-[fluorine-18]fluoro-2-deoxy-D-glucose PET. Radiology 1999;212:35–41.

210. Timmers HJ, Kozupa A, Chen CC, et al. Superiority of fluorodeoxyglucose positron emission tomography to other functional imaging techniques in the evaluation of metastatic SDHB-associated pheochromocytoma and paraganglioma. J Clin Oncol 2007;25:2262–9.

211. Wild D, Macke H, Christ E, et al. Glucagon-like peptide 1-receptor scans to localize occult insulinomas. N Engl J Med 2008;359:766–8.

212. Modlin IM, Oberg K, Chung DC, et al. Gastroenteropancreatic neuroendocrine tumours. Lancet Oncol 2008;9:61–72.

Neuroendocrine Tumors in Children and Young Adults: Rare or Not So Rare

Marie-Ellen Sarvida, MD[a],*, M. Sue O'Dorisio, MD, PhD[b]

KEYWORDS

- Neuroendocrine tumor • Neuroblastoma • Carcinoid
- Multiple endocrine neoplasia

Endocrine tumors are neoplasms arising from endocrine organs, regardless of whether the tumor secretes hormones, and tumors producing or secreting hormones, regardless of the tissue of origin. Endocrine tumors in children include germ cell tumors; adrenal and pancreatic carcinoma; thyroid, pituitary, breast, ovarian, uterine, and cervical cancers; and finally, neuroendocrine tumors (NETs). Most endocrine tumors in childhood are clinically benign or low-grade malignancies, with a small percentage of gonadal and germ cell tumors, thyroid neoplasms, and adrenocortical tumors presenting as high-grade malignancies (**Table 1**).

Although most neoplasms that occur in children are sporadic, a small portion of certain endocrine tumors are familial, some of which show mendelian inheritance. Medullary carcinomas of the thyroid gland and pheochromocytomas can occur in a familial syndrome called multiple endocrine neoplasia (MEN) type II. MEN type I is also a familial syndrome with tumors of the parathyroid glands and pituitary gland. Carney complex is a condition inherited in an autosomal dominant manner associated with skin or heart myxomas, spotty skin pigmentations, and multiple endocrine tumors. Other genetic disorders including neurofibromatosis (NF) 1 and von Hippel-Lindau (VHL) disease are frequently associated with pheochromocytoma.

Tumors arising in the neural crest, including neuroblastoma, pheochromocytoma, Ewing sarcoma, benign and malignant schwannomas, neurofibromas, and primary melanomas, are sometimes classified as NETs (see **Table 1**). Neuroblastoma, a pediatric neoplasm, is the most common cancer diagnosed during infancy. Neuroblastomas arise from neural crest–derived cells committed to sympathoadrenal

[a] Department of Pediatrics, Ronald McDonald Children's Hospital, Loyola University Medical Center, 2160 South First Avenue, Maywood, IL 60153, USA
[b] Department of Pediatrics, RJ and LA Carver College of Medicine, University of Iowa, 200 Hawkins Drive, Iowa City, IA 52242, USA
* Corresponding author.
E-mail address: msarvida@lumc.edu

Endocrinol Metab Clin N Am 40 (2011) 65–80
doi:10.1016/j.ecl.2010.12.007
0889-8529/11/$ – see front matter © 2011 Elsevier Inc. All rights reserved.

Table 1
Classification of endocrine, neuroendocrine, and neural crest tumors

Anatomic Site	Endocrine	Neuroendocrine	Neural Crest

Pituitary	Adenomas
	  Prolactin
	  Growth hormone
	  ACTH
	  TSH
	  LH/FSH
		—	—

Thyroid	Thyroid
	  carcinoma
		Medullary
		  thyroid
		  cancer
			—

Breast	Breast cancer	Medullary carcinoma NET (carcinoid)	—

Testes or
  ovary
	Germ cell tumors
	Testicular cancer
	Ovarian cancer
		Small cell
		  carcinoma
		  Ovary
		  Cervix
			—

Thymus	—	Thymic carcinoid	—
Lung	—	Small cell carcinoma Large cell carcinoma Bronchial NET (carcinoid)	—
Upper intestine	—	Esophageal NET (carcinoid) Gastric NET (carcinoid) Duodenal NET (carcinoid)	—

Pancreas	—	Islet Cell Tumors
		  Insulinoma
		  Gastrinoma
		  Verner-Morrison
		    syndrome
		  Glucagonoma
		  Somatostatinoma
		  Nonfunctional islet cell
		    tumor (Ppoma)
			—

Midgut	—	Jejunoileal NET (carcinoid) Appendiceal NET (carcinoid)	—
Hindgut	—	Colon NET (carcinoid) Rectal NET (carcinoid)	—

Adrenal
  cortex
	Adrenal
	  carcinoma
		—	—

Adrenal medulla	—	—	Pheochromocytoma Neuroblastoma

Peripheral
  ganglion
	—	—	Paraganglioma
			Benign schwannomas
			Malignant peripheral
			  nerve sheath tumors
			Melanoma

Bone	—	—	Ewing sarcoma

Abbreviations: ACTH, adrenocorticotropic hormone; FSH, follicle-stimulating hormone; LH, luteinizing hormone; TSH, thyrotropin.

development. The sites in which neuroblastomas arise correlate with normal tissues of the sympathetic nervous system, including spinal sympathetic ganglia and adrenal chromaffin cells. Because neuroblastoma can arise from any site along the sympathetic nervous system chain, the primary tumors can occur within the abdominal (adrenals), thoracic, and cervical regions (paraspinous). Because of their noradrenergic derivation, neuroblastomas have multiple components of catecholamine synthesis, including homovanillic acid (HVA) and vanillylmandelic acid (VMA).

Ewing sarcoma is the second most frequent primary malignant bone cancer derived from postganglionic parasympathetic primordial cells located throughout the parasympathetic autonomic nervous system.

Pheochromocytomas are neural crest tumors of the adrenal medulla arising from chromaffin cells. Tumors that do not develop primarily from the chromaffin cells of the adrenal medulla but from the structures of the extra-adrenal sympathetic nervous system are named paragangliomas. These tumors secrete catecholamines, including epinephrine, norepinephrine, dopamine, metanephrine, and normetanephrine.

This review focuses on NETs that arise in the diffuse neuroendocrine system; these rare tumors can develop in any organ that has dispersed single endocrine cells, for example, the intestine, or clusters of endocrine cells, for example, pancreatic islets (see **Table 1**). Previously considered benign, NETs are now recognized to recur locally or metastasize to liver and bone if not completely excised early in their course of development. Thus, even in children, 10% to 20% of these tumors are metastatic at diagnosis.[1] This article summarizes the epidemiology and reviews the diagnostic and therapeutic challenges of NETs in children and young adults, noting especially those NETs that are more prevalent in young people than in older adults.

EPIDEMIOLOGY

NETs arising from the diffuse endocrine system can occur in any organ of the body. The most common sites in adults are the ileum, pancreas, and lung, with NETs in thymus, breast, stomach, colon, ovary, and cervix being less common.[1]

The incidence of NETs has been increasing over the past 30 years as documented by Yao and colleagues,[2] who analyzed the Surveillance, Epidemiology and End Results (SEER) database in the United States, Hauso and colleagues,[3] who compared the incidence in United States and Norway, and Hegde and colleagues,[4] who analyzed the incidence in the Asia-Pacific region. This increase in NET incidence is most pronounced for midgut and pancreatic NETs.[5] Overall, the incidence rate in the United States increased from 10.9 per million to 52.4 per million from 1973 to 2004.[2] From these combined registry data, the incidence is now recognized as 38 per million persons per year referenced to 2004 in the United States. The incidence in multiple countries is shown in **Table 2**; it is to be noted that incidence seems to be lower in most early studies.

Recognizing the slower growth of most NETs, with the associated longer survival of these patients, the prevalence of NETs is significant. Survival data are not available for most of the above-mentioned studies; however, Yao and colleagues[2] estimated the US prevalence of NET at 103,000 as of January 1, 2004, and Ito and colleagues[15] estimated the prevalence of NET in Japan at 39,500. Many, if not most, patients with NETs can lead high-quality lives while being treated. Thus, a new treatment with few side effects is highly desirable in that it allows these patients to continue as productive members of the society.[17]

NETs are notorious for late diagnoses, often being diagnosed on the basis of liver or bone metastases.[18] The few published reports on NETs in children suggest that

Table 2
Estimated incidence and prevalence of NETs

Country	Population in Millions	Estimated Incidence Per Million	References
Netherlands	16	18.5	6
Australia	22	Not available	7
Sweden	9	24.3 (carcinoid only)	8
Denmark & Norway	6 + 5	11.0 (carcinoid only)	9
Italy	60	6.5 (GI carcinoid only)	10
United Kingdom	62	8.2 (carcinoid only)	11
Brazil	192	Not available	12
India	1178	Not available	4
United States	309	38.5	2
Germany	82	Not available	13
Switzerland	8	22.5 (carcinoid only)	14
Japan	127	31.1	15
Europe	830	Survival data only	16

Abbreviation: GI, gastrointestinal.

at least 10% of these young patients have metastatic disease at presentation.[19–24] These late diagnoses are due in part to the wide distribution of the diffuse neuroendocrine system[25] and to the multiple histologic diagnoses associated with NETs.[26] According to the SEER database, every NET observed in adults also occurs in children. However, epidemiologic analyses of NET incidence in young people, especially of those studies extracted from the SEER database, include several neural crest tumors as outlined in **Table 1**.

Patients who are eventually diagnosed with NETs often have a multiyear history of symptoms before identification of the malignancy, with average lag periods of 8 to 10 years.[27] Thus, a 29-year-old adult diagnosed as having a NET may well have been an adolescent when the first symptoms occurred. The incidence increases with age, and nearly 90% of NETs in the 0- to 29-year age group are diagnosed after over the age of 20 years. However, the tendency to late diagnosis, after metastases to the liver or bones, suggests that more than half of the NETs diagnosed in this age group probably occur before the age of 21 years.

The incidence of NETs in children and young adults in the United States has recently been analyzed from the SEER data. Incidence rates, observed survival rates, and 31-year limited duration prevalence counts were obtained from SEER*Stat for the diagnosis years 1975 to 2006.[1] These rates were compared between and within NETs using variables from 9 standard SEER registries for ages 0 to 29 years. The most common NET sites were lung, breast, and appendix with incidence rates of 0.6 per million, 0.6 per million, and 0.5 per million, respectively, in the 0- to 29-year age group (**Table 3**); the incidence was less than 0.1 per million for all other NETs. The estimated age-adjusted number of NETs in the United States was 1073 in 2006.

The 5-year observed survival rate for NETs was 84% for the 2000–2006 period, and the estimated 31-year limited duration prevalence for NETs as of January 1, 2006 was 7724. The age-adjusted multivariate Cox regression demonstrated small cell histology, primary location in the breast, and distant stage as the major predictors of decreased survival, with a 5-year survival of less than 24% for ovarian small cell NET.

Table 3
Distribution of NETs in children and young adults younger than 30 years

Tumor Type	Percentage of NET in This Age Group
Bronchial NET	28
Medullary Carcinoma of Breast	18
Appendiceal NET	18
Colon and rectal NET	9
Jejunal and ileal NET	5
Small Cell Carcinoma (Ovary)	5
Unknown primary NET	5
Pancreatic and gastric NET	4
Medullary carcinoma thyroid	4
Small Cell Carcinoma cervix	4

DIAGNOSIS AND THERAPY FOR NETs IN CHILDREN AND YOUNG ADULTS
Lung NET and Neuroendocrine Carcinoma (Bronchial Carcinoid)

The lung is the most common location for NET in young people, and NET is the most common childhood malignancy arising in the lung.[28] Bronchial NET should be considered in the differential diagnosis of any young person who has a culture-negative pneumonia and especially in the case of recurrent culture-negative pneumonia. A chest computed tomography (CT) should be performed, and if a lung lesion is found, Octreoscan (indium In 111 pentetreotide) single-photon emission computed tomography (SPECT) imaging should also be obtained before biopsy. In addition, plasma levels of chromogranin A, serotonin, adrenocorticotropic hormone (ACTH) and growth hormone–releasing hormone (GHRH) should be measured in these children before surgery in order to determine biomarkers to be used in follow-up. If a primary NET of lung is demonstrated on the biopsy result, a metastatic workup including triple-phase abdominal CT and a bone scan should be obtained. The pathology for both primary and metastatic lesions should be complete, including diagnosis, stage, and grade (**Table 4**).[29]

Complete excision of the tumor is curative if no detectable (or undetectable) tumor cells are left behind; thus wide excision margins or even lobectomy is the treatment of choice. Follow-up for children and young adults should include magnetic resonance imaging or ultrasonography of the original tumor site and plasma peptides (see **Table 4**) every 4 to 6 months for 3 years and yearly for an additional 5 years. The plasma peptides to be measured at follow-up are only those for which positive results were obtained at initial diagnosis. Even though bronchial NET is the most common source of extrapituitary ACTH or GHRH, these need not be measured in follow-up if not present initially.[30]

Bronchial NETs can metastasize to liver and bone. While unilateral wheezing is a common symptom in bronchial NET, carcinoid syndrome with flushing and diarrhea are rarely seen until there is significant liver metastasis. Once these NETs become metastatic, positron emission tomographic (PET) imaging with fludeoxyglucose may be of help in determining whether or not chemotherapeutic drugs such as 5-fluorouricil and doxorubicin, cisplatin and etoposide, or capecitabine and temozolomide may be useful.[31] If test results for both primary tumor and liver metastases are positive with Octreoscan, these tumors can be shrunk or be stabilized with peptide radioreceptor

Table 4
Elements of data set for pathology report on NET

	Anatomy	Histology	Immunohistochemistry	Genetics	Plasma Amines and/or Peptides
Bronchial	Location Size in 3-D Multicentric Invasion Node positivity	Clear cell vs glandular Grade & stage Necrosis Mitotic index	Chromogranin A Synaptophysin Ki-67	Menin	Chromogranin A Serotonin ACTH GHRH Pancreastatin
Breast	Location Size in 3-D Multicentric Invasion Node positivity	Syncytial vs glandular Grade & stage Necrosis Mitotic index	Estrogen R Progesterone R HER2 CDK5/6, 14, 17 VEGFR Ki-67 Synaptophysin Chromogranin A	TP53	Calcitonin CEA
Thyroid	Location Size in 3-D Multicentric Invasion Node positivity	Papillary vs follicular vs medullary Grade & stage Necrosis Mitotic index	Calcitonin CEA Synaptophysin Chromogranin A	RET	Calcitonin CEA Chromogranin A Pancreastatin
Upper GI Tract	Location Size in 3-D Multicentric Invasion Node positivity	Gastric vs adenocarcinoma Grade & stage Necrosis Mitotic index	Synaptophysin Chromogranin A Serotonin		Serotonin Substance P Chromogranin A Pancreastatin

Pancreatic	Location Size in 3-D Multicentric Invasion Node positivity	Exocrine vs endocrine Grade & stage Necrosis Mitotic index	Synaptophysin Chromogranin A Insulin Glucagon Somatostatin Gastrin Pancreatic polypeptide	Menin	Insulin Glucagon Somatostatin Gastrin Pancreatic polypeptide Chromogranin A Pancreastatin
Midgut	Location Size in 3-D Multicentric Invasion Node positivity	Grade & stage Necrosis Mitotic index	Synaptophysin Chromogranin A Serotonin		Neurokinin A Substance P Chromogranin A Pancreastatin
Hindgut	Location Size in 3-D Multicentric Invasion Node positivity	Adeno vs endocrine Grade & stage Necrosis Mitotic index	Synaptophysin Chromogranin A		GLP-1 Peptide YY Chromogranin A Pancreastatin
Ovarian	Location Size in 3-D Multicentric Invasion Node positivity	Adeno vs endocrine Grade & stage Necrosis Mitotic index	Synaptophysin Chromogranin A	BRCA 1,2 TP53	Chromogranin A Pancreastatin Substance P

Abbreviations: 3-D, 3-dimension; BRCA, breast cancer gene; CDK, cyclin-dependent kinase; CEA, carcinoembryonic antigen; GI, gastrointestinal; GLP, glucagon-like peptide; TP53, tumor protein p53; VEGFR, vascular endothelial cell growth factor receptor.

nuclide therapy (PRRNT) using octreotate labeled with lutetium 177 or edotreotide labeled with yttrium 90 as discussed further in the section future directions.[32,33]

Medullary Carcinoma of Breast and Thyroid Gland

Recent analysis of the SEER database in the United States demonstrated that medullary carcinoma occurs more often in breast than in thyroid gland in people younger than 30 years.[1] The primary breast lesion is often found by the patient, but medullary carcinoma of breast should also be considered in the case of metastatic disease of bone that is found on pathologic examination to be medullary carcinoma. Medullary carcinoma of breast is classified in the basal-like subtype of triple-negative breast cancers (ER−, PgR−, Her2−).[34] This cancer is a high-grade tumor without glandular structures but instead is histologically a solid tubular carcinoma with large sheets of poorly differentiated cells giving it a syncytial appearance, which may have central necrosis; these tumors may be invasive and may have prominent inflammatory cells.[35] Greater extent of inflammatory cells is associated with both higher histologic grade and, paradoxically, a better prognosis.[36]

Medullary thyroid carcinoma is a component of MEN. MEN type IIA tumors occur in parathyroid (adenoma), thyroid (medullary thyroid, [MTC]), and adrenal medulla (pheochromocytoma), whereas MEN type IIB includes MTC and neural crest tumors (pheochromocytoma and paraganglioma). Family history and blood pressure measurements are the most important screening tools. Children can be tested and the diagnosis made as early as 4 years of age with blood calcitonin levels; the pentagastrin stimulation test is available but rarely performed. Levels of urine catecholamines are also important, and a 24-hour urine test with plasma metanephrine measurement is an alternative in young children for whom 24-hour urine test is not practical. Specific screening tests for MEN types IIA and IIB therefore depend on the family history and the precise RET mutation.[37] The decision as to how early a complete thyroidectomy should be performed is controversial, but recent observations suggest that thyroid removal can be safely delayed until late adolescence in some families.[38]

As is true for most other NETs, complete excision is curative if performed before metastasis. Nodal sampling is imperative to look for regional spread. If adjuvant therapy is necessary, the combination of an anthracycline and a taxane, for example, doxorubicin + docetaxel, has been shown to be effective in 30% of triple-negative breast tumors, including medullary breast cancer, whereas cisplatin as a single agent induced partial remission in 22% of patients.[35] PRRNT would only be considered if the test results for primary tumor and any metastatic lesions were positive on ^{111}In-diethylene·triamine pentaaceticacid (DTPA)-octreotide SPECT scan.

Appendiceal, Jejunal, and Ileal NETs (Carcinoids)

Gastric, jejunoileal, and appendiceal NETs together constitute another major type of NET in children, with the appendix being the most frequent site (see **Table 2**). Diagnosis of an appendiceal carcinoid is often an incidental finding by the pathologist after acute appendicitis or removal of appendix when another surgical procedure exposes the area. The minimal data set (see **Table 3**) is extremely important for appendiceal NET because a tumor of size less than 1 cm at the tip of the appendix without any invasion into the periappendiceal tissue and with no regional node involvement has a 5-year disease-free survival rate of 95% without further therapy. On the other hand, right hemicolectomy is recommended for tumors larger than 2 cm for tumors at the base of the appendix, for tumors with goblet cell histology, and when tests results for regional lymph node involvement are positive.[39] Tumors of intermediate size between 1 and 2 cm diameter must be carefully evaluated based on all the above-mentioned factors to determine the best treatment.

Tumors of the stomach, duodenum, jejunum, ileum, and cecum constitute 5% of NETs in children and young adults (see **Table 2**). These tumors are among the most difficult to diagnose because of their small size and vague symptoms of abdominal pain with or without intermittent diarrhea.

Gastrinoma has been reported as early as 6 years of age.[22] Normal fasting gastrin levels are similar in children and adults, making this an easy and extremely useful test. However, even short-term use of proton pump inhibitors (PPIs) can significantly increase gastrin and chromogranin A levels. PPIs should be discontinued for at least 72 hours before measuring neuropeptide levels in serum, and some patients may require PPIs to be discontinued for at least 4 weeks before testing for peptide levels to return to normal.[40]

Pancreatic Islet Cell Tumors

Both functioning and nonfunctioning pancreatic NETs occur in children. Biomarkers are also useful in the diagnosis and follow-up of these tumors because specific markers can be used to indicate the likely location of the primary tumor and follow the response to therapy (eg, gastrin, insulin, glucagon, substance P, neurokinin A, pancreatic polypeptide, somatostatin) as well as to follow liver metastases (pancreastatin).

Nisidioblastosis is the result of an overactive pancreas (hypertrophy and hyperplasia of the islet cells) and most often presents at birth as hypoglycemia unresponsive to feeding or intravenous glucose. This condition most often resolves with close follow-up and octreotide therapy but may resurface when these children reach puberty.[41] Insulinoma has been seen in children as young as 5 years.[42–46] Insulin and C peptide levels are measured in blood, and normal levels are similar to those in adults.

MEN type I occurs in parathyroid, pancreas, and pituitary. The pancreatic tumors most often secrete gastrin (although gastrin-secreting cells have not been identified in normal pancreatic islets). Families with MEN type I can also have gastrin-secreting tumors of the duodenum.

These tumors do not respond well to conventional chemotherapeutic agents such as platinum compounds or anthracyclines; however, they do respond to an oral-based therapeutic combination of temozolomide and capecitabine.[47] These tumors also have high somatostatin receptor expression and have an excellent[48] response to PRRNT.[49] PRRNT may render previously unresectable tumors amenable to surgery. Whether PRRNT should be the initial therapy followed by surgery and/or chemotherapy with drugs such as temozolomide and capecitabine must be decided on an individual basis.

Colon and Rectal NETs (Carcinoids)

With the increased use of colonoscopy and capsule endoscopy, NETs in the colon and rectum are more easily identified and biopsied; this may account for a significant proportion of the observed increase in incidence among children and young adults[1] in whom asymptomatic disease is much more common than presentation with hematochezia and change in bowel habits. Incidence is higher among Asians and African Americans than in Whites.[2] If identified early, before invasion of the deeper layers of muscularis propria, NETs of the colon and rectum are easily removed with excisional biopsy. However, once these NETs have metastasized to bone or liver, they are very aggressive. This aggressiveness makes the pathologic grade and stage important prognostic indicators. The TNM staging system along with grading based on mitotic rate and/or Ki-67 index is endorsed by both the European Neuroendocrine Tumor Society and North American Neuroendocrine Tumor Society.[47,50] For both grading/staging systems, a mitotic rate or Ki-67 index greater than 20% indicates a highly aggressive tumor regardless of the TNM stage. Chromogranin A, glucagon-like peptide, and peptide YY are the primary biomarkers in colon and rectal NETs; however, only chromogranin A is readily available as a plasma biomarker. Furthermore, test results for chromogranin A may be negative in more aggressive tumors,[51] again emphasizing the importance of pathologic grading and TNM staging in the decision for treatment strategy.

Tumors that are confined to the submucosa and are less than 1 cm of the largest diameter with no lymph node involvement or other metastatic disease can be treated with surgery alone and yearly follow-up. However, no controlled trials of other therapies have included sufficient colon or rectal NETs on which to base a firm recommendation, although a recent abstract[52] suggests that PRRNT may be beneficial.

Small Cell Carcinoma of Ovary and Cervix

Small cell carcinoma of the cervix and ovary is more common in children and young adults than that of the lung.[1] Diagnosis is made on the basis of an abnormal Papanicolaou test or biopsy of a presumed ovarian cyst. Ovarian small cell carcinoma can be familial[53,54] and has a poor prognosis. These tumors, like small cell carcinoma of the lung, are unresponsive to conventional chemotherapy.[55] There is very little information on somatostatin receptor type 2 (sstr2) expression in these tumors, and thus, the use of PRRNT must be based on positive results for sstr2 SPECT or PET imaging.

Pheochromocytoma and Paraganglioma

Pheochromocytoma is associated with MEN types IIA and IIB, VHL syndrome, and NF 1. With the peak incidence between 9 and 12 years of age, nearly 10% of all pheochromocytomas occur in children and 10% of these are malignant. Headaches, palpitations, diaphoresis, and hypertension are the most common symptoms. Diagnostic testing should include a 24-hour urine test for measuring levels of creatinine, VMA, catecholamines, metanephrine as well as free plasma metanephrine, and chromogranin A. Because pheochromocytoma can be seen in adolescents and young adults, drug interference with metanephrine testing should be ruled out with a careful medication and illicit drug history. False-positive result for metanephrines can be caused by buspirone, benzodiazepines, methyldopa, labetalol, tricyclic antidepressants, levodopa, ethanol, amphetamines, sotalol, and chlorpromazine. Surgery is curative if performed before metastatic disease. Once metastasis occurs, surgical extirpation of the primary tumor is recommended with additional systemic treatment using [131I]metaiodobenzylguanidine (MIBG) if an MIBG scan demonstrates that the required catecholamine transporters (VMAT1/2) are expressed on the tumors. Those pheochromocytomas and paragangliomas that yield positive result on 111In-DPTA-octreotide scan may be amenable to PRRNT.[49,56]

Neuroblastoma

This neural crest tumor shares multiple biomarkers with NETs, including chromogranin A, synaptophysin, neuron-specific enolase, and sstr2.[57] About 90% of all neuroblastomas can be imaged with either 111In-DPTA-octreotide or DOTA-octreotate labeled with gallium 68,[58,59] supporting the use of PRRNT in the treatment of neuroblastoma. Individual case studies validate this theoretical consideration, including minor responses (MRs) in 2 subjects with neuroblastoma who participated in a phase 1 trial of DOTA-tyr^3-octreotide labeled with yttrium 90 in children.[49] Diagnostic testing should include VMA and HVA in urine, serum chromogranin A, and either SPECT/CT or PET/CT to localize sstr2-positive disease.

FUTURE DIRECTIONS
Molecular Diagnostics

While more than 90% of all NETs are thought to be sporadic, the increased incidence of NETs in families with MEN type I, VHL syndrome, NF 1, or tuberous sclerosis (TSC1, TSC2) syndrome has been well documented.[60] Moreover, abnormalities of chromosomes 1, 11q, and 9p in pancreatic NET and of chromosome 18 in gastrointestinal NET are recognized,[61] but the causal gene mutations have not yet been identified. Gene expression studies are now being used in predicting tumor aggressiveness.[62] However, genetic tests that will identify NETs and predict prognosis are not yet available.

With multiple targeted therapies such as mammalian target of rapamycin inhibitors, other tyrosine kinase inhibitors, and growth factor receptor antibodies, we should be able to individualize therapies based on tumor genetics in the future.[63] However, most pharmacogenetic testing is based on genome-wide association studies of tumor tissue[64] in addition to knowledge of tumor susceptibility genes, such as breast cancer gene BRCA1/2. Such rational use of pharmacogenetic data can decrease the number of subjects required to definitively test outcomes with new drugs.[65]

Our understanding of susceptibility to NET is limited to the inherited cancer genes noted earlier and thus of limited utility in predicting the response of NET to individual drugs. However, the use of molecularly targeted imaging using somatostatin analogues to identify and quantify somatostatin receptor expression as a predictor of response to PRRNT is an example of pharmacogenetic imaging[59] that has led to important advances in therapy for patients with NETs.[66] We therefore, conclude this review of NET in children and young adults with the analysis of a phase 1 clinical trial of PRRNT in this age group.

Peptide Radioreceptor Therapy

PRRNT is the systemic or local-regional administration of unsealed radionuclides chelated to a peptide for the purpose of delivering cytotoxic radiations to a tumor. The peptide agents are designed to target cellular proteins, usually cell surface receptors that are overexpressed in a tumor-specific pattern, thus providing specificity to the radiation delivery.

NETs have proved to be ideal neoplasms in which to exploit PRRNT because the majority of these slow-growing malignancies overexpress somatostatin receptors. Furthermore, the endogenous ligand, somatostatin, is a small cyclic peptide, which lends itself to both chemical stabilization through substitution of D-amino acids and attachment of a chelating moiety to bind radionuclides while retaining high affinity for the target receptor.[67] Initial attempts at functional nuclear medicine imaging of NETs provided clear demonstrations of the specificity and sensitivity of ^{111}In-DTPA-octreotide for the somatostatin receptor in gastroenteropancreatic tumors[68] and paved the way for PRRNT using ^{90}Y-DOTA-tyr^3-octreotide and ^{177}Lu-DOTA-octreotate.[69,70] These 2 radiopharmaceuticals remain the primary PRRNT agents in current practice.

PRRNT is molecularly targeted internal radiation in contrast to electronically targeted external beam radiation. Peptides that target sstr2 are the prototype and are currently in use in Europe for adults with NETs.

NETs and neural crest tumors in children also express high levels of somatostatin receptors and can potentially be treated with PRRNT; however, children younger than 18 years have been excluded from participation in most PRRNT trials, resulting in a lack of information on safety, toxicity, and efficacy in this age group.

Only 1 controlled clinical trial of PRRNT has ever been conducted in children and young adults; this was a phase 1 trial of ^{90}Y-DOTA-tyr^3-Octreotide to determine the dose/toxicity profile in subjects younger than 25 years with somatostatin receptor–positive tumors.[49] A dose-escalation design was used to determine the highest tolerable dose of ^{90}Y-DOTA-tyr^3-octreotide while limiting renal radiation dose to less than or equal to 21 Gy. The activity levels of the administered ^{90}Y-DOTA-tyr^3-octreotide were 1.11, 1.48, and 1.85 GBq/m^2/cycle in 3 cycles at 6-week intervals, coadministered with an amino acid infusion for renal protection. Eligibility criteria included age 2 to 25 years, progressive disease (PD), positive lesion on ^{111}In-DTPA-octreotide scan, glomerular filtration rate greater than or equal to 80 mL/min/m^2, bone marrow cellularity greater than or equal to 40% or stored autologous hematopoietic stem cells, Lansky play scale greater than or equal to 60%, and informed consent.

Seventeen subjects, aged 2 to 24 years, received at least 1 dose of ^{90}Y-DOTA-tyr^3-octreotide; diagnoses included neuroblastoma, embryonal and astrocytic brain tumors, paraganglioma, MEN type IIB, and gastroenteropancreatic NETs. There were no dose-limiting toxicities and no individual dose reductions caused by renal or hematologic toxicity. The most frequent toxicity was reversible nausea in 70%, even in the presence of antiemetics. There were no complete responses; 3 subjects had partial response (PR), 5 had MRs, 5 had stable disease, 2 had PD, and 2 subjects withdrew. Dosimetry performed on subjects in the 1.85 GBq/m^2/cycle cohort demonstrated an average 2.24 mGy/MBq dose to kidneys, similar to the dosimetry estimates in adults. PRRNT with ^{90}Y-DOTA-tyr^3-octreotide demonstrated an 18% PR plus 29% MR rate in children and young adults with somatostatin receptor–positive tumors. The recommended phase 2 dosing is 3 cycles of 1.85 GBq/m^2/dose ^{90}Y-DOTA-tyr^3-octreotide coadministered with amino acids. In the future, higher doses may be attainable through the use of dosimetry-guided therapy.

Although there has been only 1 clinical trial in children, the observations in that trial of ^{90}Y-DOTA-tyr^3-octreotide together with the combined experience of several centers using ^{177}Lu-octreotate in children and young adults allow us to offer several recommendations for PRRNT in this age group:

1. PRRNT is safe in children and young adults when given with renal protection.
2. Dosing of ^{90}Y-DOTA-tyr^3-octreotide is recommended at 1.85 GBq/m^2 in all children and at less than 1.73 GBq/m^2 in young adults. No dosing recommendations are currently available for ^{177}Lu-octreotate in the pediatric population because of a lack of clinical trials in this age group.
3. Total dose to kidneys should be limited to 23 Gy until further controlled trials have been performed to demonstrate safety at higher doses.
4. Renal protection with amino acid infusion 30 to 60 minutes before and at least 3 hours 30 minutes after PRRNT administration is mandatory. Recent trials suggest that such protection should be continued for 24 to 48 hours after PRRNT administration.[71]

SUMMARY

NETs, although rare, do occur in children as young as 4 to 6 years and are often diagnosed late because of the lack of recognition of the signs and symptoms. The incidence and prevalence of NET in this population are comparable to other solid tumors of childhood such as neuroblastoma and Ewing sarcoma. NET of the lung, breast, and appendix are the most common in this age group followed by gastroenteropancreatic NET. Complete pathologic characterization, including grade, stage, and biomarkers, are critical for determining the appropriate treatment and follow-up. More complete genetic analysis of this family of tumors should allow the rational employment of pharmacogenetics and molecularly targeted therapy in order to increase the length and improve the quality of life for children and young adults with NETs.

REFERENCES

1. Navalkele P, O'Dorisio MS, O'Dorisio TM. Incidence, survival and prevalence of neuroendocrine tumors versus neuroblastoma in children and young adults: nine standard SEER registries, 1975–2006. Pediatr Blood Cancer 2011;56(1): 50–7.
2. Yao JC, Hassan M, Phan A, et al. One hundred years after "carcinoid": epidemiology of and prognostic factors for neuroendocrine tumors in 35,825 cases in the United States. J Clin Oncol 2008;26:3063–72.
3. Hauso O, Gustafsson BI, Kidd M, et al. Neuroendocrine tumor epidemiology: contrasting Norway and North America. Cancer 2008;113(10):2655–64.
4. Hegde V, Mohandas KM, Ramadwar M, et al. Gastric carcinoids–a changing trend. Indian J Gastroenterol 2003;22:209–11.
5. Modlin IM, Oberg K, Chung DC, et al. Gastroenteropancreatic neuroendocrine tumours. Lancet Oncol 2008;9:61–72.
6. Taal BG, Visser O. Epidemiology of neuroendocrine tumours. Neuroendocrinology 2004;80(Suppl 1):3–7.
7. Rangiah DS, Cox M, Richardson M, et al. Small bowel tumours: a 10 year experience in four Sydney teaching hospitals. ANZ J Surg 2004;74:788–92.
8. Hemminki K, Li X. Incidence trends and risk factors of carcinoid tumors: a nationwide epidemiologic study from Sweden. Cancer 2001;92:2204–10.
9. Westergaard T, Frisch M, Melbye M. Carcinoid tumors in Denmark 1978–1989 and the risk of subsequent cancers. A population-based study. Cancer 1995; 76:106–9.
10. Crocetti E, Buiatti E, Amorosi A. Epidemiology of carcinoid tumours in central Italy. Eur J Epidemiol 1997;13:357–9.
11. Newton JN, Swerdlow AJ, dos Santos Silva IM, et al. The epidemiology of carcinoid tumours in England and Scotland. Br J Cancer 1994;70:939–42.
12. Younes RN. Neuroendocrine tumors: a registry of 1,000 patients. Rev Assoc Med Bras 2008;54:305–7.
13. Ploeckinger U, Kloeppel G, Wiedenmann B, et al. The German NET-registry: an audit on the diagnosis and therapy of neuroendocrine tumors. Neuroendocrinology 2009;90:349–63.
14. Levi F, Randimbison L, Franceschi S, et al. Descriptive epidemiology of malignant carcinoids in the Swiss Canton of Vaud. Int J Cancer 1993;53:1036–7.
15. Ito T, Sasano H, Tanaka M, et al. Epidemiological study of gastroenteropancreatic neuroendocrine tumors in Japan. J Gastroenterol 2010;45:234–43.
16. Lepage C, Ciccolallo L, De Angelis R, et al. European disparities in malignant digestive endocrine tumours survival. Int J Cancer 2010;126(12):2928–34.
17. Bloom D, Canning D, Sevilla J. The effect of health on economic growth: a production function approach. World Dev 2004;32:1–13.

18. Hassan MM, Phan A, Li D, et al. Risk factors associated with neuroendocrine tumors: a U.S.-based case-control study. Int J Cancer 2008;123:867–73.

19. Corpron CA, Black CT, Herzog CE, et al. A half century of experience with carcinoid tumors in children. Am J Surg 1995;170:606–8.

20. Ladd AP, Grosfeld JL. Gastrointestinal tumors in children and adolescents. Semin Pediatr Surg 2006;15:37–47.

21. Broaddus RR, Herzog CE, Hicks MJ. Neuroendocrine tumors (carcinoid and neuroendocrine carcinoma) presenting at extra-appendiceal sites in childhood and adolescence. Arch Pathol Lab Med 2003;127:1200–3.

22. Khanna G, O'Dorisio MS, Menda Y, et al. Gastroenteropancreatic neuroendocrine tumors in children and young adults. Pediatr Radiol 2008;38:251–9.

23. Parham DM. Neuroectodermal and neuroendocrine tumors principally seen in children. Am J Clin Pathol 2001;115(Suppl):S113–28.

24. Spunt SL, Pratt CB, Rao BN, et al. Childhood carcinoid tumors: the St Jude Children's Research Hospital experience. J Pediatr Surg 2000;35:1282–6.

25. Modlin IM, Champaneria MC, Bornschein J, et al. Evolution of the diffuse neuroendocrine system—clear cells and cloudy origins. Neuroendocrinology 2006;84: 69–82.

26. Papotti M, Rosas R, Longo M, et al. [Spectrum of neuroendocrine tumors in non-endocrine organs]. Pathologica 2005;97:215 [in Italian].

27. Vinik A, Moattari AR. Use of somatostatin analog in management of carcinoid syndrome. Dig Dis Sci 1989;34:14S–27S.

28. Gustafsson BI, Kidd M, Chan A, et al. Bronchopulmonary neuroendocrine tumors. Cancer 2008;113:5–21.

29. Klimstra DS, Modlin IR, Adsay NV, et al. Pathology reporting of neuroendocrine tumors: application of the Delphic consensus process to the development of a minimum pathology data set. Am J Surg Pathol 2010;34:300–13.

30. Phan AT, Oberg K, Choi J, et al. NANETS concensus guideline for the diagnosis and management of neuroendocrine tumors: well-defined neuroendocrine tumors of the thorax (includes lung and thymus). Pancreas 2010;39(6): 784–98.

31. Clark OH, Benson AB 3rd, Berlin JD, et al. NCCN clinical practice guidelines in oncology: neuroendocrine tumors. J Natl Compr Canc Netw 2009;7:712–47.

32. van EM, Krenning EP, Bakker WH, et al. Peptide receptor radionuclide therapy with (177)Lu-octreotate in patients with foregut carcinoid tumours of bronchial, gastric and thymic origin. Eur J Nucl Med Mol Imaging 2007;34(8):1219–27.

33. Bushnell DL Jr, O'Dorisio TM, O'Dorisio MS, et al. 90Y-edotreotide for metastatic carcinoid refractory to octreotide. J Clin Oncol 2010;28(10):1652–9.

34. Kleer CG. Carcinoma of the breast with medullary-like features: diagnostic challenges and relationship with BRCA1 and EZH2 functions. Arch Pathol Lab Med 2009;133:1822–5.

35. Sasaki Y, Tsuda H. Clinicopathological characteristics of triple-negative breast cancers. Breast Cancer 2009;16:254–9.

36. Rakha EA, Aleskandarany M, El-Sayed ME, et al. The prognostic significance of inflammation and medullary histological type in invasive carcinoma of the breast. Eur J Cancer 2009;45:1780–7.

37. Skinner MA, Moley JA, Dilley WG, et al. Prophylactic thyroidectomy in multiple endocrine neoplasia type 2A. N Engl J Med 2005;353:1105–13.

38. Calva D, O'Dorisio TM, Sue O'Dorisio M, et al. When is prophylactic thyroidectomy indicated for patients with the RET codon 609 mutation? Ann Surg Oncol 2009;16:2237–44.

39. Boudreaux JP, Putty B, Frey DJ, et al. Surgical treatment of advanced-stage carcinoid tumors: lessons learned. Ann Surg 2005;241:839–45.

40. Giusti M, Sidoti M, Augeri C, et al. Effect of short-term treatment with low dosages of the proton-pump inhibitor omeprazole on serum chromogranin A levels in man. Eur J Endocrinol 2004;150:299–303.

41. Glaser B, Landau H, Smilovici A, et al. Persistent hyperinsulinaemic hypoglycaemia of infancy: long-term treatment with the somatostatin analogue Sandostatin. Clin Endocrinol (Oxf) 1989;31:71–80.

42. Manabe M, Morimatsu H, Egi M, et al. [Anesthetic management of pediatric patients with insulinoma using continuous glucose monitoring]. Masui 2009;58:757–9 [in Japanese].

43. Lodish MB, Powell AC, Abu-Asab M, et al. Insulinoma and gastrinoma syndromes from a single intrapancreatic neuroendocrine tumor. J Clin Endocrinol Metab 2008;93:1123–8.

44. Bonfig W, Kann P, Rothmund M, et al. Recurrent hypoglycemic seizures and obesity: delayed diagnosis of an insulinoma in a 15 year-old boy–final diagnostic localization with endosonography. J Pediatr Endocrinol Metab 2007;20:1035–8.

45. Bax KN, van der Zee DC. The laparoscopic approach toward hyperinsulinism in children. Semin Pediatr Surg 2007;16:245–51.

46. de Vogelaere K, De Schepper J, Vanhoeij M, et al. Laparoscopic management of insulinoma in a child with multiple endocrine neoplasia type 1. J Laparoendosc Adv Surg Tech A 2006;16:335–8.

47. Karachaliou F, Vlachopapadopoulou E, Kaldrymidis P, et al. Malignant insulinoma in childhood. J Pediatr Endocrinol Metab 2006;19:757–60.

48. Menda Y, O'Dorisio MS, Kao S, et al. Phase I trial of 90Y-DOTATOC therapy in children and young adults with refractory solid tumors that express somatostatin receptors. J Nucl Med 2010;51(10):1524–31.

49. Rindi G, Kloppel G, Couvelard A, et al. TNM staging of midgut and hindgut (neuro) endocrine tumors: a consensus proposal including a grading system. Virchows Arch 2007;451:757–62.

50. Anthony LB, Strosberg JR, Klimstra DS, et al. The NANETS consensus guidelines for the diagnosis and management of gastrointestinal neuroendocrine tumors (NETs): well-differentiated NETs of the distal colon and rectum. Pancreas 2010;39:767–74.

51. Vinik AI, Anthony L, Boudreaux JP, et al. Neuroendocrine tumors: a critical appraisal of management strategies. Pancreas 2010;39(6):801–18.

52. Prasad V, Kaemmerer D, Hommann M, et al. Management of neuroendocrine tumors of the rectum (rNET) using Ga-68 somatostatin receptor PET/CT (SR-PET/CT) and Peptide Receptor Radionuclide Therapy (PRRT). Proceedings: 6th Annual European Neuroendocrine Tumor Society (ENETS) Conference. Granada (Spain), March 5–7, 2009.

53. Martinez-Borges AR, Petty JK, Hurt G, et al. Familial small cell carcinoma of the ovary. Pediatr Blood Cancer 2009;53:1334–6.

54. Christin A, Lhomme C, Valteau-Couanet D, et al. Successful treatment for advanced small cell carcinoma of the ovary. Pediatr Blood Cancer 2008;50:1276–7.

55. Shrimali RK, Correa PD, Reed NS. Dose-dense and dose-intense chemotherapy for small cell ovarian cancer: 2 cases and review of literature. Med Oncol 2010;1–5. [Epub ahead of print].

56. Fanti S, Ambrosini V, Tomassetti P, et al. Evaluation of unusual neuroendocrine tumours by means of 68Ga-DOTA-NOC PET. Biomed Pharmacother 2008;62:667–71.

57. Khanna G, Bushnell D, O'Dorisio MS. Utility of radiolabeled somatostatin receptor analogues for staging/restaging and treatment of somatostatin receptor-positive pediatric tumors. Oncologist 2008;13(4):382–9.

58. Juweid ME, Menda Y, O'Dorisio MS, et al. 111In-pentetreotide versus bone scintigraphy in the detection of bony metastases of neuroblastoma. Nucl Med Commun 2002;23:983–9.

59. Baum RP, Prasad V, Hommann M, et al. Receptor PET/CT imaging of neuroendocrine tumors. Recent Results Cancer Res 2008;170:225–42.

60. Starker LF, Carling T. Molecular genetics of gastroenteropancreatic neuroendocrine tumors. Curr Opin Oncol 2009;21:29–33.

61. Oberg K. Genetics and molecular pathology of neuroendocrine gastrointestinal and pancreatic tumors (gastroenteropancreatic neuroendocrine tumors). Curr Opin Endocrinol Diabetes Obes 2009;16:72–8.

62. Drozdov I, Kidd M, Nadler B, et al. Predicting neuroendocrine tumor (carcinoid) neoplasia using gene expression profiling and supervised machine learning. Cancer 2009;115:1638–50.

63. August J. Market watch: emerging companion diagnostics for cancer drugs. Nat Rev Drug Discov 2010;9:351.

64. Schork NJ, Topol EJ. Genotype-based risk and pharmacogenetic sampling in clinical trials. J Biopharm Stat 2010;20:315–33.

65. Chen S, Chen J, Ma G, et al. Clinical therapeutic effect and biological monitoring of p53 gene in advanced hepatocellular carcinoma. Am J Clin Oncol 2011. [Epub ahead of print].

66. Kwekkeboom DJ, de Herder WW, van Eijck CH, et al. Peptide receptor radionuclide therapy in patients with gastroenteropancreatic neuroendocrine tumors. Semin Nucl Med 2010;40:78–88.

67. Otte A, Jermann E, Behe M, et al. DOTATOC: a powerful new tool for receptor-mediated radionuclide therapy. Eur J Nucl Med 1997;24:792–5.

68. Krenning EP, Kwekkeboom DJ, Bakker WH, et al. Somatostatin receptor scintigraphy with [111In-DTPA-D-Phe1]- and [123I-Tyr3]-octreotide: the Rotterdam experience with more than 1000 patients. Eur J Nucl Med 1993;20:716–31.

69. Waldherr C, Pless M, Maecke HR, et al. The clinical value of [90Y-DOTA]-D-Phe1-Tyr3-octreotide (90Y-DOTATOC) in the treatment of neuroendocrine tumours: a clinical phase II study. Ann Oncol 2001;12:941–5.

70. Kwekkeboom DJ, Mueller-Brand J, Paganelli G, et al. Overview of results of peptide receptor radionuclide therapy with 3 radiolabeled somatostatin analogs. J Nucl Med 2005;46(Suppl 1):62S–6S.

71. Bodei L, Cremonesi M, Ferrari M, et al. Long-term evaluation of renal toxicity after peptide receptor radionuclide therapy with 90Y-DOTATOC and 177Lu-DOTA-TATE: the role of associated risk factors. Eur J Nucl Med Mol Imaging 2008;35:1847–56.

Update: Metabolic and Cardiovascular Consequences of Bariatric Surgery

Donald W. Richardson, MD[a],*, Mary Elizabeth Mason, MD[a],
Aaron I. Vinik, MD, PhD, FCP, MACP[b]

KEYWORDS

• Obesity • Weight loss • Bariatric surgery • Diabetes mellitus

METABOLIC HEALTH EFFECT OF OBESITY

The US and worldwide prevalence of obesity is accelerating and has doubled in the last 20 years.[1] The latest National Health and Nutrition Examination Survey shows that more than two-thirds of adult Americans are obese or overweight.[1]

This rapid increase in adiposity in the United States and elsewhere has generated a secondary epidemic of the syndrome variously labeled metabolic, dysmetabolic, or cardiometabolic risk,[2,3] which includes not only type 2 diabetes mellitus (T2DM)[4–10] but also hypertension and dyslipidemia[5,10] and is directly associated with body weight.[2–5,8–10] In a national sample of adults, a 1-kg increase in measured weight increased the risk of diabetes by 4.5%.[10] Even in the top half of the normal healthy weight range (body mass index [BMI] 22.0–24.9, calculated as the weight in kilograms divided by the height in meters squared), women in the Nurses' Health Study and men in the Health Professionals Follow-up Study doubled their risk of developing diabetes or hypertension.[5] The etiologic connections between obesity and diabetes continue to multiply, with new discoveries concerning the adipose organ. A partial list now includes elevated levels of free fatty acids (FFAs), suppressed adiponectin, elevated levels of inflammatory cytokines, and increased triglyceride content in the pancreas, liver, and skeletal and heart muscles.[6,7]

The cardiometabolic risk syndrome (CMRS) has most recently been defined as the constellation of insulin resistance (manifested by fasting blood glucose levels

[a] Department of Medicine, L.R. Strelitz Diabetes Center for Endocrinology and Metabolism, L.R. Strelitz Diabetes Research Institute, Eastern Virginia Medical School, 855 West Brambleton Boulevard, Norfolk, VA 23510, USA
[b] Eastern Virginia Medical School, Strelitz Diabetes Center, 855 West Brambleton Avenue, Norfolk, VA 23510, USA
* Corresponding author.
E-mail address: richardw@evms.edu

Endocrinol Metab Clin N Am 40 (2011) 81–96
doi:10.1016/j.ecl.2010.12.009
0889-8529/11/$ – see front matter © 2011 Published by Elsevier Inc.

>110 mg/dL or a diagnosis of T2DM), visceral adiposity (resulting in abdominal obesity and increased waist circumference), high blood pressure (BP), and dyslipidemia (hypertriglyceridemia or low levels of high-density lipoprotein [HDL] cholesterol).[11] The CMRS is also associated with nontraditional risk factors, which include microalbuminuria,[12] endothelial and neurovascular dysfunction,[13] and a proinflammatory/prothrombotic state including elevated levels of C-reactive protein (CRP), tumor necrosis factor (TNF) α, interleukin (IL) 6, fibrinogen, and plasminogen activator inhibitor (PAI) 1.[2] First associated by Reaven[14,15] as a syndrome with components that were related by insulin resistance, the cluster of risk factors that define CMRS increases cardiovascular disease morbidity by 2- to 3-fold.[2,5,14] About 34% of all US adults now have CMRS, whereas up to 54.4% of adults older than 60 years are afflicted and 65% of obese Americans qualify.[3]

Additional metabolic abnormalities associated with obesity (and CMRS) include polycystic ovary syndrome (PCOS), the most common chronic disorder in women,[16] and nonalcoholic steatohepatitis (NASH), which is arguably the most common cause of chronic liver disease in the United States, Europe, and Japan.[17,18] PCOS affects approximately 4% to 10% of women and is associated with hyperandrogenism, hirsutism, anovulation, infertility, and increased cardiovascular and cancer risk (see PCOS section). NASH occurs in 2% to 4% of the population,[2] with its precursor, nonalcoholic fatty liver disease (NAFLD or hepatic steatosis), occurring in 16% to 23%. Both PCOS and NASH are increasing with the obesity tide.

Nonmetabolic but equally distressing chronic conditions engendered or aggravated by obesity include osteoarthritis of the spine, hips, knees, and feet; hypoventilation and sleep apnea (which have been associated with atrial fibrillation and cor pulmonale); and obesity-induced hypogonadism in men. Sleep apnea and sleep disturbance have also been associated with insulin resistance per se, and treatment of sleep apnea may even result in improvements in insulin-mediated glucose disposal.[19]

CAUSES OF OBESITY EPIDEMIC

The long present but ill supported (especially by at-risk financial entities such as the Federal government and private health insurance agencies) notion that corpulence might best be categorized as a chronic disease state rather than as evidence of a sinful nature, moral turpitude, or failure of will power began to advance with the discovery of leptin in 1994, the absence of which produces extreme obesity in affected rodents and (rarely) humans.[20–24]

The centrally mediated component that defends body fat mass after weight loss has long been known from observation of human weight regain in controlled trials of diet, exercise, and pharmacologic weight loss and from animal experiments. In addition, much has been found about the peripheral (mostly gastric) secretion of the potent orexigenic hormone ghrelin, which is implicated in mealtime hunger and the initiation of feeding behavior mediated by the arcuate nucleus of the ventral medial hypothalamus. Concentrations of this hormone decrease with feeding and increase to levels sufficient to stimulate hunger and food intake after fasting and before meals. Ghrelin infusions stimulate food intake, and ghrelin gene knockout mice are resistant to diet-induced obesity.[25] Overweight and obese individuals' efforts to lose weight are stymied by their own physiology. Systems that regulate body weight defend body fat stores by compensatory changes in appetite and energy expenditure that counter any weight loss.

A recent evaluation of the lean offspring of patients with T2DM also suggests that those at risk for obesity and insulin resistance may have inherited a defect in mitochondrial oxidative phosphorylation, resulting in impaired intramyocellular fatty acid metabolism[26] and provides further support for the view of obesity and the propensity to it as biologic.

Thus, there is strong and increasing evidence that obesity as a disease has a major biologic underpinning and is resistant to diet-based therapy.[27] An obvious corollary should be that obesity should be treated as any other chronic health disorder, using an increasingly aggressive treatment plan as the severity of the disease (increasing obesity) indicates. The treatment should start with therapeutic lifestyle change, escalate through monopharmacologic and polypharmacologic therapies, and end in surgical intervention when required because of failure of previous efforts or the magnitude of the obesity, which is beyond the capabilities of the early line treatments to manage. Similarly, agencies charged with paying for medical costs should be required to include coverage for this disease state, as for hypertension, diabetes, and other diseases.[28,29]

While it seems clear that up to 75% of the population is capable of developing excess adipose tissue if provided with plenty of tasty food and no reason to exercise, there are clearly recent environmental factors in the civilization that have created just these conditions. Larger portion size, carbonated beverages, higher fat and fructose sweetener content, and lower fiber intake (ie, more refined, processed foods) have all been implicated.[30,31] Increase in television watching or video game playing time and decline in exercising during leisure time have been legitimate targets in the search for alterations in the environment.[32]

SUMMARY OF PATHOPHYSIOLOGY

The pathophysiologic underpinning of CMRS, which accompanies abdominal obesity, is the hypertrophied fat cell and the attendant increased secretion of multiple factors, which accompanies the triglyceride-engorged adipocyte.[33–35] As these cells become filled with fat, they release increasing amounts of aforementioned cytokines (except the protective adiponectin, the secretion of which is inversely related to the size of the adipocytes). Other than adiponectin and possibly leptin, all aforementioned cytokines have deleterious effects on glucose and lipid metabolism, increase insulin resistance, and produce inflammation in the liver and vascular system. The increasing release of FFAs from enlarged fat cells increases the delivery of fatty acids to the liver, muscle, and other tissues. Increased FFA levels reduce glucose utilization by all these tissues by mechanisms that are only now being elucidated.[34,35] One of the consequences of this increased delivery of fatty acids is storage of fat in nonadipose tissues, including muscle, liver, and pancreas. The storage of fat in nonadipose tissues may play a role in the development of insulin deficiency and overt diabetes mellitus.[36–38]

TREATMENT

There are 2 separate goals worth achieving in persons with obesity with CMRS/ diabetes: reduction of cardiovascular risk to the same as those without these risk factors and reduction of weight to avoid the direct effects on respiration, joints, income, and psychosocial well-being. The former can be achieved by non–weight-loss methods to correct dyslipidemia, hypertension, and hyperglycemia. However, such methods require onerous and financially burdensome pill (or insulin) taking, 2 to 3 or more of each antidiabetic, lipid-lowering, and hypotensive agents.[39,40] Thus, a method of meeting metabolic and nonmetabolic goals via weight loss, although so far mostly elusive, would be thoroughly worthwhile, if followed only to reduce the numbers and expense of drugs required to meet target levels of glucose and lipids and BP.

Lifestyle

Trials of lifestyle intervention including nutritional and behavior counseling, prescribed exercise, and meal replacement interventions have been successful but weight loss has generally been modest (2–7 kg more than that of control groups) and was not sustained (only 20% maintained a 10% weight loss after 12 months),[41] except for the Diabetes Prevention Program,[42] in which the intensive lifestyle arm members regained only 43% of their lost weight over 4 years.

Herbal Therapy

Some randomized trial data are available in the scientific literature about the use of herbal therapies for weight loss, and of these data, the majority deal with ephedrine and caffeine or closely related substances derived from plants. This combination, used pharmaceutically, has a long track record of modest success but is now banned because of concerns about the cardiovascular safety of ephedrine alkaloids.[43–48]

Pharmacologic Therapy

Several meta-analyses suggest that antiobesity agents are effective and can produce a modest improvement in some of the key cardiovascular risk factors (diabetes, hypertension, and dyslipidemia).[49–51] Although several entirely new or combination products are in final stages of Food and Drug Administration evaluation, only 2 weight-loss drugs, orlistat, a lipase inhibitor, and sibutramine, a combined serotonin-norepinephrine reuptake inhibitor, are approved for long-term use. Sibutramine has been removed from the market because of concerns with cardiovascular effects (hypertension, arrhythmias, stroke, death). Although treatment with orlistat is more effective than most behavioral interventions in terms of weight loss, the mean decrease is still dissatisfying: 2.7 kg more weight loss in those on orlistat versus 2.2 kg in those on acarbose, not marketed as a weight-loss drug, than the control groups, who were essentially on behavioral intervention therapies.[50,51] Orlistat therapy had minor positive effects on other components of the CMRS.[52,53] The effects include waist circumference decreased by 0.7 to 3.4 cm, the total low-density lipoprotein cholesterol level declined by about 0.3 mmol/L, and the triglyceride level decreased by 0.05 mmol/L. Systolic BP was reduced on average by 1.8 mm Hg and the fasting blood glucose level by 1.3 mmol/L as well as glycated hemoglobin (HbA_{1c}) levels declined by 0.2%. Sibutramine had no positive metabolic effect on any glucose or lipid parameter, besides a 0.13-mmol/L increase in HDL levels and overall, had a negative effect on BP by increasing both systolic and diastolic BP by 1.8 mm Hg.[54] Metformin has been used for weight loss but is relatively impotent, results in 3% weight loss after 1 year and 2% after 4 years,[42] as a weight-loss drug as opposed to its more evident effects on glucose and insulin concentrations and menstrual cyclicity in patients with PCOS. The α-glucosidase inhibitor (starch blocker) acarbose has also been shown to reduce the frequency of conversion of prediabetes to diabetes.[51] Older catecholaminergic agents, such as phentermine, mazindol, and diethylpropion, are not approved for long-term use.

Bariatric surgery

In stark contrast to the average 4% to 8% drop in body weight found with lifestyle change or pharmaceuticals, the effect of bariatric surgery, whether vertical banded gastroplasty (VBG), laparoscopic adjustable gastric banding (LAGB), or (laparoscopic)

Roux-en-Y gastric bypass (RYGBP), is spectacular, with typical weight losses of 25 to 60 kg (gastric banding) or up to 50% of the initial body weight (RYGBP). Gastric banding procedures produce less initial weight loss and therefore diminished reduction in CMRS-related parameters; weight also tends to return more over time with VBG. Thus, although most US surgeons prefer RYGBP[52,55] for patients with diabetes, the LAGB procedure is rapidly gaining favor in the United States because of reduced hospital length of stay, surgical complications, mortality, and long-term nutritional complexities.

Originally thought to result in weight loss by limiting gastric capacity and causing mild malabsorption, accumulating evidence suggests that both the reduction in appetite and the amelioration of diabetes mellitus result from hormonal changes induced by bariatric surgery, especially RYGBP. Both reductions in ghrelin concentrations, caused by vagotomy or delivery of osmotic load to the distal gut, and increments in glucagon-like peptide 1 (GLP-1) levels, which delays gastric emptying and reduces hunger, possibly by an effect on the area postrema, have been implicated in the weight loss from RYGBP. The latter has been implicated in the rapid amelioration of diabetes long before significant weight loss because it suppresses glucagon and stimulates insulin secretion from the alpha and beta cells, respectively, in the islets of Langherhans.[56–58]

Benefits of weight loss on CMRS, diabetes complications, and mortality

There is abundant evidence that just as excess adiposity increases the risk of diabetes, hypertension, dyslipidemia, and mortality, so does intentional weight loss reduce these risks. Weight loss after gastric bypass, maintained for up to 15 years, reduces BP, improves abnormal lipid levels, and reduces the risk of diabetes by approximately 75%. Gastric bypass and non–surgically induced weight loss lowers mortality rate by 24% (hazard ratio, 0.76; 95% confidence interval, 0.60–0.97), including from both myocardial infarction and cancer.[53,54,59,60] It seems that the metabolic and endocrine consequences of obesity are, at least partly, reversible.

Large controlled intervention trials in Finland (Finnish Diabetes Prevention Study Group)[61] and the United States[42] have proved that weight loss due to lifestyle intervention (and less successfully, metformin) can reduce the risk of developing T2DM, reduce BP and triglyceride levels, and increase HDL cholesterol levels in high-risk individuals with well-categorized CMRS. These results were accomplished by the loss of about 4.5% and 7.5%, respectively, of body weight in high-risk subjects. Conversion rates from impaired fasting blood glucose tolerance to diabetes were reduced by 58% (34% by metformin). Fasting and 2-hour post–glucose load blood glucose and insulin levels, triglyceride and total cholesterol levels, systolic and diastolic BP, and waist circumference were all reduced (most parameters had less than or nearly 0.05% significance), and HDL cholesterol levels were increased slightly (and nonsignificantly).

Although no statistically significant improvement in cardiovascular events (CVEs) or cardiac-related or total mortality was noted in the Diabetes Prevention Program or Finnish Diabetes Prevention Study, these studies were not powered to detect small changes in these end points. In contrast, all these parameters have favored bariatric surgery in both randomized controlled trials and meta-analyses.[59–65]

However, only about 40% of the subjects in the intensive lifestyle treatment groups met the lifestyle goals, and the benefits diminished over 4 years. These results were, of course, obtained in interested subjects who had volunteered and they were then subjected to much better dietary counseling and exercise supervision than available to most people. This situation is somewhat depressing because the standard recommendation for overweight or obese patients with diabetes, hypertension, or other comorbidities of CMRS is to lose 5% to 10% of their body weight by maintaining a daily 700-cal deficit and exercising 1 h/d 6 to 7 days a week. According to the 2010 position statement of the American Diabetes Association: Nutrition Recommendations and Interventions for Diabetes: "Although structured lifestyle programs have been effective when delivered in well-funded clinical trials, it is not clear how the results should be translated into clinical practice. Organization, delivery, and funding of lifestyle interventions are all issues that must be addressed. Third-party payers may not provide adequate benefits for sufficient Medical Nutritional Therapy (MNT) frequency and time to achieve weight loss goals." Randomized assignment to lifestyle intervention versus diabetes support and education is the subject of the Look AHEAD (Action for Health in Diabetes) trial, which has finished recruiting 5145 people to be followed up for 11.5 years to study the effects of the 2 interventions on the major CVEs such as heart attack, stroke, and cardiovascular-related death.[66] A positive outcome might stimulate Centers for Medicare & Medicaid Services, and subsequently other payers, to fund medical nutritional therapy and lifestyle interventions.

RESULTS OF BARIATRIC SURGERY: CMRS

Because of (1) poor long-term results with behavioral, exercise, and pharmacologic therapy for the great majority of overweight patients, (2) the magnitude of the needed weight loss in many severely or morbidly obese persons with risk factors for cardiovascular disease, and (3) the major long-term salutary effect of surgically induced weight loss on diabetes, hypertension, and dyslipidemia, bariatric surgery has emerged as an important therapy for CMRS in patients starting with BMIs greater than 35.[52,53,59,67–74] At 1-year follow-up, CMRS resolved in 89% of women who underwent LAGB.[71] It has been reported that after undergoing bariatric surgery, patients with prediabetes are uniformly rendered euglycemic[70]; 60% to 80% of patients with T2DM resolved their requirement for insulin, 90% required less oral hypoglycemic therapy, and all patients achieved an average HbA_{1c} level of 6% in contrast to only 58% of patients in the lifestyle interventions (which were in less-obese people).

Hypertension

Hypertension resolves or improves at 1 to 2 years in 80% to 90% of diabetic patients undergoing laproscopic RYGPB,[53] although with time it tends to become reestablished.[69]

Dyslipidemia

As expected from epidemiologic and interventional trials of weight loss for dyslipidemia, RYGBP resulted in the resolution of hypercholesterolemia in 37% and amelioration of the condition in 41% of 107 patients, along with a reduction of myocellular lipid content, which correlates highly with insulin resistance, as opposed to an increase in adiponectin concentrations, which is a marker for insulin sensitivity.[74–76]

Levels of the inflammatory markers IL-6, TNF-α, CRP, and leptin; the procoagulant PAI-1; and angiotensinogen decrease after RYGBP.[77,78]

NAFLD

Although much liver biopsy data have been generated, confirming the high prevalence of hepatic steatosis and steatohepatitis, with unsuspected fibrosis found in up to 10% of patients,[79] the hepatic outcome of bariatric surgery is unknown, even though the presence of cirrhosis does not seem to worsen the immediate outcome.[80,81]

Jejunoileal bypass was associated with worsening of previous liver injury, which led to its becoming outmoded.[82]

PCOS

Two prospective trials of surgically induced weight loss have been performed in women with PCOS.[83,84] The expectation that bariatric surgery would be helpful in reinitiating ovulatory menstrual cycles based on (fairly ineffective) attempts to reduce weight using lifestyle change, meal replacement, and metformin[85–87] was supported by both these trials. The possibility of interference with reproduction by the surgery itself (such as tubal adhesions) seems not to be overly concerning.[88,89]

Complications of T2DM

The incidence of diabetic sensory neuropathy is reduced by the reduction of blood glucose level to near normal.[39,90] Cure of type 1 diabetes by pancreas transplant has similar effects on sensory and autonomic neuropathy.[91,92] It is, therefore, not too surprising that at least 1 group has discerned an improvement in neuropathy in patients who underwent gastric bypass, all of whom were rendered euglycemic. Diabetic neuropathy was present in 25% of patients preoperatively, and symptomatic improvement was reported by 50% of patients after surgery: 33% much improved and 17% improved.[69] In the same study, patient-reported erectile dysfunction was present in 11 of 48 men before gastric bypass; 2 men noted improvement after surgery.

Prevention or reversal of established nephropathy and retinopathy have yet to be addressed in patients whose diabetes has been cured by bariatric surgery. Using the same models of prevention and cure in type 1 diabetes mellitus as for neuropathy, it can be hoped that renal disease will stabilize or improve after weight loss surgery.[90]

Finally, economically, the use of weight loss surgery seems attractive,[93] with a price per quality-adjusted life-year of approximately $7000 only.[91]

METABOLIC COMPLICATIONS AFTER BARIATRIC SURGERY

There are well-described nutritional complications of bariatric (especially gastric bypass) surgery, which are thoroughly reviewed,[94] and they are not addressed in this article. More recently, there is increasing recognition of severe hypoglycemia as a complication of bariatric surgery, although the overall incidence of this problem is not known. Hypoglycemia occurs both with RYGBP and LAGB. An incidence of 3% to 4% asymptomatic hypoglycemia was reported in a series of patients after LAGB.[95]

Episodes of hypoglycemia are typically postprandial and often severe, characterized by rapid development of neuroglycopenia (defined by documented hypoglycemia associated with altered mental status requiring assistance of others). Patients experience confusion, tunnel vision, and sometimes loss of consciousness, which usually begin between 6 months and 8 years after surgery.[96] These episodes intrude significantly, unpredictably, and dangerously into patients' lives. Motor vehicle accidents and grand mal seizures are among the reported consequences.[97,98]

Asymptomatic hypoglycemia may also occur more frequently in the postprandial state in patients who underwent RYGBP. This observation was recently reported in 33% of a small group of carefully tested patients.[99]

Compared with men, women are affected more frequently with hypoglycemia after gastric bypass surgery, but more women undergo gastric bypass surgery.

The clinical syndrome overlaps noninsulinoma pancreatogenous hypoglycemia syndrome as described by Service and colleagues[100] originally in a non–gastric bypass surgery population.

Pathophysiology

The pathophysiology of this form of hypoglycemia is likely because of more than one alteration in normal carbohydrate metabolism.

Hypoglycemia may be part of a late-phase dumping syndrome.[101] This phase of dumping is different from the familiar early phase, when symptoms of sweating, dizziness, nausea, and diarrhea occur, which is attributed to the rapid entry of hyperosmotic foods into the jejunum, drawing isotonic fluids from plasma into the intestinal lumen, with a decrease in blood volume and sympathetic stimulation, typically at about 15 minutes after eating. In contrast, the late phase occurs 1.5 to 3.0 hours after eating and is characterized by neuroglycopenic symptoms only. It can be provoked by meals containing foods that have large quantities of rapidly absorbed carbohydrates. The glucose load presented abruptly to the jejunum is rapidly absorbed, causing hyperglycemia, and an excessive insulin response occurs, resulting in hypoglycemia. Some patients who are severely affected also describe the ability of very minor carbohydrate loads to provoke hypoglycemia. All 3 authors followed up patients post–bariatric surgery, who have reliably developed a glucose level of less than 40 mg/dL after ingestion of trivial amounts of carbohydrate, for example, a single Triscuit cracker.

Reinforcing the concept that dumping is an important part of the cause of hypoglycemia after gastric bypass surgery, Z'graggen and colleagues[102] observed 12 patients and noted that restoring gastric restriction surgically (for pouches larger than 30 mL) was curative in most, presumably by slowing down nutrient entry into the jejunum.

However, some patients with hypoglycemia clearly have extra insulin secretion because of the expanded islet cell mass unrelated to the path of nutrient delivery.

For example, a patient with severe hypoglycemia was treated with reversal of the gastric bypass and gained back the pre–gastric bypass weight but continued to experience hypoglycemia until pancreatectomy was performed. Pancreas from some patients so treated showed diffuse islet hyperplasia and expansion of beta cell mass and sometimes, islets adjacent to and budding from ducts.[97,98,103] In contrast, other patients have undergone partial or complete pancreatectomy and no abnormality of islets could be demonstrated.[104]

Systematic examinations of islets has revealed increased expression of insulinlike growth factor 2, insulinlike growth factor receptor 1, receptor X, and transforming growth factor β receptor 3.[105]

The incretin hormone GLP-1 is produced in increased amounts after bariatric surgery, 5 to 10 fold higher than in overweight or morbidly obese patients.[99] Although this overproduction is sometimes suggested as a cause of islet cell expansion, evidence is scant. GLP-1 itself may possibly contribute to overt hypoglycemia, as has been observed in a patient with a GLP-1–producing tumor[106] or when high levels of GLP-1 are infused. There is no certainty that GLP-1 causes the hypoglycemic syndrome.

High levels of insulin production, causing hypoglycemia, seems to be specifically stimulated by the passage of nutrients through the bypassed gastrointestinal tract. This condition has been observed in an individual patient who had recurrent hypoglycemia with oral alimentation after RYGBP. When this patient was given the same nutrient mix via gastrotomy tube feeding into the original stomach, no hypoglycemia/hyperinsulinemia occurred.[107]

Insulinoma has occasionally been reported in the post–gastric bypass setting as well and should be excluded.[108] Hypoglycemia occurred soon after gastric bypass surgery in this instance.

Some patients may have an unrecognized predisposition to hyperinsulinemic hypoglycemia, perhaps masked before surgery by obesity and insulin resistance.

Evaluation

Establishing that low–blood glucose levels truly occurs at the time of symptoms and that the condition is relieved with the administration of food or glucose is a critical step, which can be done when an episode occurs spontaneously. Measurement of glucose, C-peptide, and insulin levels, along with screening for the presence of sulfonylureas is indicated. Hyperinsulinemic hypoglycemia is confirmed by observing a blood glucose level of less than 55 mg/dL, a C-peptide level of at least 0.6 ng/mL, an insulin level of 3 U/mL, and the absence of sulfonylurea in plasma.

A 72-hour fast is usually not required and typically does not provoke hypoglycemia in these patients, in contrast to those with insulinoma.[102]

An alternative approach is to provoke an episode of hypoglycemia by administering Ensure (Abbott Nutrition Consumer Relations, Columbus, OH, USA) as a liquid mixed meal and collecting blood at 10, 20, 30, 60, and 120 minutes for measuring glucose, insulin, and C-peptide levels. Including a sulfonylurea screen on one of these specimens excludes ingestion of the drug as a cause of the episode.[97]

Imaging of the abdomen for insulinoma is done with triple-phase computed tomographic scan, and transabdominal ultrasonography.[97]

More detailed testing in those being considered for pancreatic resection can be performed at specialized centers.

The calcium stimulation test is performed by infusion of 0.025 mEq of calcium gluconate (an insulin secretogogue) per kg weight into the splenic, superior mesenteric, and gastroduodenal arteries. Insulin and C-peptide levels are measured before and after the infusion; a 2-fold increase in the 30- or 60-second postinfusion sample in the region injected indicates beta cell hyperfunction. This information may indicate diffuse or more localized insulin hypersecretion and can be used to guide pancreatic resection.[97]

Treatment

Treatment of this condition is difficult, and there are no clinical trials comparing efficacy. In general, the most severely affected patients require the most invasive interventions.

1. Diet: reduction in carbohydrate load is the primary emphasis, and rapidly digested and absorbed carbohydrates (soda, juice) are especially to be avoided.[109]
2. Pharmacologic: in general, pharmacologic treatments have unimpressive results. The following medications have occasionally been reported to be successful in individual patients:
   Verapamil (80 mg twice daily) and acarbose (50 mg 3 times daily before meals)[110]
   Octreotide by subcutaneous injection has been used successfully for early-phase dumping syndrome and with occasional success for hypoglycemia[111]
   Diazoxide (50 mg twice daily).[112]
3. Surgical: approaches to restore restriction have included stapling, silastic ring insertion, or use of an adjustable gastric band.[102] Placement of a gastric feeding tube into the remnant stomach has also been successful.[108] The most drastic but sometimes necessary intervention is pancreatic resection.[97,98,103]

Prognosis

There are patients in whom hypoglycemia is severely symptomatic, frequent, and disabling. Those individuals do not seem to experience any natural remission over time and require long-term management and support.

SUMMARY

As presciently described by Pories and colleagues[113] 15 years ago, T2DM, along with the other components of CMRS, and associated cardiovascular risk markers (elevated BP, dyslipidemia, and serum markers of inflammation and hypercoaguability) are ameliorated or resolved after RYGBP and to a lesser extent after LAGB.[69,72–80] Randomized trials have shown that rates of CVEs, total mortality, and even cancer-related mortality are reduced when compared with those in similar unoperated patients in a well-designed cohort-controlled study.[59] Surgical therapy seems to be cost-effective when compared with conventional therapeutic lifestyle and pharmacologic interventions, with at least twice the weight loss that is generally maintained for up to 15 years.

REFERENCES

1. Flegal K, Carroll M, Ogden C, et al. Prevalence and trends in obesity among US adults, 1999–2008. JAMA 2010;303(3):235–41.
2. Haffner S, Taegtmeyer H. Epidemic obesity and the metabolic syndrome. Circulation 2003;108:1541–5.
3. Ervin RB. Prevalence of metabolic syndrome among adults 20 years of age and over, by sex, age, race and ethnicity, and body mass index: United States, 2003–2006. Natl Health Stat Report 2009;13:1–5.
4. Cowie C, Rust K, Ford E, et al. Full accounting of diabetes and pre-diabetes in the U.S. population in 1988–1994 and 2005–2006. Diabetes Care 2009;32(2):287–94.
5. Field AE, Coakley EH, Must A, et al. Impact of overweight on the risk of developing common chronic diseases during a 10-year period. Arch Intern Med 2001;161(13):1581–6.
6. Bays H, Mandarino L, DeFronzo RA. Adipocyte, FFAs, and ectopic fat in pathogenesis of type 2 diabetes mellitus- peroxisomal proliferator-activated receptor agonists provide a rational therapeutic approach. J Clin Endocrinol Metab 2004; 89(2):463–78.
7. der Zijl NJ, Goossens GH, Moors CC, et al. Ectopic fat storage in the pancreas, liver, and abdominal fat depots: impact on {beta}-cell function in individuals with impaired glucose metabolism. J Clin Endocrinol Metab 2011;96(2).
8. Ford ES, Williamson DF, Liu S. Weight change and diabetes incidence: findings from a national cohort of US adults. Am J Epidemiol 1997;146:214–22.
9. Centers for Disease Control and Prevention. Prevalence of diabetes and impaired fasting glucose in adults–United States, 1999–2000. MMWR Morb Mortal Wkly Rep 2003;52(35):833–7.
10. Willett WC, Dietz WH, Colditz GA. Guidelines for healthy weight. N Engl J Med 1999;341(6):427–34.
11. Grundy SM, Brewer HB, Cleeman JI, et al. Definition of metabolic syndrome. Report of the National Heart, Lung, and Blood Institute/American Heart Association conference on scientific issues related to definition. Circulation 2004;109: 433–8.

12. Chen J, Muntner P, Hamm L, et al. The metabolic syndrome and chronic kidney disease in US adults. Ann Intern Med 2004;140:167–74.
13. Vinik AI, Erbas T, Park TS, et al. Dermal neurovascular dysfunction in type 2 diabetes. Diabetes Care 2001;24(8):1468–75.
14. Reaven GM. Banting lecture 1988. Role of insulin resistance in human disease. Diabetes 1988;37:1595–602.
15. Isomaa B, Almgren P, Lahti K, et al. Cardiovascular morbidity and mortality associated with the CMRS. Diabetes Care 2001;24:683–9.
16. Glueck C, Papanna R, Wang P, et al. Incidence and treatment of CMRS in newly referred women with confirmed polycystic ovarian syndrome. Metabolism 2003; 52(7):908–15.
17. Dixon JB, Bhathal PS, O'Brien PE. Nonalcoholic fatty liver disease: predictors of nonalcoholic steatohepatitis and liver fibrosis in the severely obese. Gastroenterology 2001;121(1):91–100.
18. Medina J, Garcia-Buey L, Fernandez-Salazar L, et al. Approach to the pathogenesis and treatment of nonalcoholic steatohepatitis. Diabetes Care 2004;27: 2057–66.
19. Harsch IA, Schahin SP, Bruckner K, et al. The effect of continuous positive airway pressure treatment on insulin sensitivity in patients with obstructive sleep apnea syndrome and type 2 diabetes. Respiration 2004;71(3):252–9.
20. Zhang Y, Proenca R, Maffei M, et al. Positional cloning of the mouse obese gene and its human homologue. Nature 1994;372:425–32.
21. Weigle DS, Bukowski TR, Foster DC, et al. Recombinant ob protein reduces feeding and body weight in the ob/ob mouse. J Clin Invest 1995;96(4):2065–70.
22. Licinio J, Caglayan S, Ozata M, et al. Phenotypic effects of leptin replacement on morbid obesity, diabetes mellitus, hypogonadism, and behavior in leptin-deficient adults. Proc Natl Acad Sci U S A 2004;101(13):4531–6.
23. Cummings DE, Schwartz MW. Genetics and pathophysiology of human obesity. Annu Rev Med 2003;54:453–71.
24. Bray GA. Obesity is a chronic, relapsing neurochemical disease. Int J Obes Relat Metab Disord 2004;28(1):34–8.
25. Murphy KG, Dhillo WS, Bloom SR. Gut peptides in the regulation of food intake and energy homeostasis. Endocr Rev 2006;27(7):719–27.
26. Befroy DE, Petersen KF, Dufour S, et al. Impaired mitochondrial substrate oxidation in muscle of insulin-resistant offspring of type 2 diabetic patients. Diabetes 2007;56(5):1376–81.
27. Majdan JF. On being a doctor: memoirs of an obese physician. Ann Intern Med 2010;153(10):686–7.
28. Marks JB. The disappearance of insurance coverage for weight reduction surgery. Clin Diabetes 2004;22(3):105–6.
29. Flum DR, Khan TV, Dellinger EP. Toward the rational and equitable use of bariatric surgery. JAMA 2007;298:1442–4.
30. Gross LS, Li L, Ford ES, et al. Increased consumption of refined carbohydrates and the epidemic of type 2 diabetes in the United States: an ecologic assessment. Am J Clin Nutr 2004;79(5):774–9.
31. Bray GA, Nielsen SJ, Popkin BM. Consumption of high-fructose corn syrup in beverages may play a role in the epidemic of obesity. Am J Clin Nutr 2004; 79(4):537–43.
32. Marshall SJ, Biddle SJ, Gorely T, et al. Relationships between media use, body fatness and physical activity in children and youth: a meta-analysis. Int J Obes Relat Metab Disord 2004;28(10):1238–46.

33. Bjørbæk C, Kahn BB. Leptin signaling in the central nervous system and the periphery. Recent Prog Horm Res 2004;59:305–31.
34. Kershaw EE, Flier JS. Adipose tissue as an endocrine organ. J Clin Endocrinol Metab 2004;89:2548–56.
35. Díez JJ, Iglesias P. The role of the novel adipocyte-derived hormone adiponectin in human disease. Eur J Endocrinol 2003;148(3):293–300.
36. Carr MC, Brunzell JD. Abdominal obesity and dyslipidemia in the metabolic syndrome: importance of type 2 diabetes and familial combined hyperlipidemia in coronary artery disease risk. J Clin Endocrinol Metab 2004;89:2601–7.
37. Dresner A, Laurent D, Marcucci M, et al. Effects of free fatty acids on glucose transport and IRS-1-associated phosphatidylinositol 3-kinase activity. J Clin Invest 1999;103:253–9.
38. Randle PJ, Garland PB, Hales CN, et al. The glucose fatty-acid cycle: its role in insulin sensitivity and the metabolic disturbances of diabetes mellitus. Lancet 1963;I:785–9.
39. UK Prospective Diabetes Study (UKPDS) Group. UKPDS Intensive blood-glucose control with sulphonylureas or insulin compared with conventional treatment and risk of complications in patients with type 2 diabetes (UKPDS 33). Lancet 1998;352:837–53.
40. ALLHAT Officers and Coordinators for the ALLHAT Collaborative Research Group. The Antihypertensive and Lipid-Lowering Treatment to Prevent Heart Attack Trial. Major outcomes in high-risk hypertensive patients randomized to angiotensin-converting enzyme inhibitor or calcium channel blocker vs diuretic: the Antihypertensive and Lipid-Lowering Treatment to Prevent Heart Attack Trial (ALLHAT). JAMA 2002;288:2981–97.
41. Wing RR, Phelan S. Long-term weight loss maintenance. Am J Clin Nutr 2005; 82(1):222S–5S.
42. Knowler WC, Barrett-Connor E, Fowler SE, et al. Reduction in the incidence of type 2 diabetes with lifestyle intervention or metformin. N Engl J Med 2002; 346(6):393–403.
43. Padwal R, Li SK, Lau DC. Long-term pharmacotherapy for obesity and over-weight. Cochrane Database Syst Rev 2004;3:CD004094.
44. McTigue KM, Harris R, Hemphill B, et al. Screening and interventions for obesity in adults: summary of the evidence for the U.S. Preventive Services Task Force. Ann Intern Med 2003;139(11):933–49.
45. Shekelle PG, Hardy ML, Morton SC, et al. Efficacy and safety of ephedra and ephedrine for weight loss and athletic performance: a meta-analysis. JAMA 2003;289(12):1537–45.
46. Coffey CS, Steiner D, Baker BA, et al. A randomized double-blind placebo-controlled clinical trial of a product containing ephedrine, caffeine, and other ingredients from herbal sources for treatment of overweight and obesity in the absence of lifestyle treatment. Int J Obes Relat Metab Disord 2004;28(11): 1411–9.
47. Sindler BH. Herbal therapy for management of obesity: observations from a clinical endocrinology practice. Endocr Pract 2001;7(6):443–7.
48. Bent S, Tiedt TN, Odden MC, et al. The relative safety of ephedra compared with other herbal products. Ann Intern Med 2003;138(6):468–71.
49. Norris SL, Zhang X, Avenell A, et al. Efficacy of pharmacotherapy for weight loss in adults with type 2 diabetes mellitus: a meta-analysis. Arch Intern Med 2004; 164(13):1395–404.

50. Guy-Grand B, Drouin P, Eschwege E, et al. Effects of orlistat on obesity-related diseases- a six-month randomized trial. Diabetes Obes Metab 2004;6(5): 375–83.
51. Chiasson JL, Josse RG, Gomis R, et al. Acarbose treatment and the risk of cardiovascular disease and hypertension in patients with impaired glucose tolerance: the STOP-NIDDM trial. JAMA 2003;290(4):486–94.
52. Howard L, Malone M, Michalek A, et al. Gastric bypass and vertical banded gastroplasty- a prospective randomized comparison and 5-year follow-up. Obes Surg 1995;5(1):55–60.
53. Sjostrom CD, Peltonen M, Wedel H, et al. Differentiated long-term effects of intentional weight loss on diabetes and hypertension. Hypertension 2000; 36(1):20–5.
54. Gregg EW, Gersoff RB, Thompson TJ, et al. Intentional weight loss and death in overweight and obese U.S., adults 35 years of age and older. Ann Intern Med 2003;138(5):383–9.
55. Capella JF, Capella RF. An assessment of vertical banded gastroplasty-Roux-en-Y gastric bypass for the treatment of morbid obesity. Am J Surg 2002;183(2): 117–23.
56. Cummings DE, Weigle DS, Frayo RS, et al. Plasma ghrelin levels after diet-induced weight loss or gastric bypass surgery. N Engl J Med 2002;346: 1623–30.
57. Cummings DE, Shannon MH. Ghrelin and gastric bypass: is there a hormonal contribution to surgical weight loss? J Clin Endocrinol Metab 2003;88: 2999–3002.
58. Borg CM, le Roux CW, Ghatei MA, et al. Progressive rise in gut hormone levels after Roux-en-Y gastric bypass suggests gut adaptation and explains altered satiety. Br J Surg 2006;93:210–5.
59. Sjöström L, Narbro K, Sjostrom CD, et al. Effects of bariatric surgery on mortality in Swedish obese subjects. N Engl J Med 2007;357:741–75.
60. Bray GA. Medical consequences of obesity. J Clin Endocrinol Metab 2004;89: 2583–9.
61. Tuomilehto J, Lindstrom J, Eriksson JG, et al. Prevention of type 2 diabetes mellitus by changes in lifestyle among subjects with impaired glucose tolerance. N Engl J Med 2001;344:1343–50.
62. Buchwald H, Avidor Y, Braunwald E, et al. Bariatric surgery: a systematic review and meta-analysis. JAMA 2004;292(14):1724–37.
63. Buchwald H, Estok R, Fahrbach K, et al. Weight and type 2 diabetes after bariatric surgery: systematic review and meta-analysis. Am J Med 2009;122(3): 248.e5–256.e5.
64. Garb J, Welch G, Zagarins S, et al. Bariatric surgery for the treatment of morbid obesity: a meta-analysis of weight loss outcomes for laparoscopic adjustable gastric banding and laparoscopic gastric bypass. Obes Surg 2009;19(10): 1447–55.
65. Cunneen SA. Review of meta-analytic comparisons of bariatric surgery with a focus on laparoscopic adjustable gastric banding. Surg Obes Relat Dis 2008;4(3):S47–55.
66. Ryan DH, Espeland MA, Foster GD, et al. Look AHEAD (Action for Health in Diabetes): design and methods for a clinical trial of weight loss for the prevention of cardiovascular disease in type 2 diabetes. Control Clin Trials 2003;24:610–28.

67. Balsiger BM, Kennedy FP, Abu-Lebdeh HS, et al. Prospective evaluation of Roux-en-Y gastric bypass as primary operation for medically complicated obesity. Mayo Clin Proc 2000;75(7):673–80.
68. Sugerman HJ, DeMaria EJ, Kellum JM, et al. Effects of bariatric surgery in older patient. Ann Surg 2004;240(2):243–7.
69. Sugerman HJ, Wolfe LG, Sica DA, et al. Diabetes and hypertension in severe obesity and effects of gastric bypass-induced weight loss. Ann Surg 2003; 237(6):751–8.
70. Giusti V, Suter M, Heraief E, et al. Effects of laparoscopic gastric banding on body composition, metabolic profile and nutritional status of obese women: 12-months follow-up. Obes Surg 2004;14(2):239–45.
71. Schauer PR, Burguera B, Ikramuddin S, et al. Effect of laparoscopic Roux-en Y gastric bypass on type 2 diabetes mellitus. Ann Surg 2003;238:467–84.
72. Greenway SE, Greenway FL 3rd, Klein S. Effects of obesity surgery on non-insulin-dependent diabetes mellitus. Arch Surg 2002;137:1109–17.
73. Pories WJ. Diabetes: the evolution of a new paradigm. Ann Surg 2004;239(1): 12–3.
74. Christou NV, Sampalis JS, Liberman M, et al. Surgery decreases long-term mortality, morbidity, and health care use in morbidly obese patients. Ann Surg 2004;240:416–23.
75. Letiexhe MR, Desaive C, Lefebvre PJ, et al. Intact cross-talk between insulin secretion and insulin action after postgastroplasty recovery of ideal body weight in severely obese patients. Int J Obes Relat Metab Disord 2004;28:821–3.
76. Kelley DE. Influence of weight loss and physical activity interventions upon muscle lipid content in relation to insulin resistance. Curr Diab Rep 2004;4: 165–8.
77. Pender C, Goldfine ID, Tanner CJ, et al. Muscle insulin receptor concentrations in obese patients post bariatric surgery: relationship to hyperinsulinemia. Int J Obes Relat Metab Disord 2004;28:363–9.
78. Cottam DR, Mattar SG, Barinas-Mitchell E, et al. The chronic inflammatory hypothesis for the morbidity associated with morbid obesity: implications and effects of weight loss. Obes Surg 2004;14:589–600.
79. van Dielen FM, Buurman WA, Hadfoune M, et al. Macrophage inhibitory factor, plasminogen activator inhibitor-1, other acute phase proteins, and inflammatory mediators normalize as a result of weight loss in morbidly obese subjects treated with gastric restrictive surgery. J Clin Endocrinol Metab 2004;89: 4062–8.
80. Crespo J, Fernandez-Gil P, Hernandez-Guerra M, et al. Are there predictive factors of severe liver fibrosis in morbidly obese patients with non-alcoholic steatohepatitis? Obes Surg 2001;11:254–7.
81. Spaulding L, Trainer T, Janiec D. Prevalence of non-alcoholic steatohepatitis in morbidly obese subjects undergoing gastric bypass. Obes Surg 2003;13: 347–9.
82. Shalhub S, Parsee A, Gallagher SF, et al. The importance of routine liver biopsy in diagnosing nonalcoholic steatohepatitis in bariatric patients. Obes Surg 2004; 14:54–9.
83. Vyberg M, Ravn V, Andersen B. Pattern of progression in liver injury following jejunoileal bypass for morbid obesity. Liver 1987;7(5):271–6.
84. Escobar-Morreale HF, Botella-Carretero JI, Álvarez-Blasco F, et al. The poly-cystic ovary syndrome associated with morbid obesity may resolve after weight loss induced by bariatric surgery. J Clin Endocrinol Metab 2005;90(12):6364–9.

85. Eid G, Cottam D, Velcu L, et al. Effective treatment of polycystic ovarian syndrome with Roux-en-Y gastric bypass. Surg Obes Relat Dis 2005;1(2):77–80.

86. Huber-Buchholz MM, Carey DG, Norman RJ. Restoration of reproductive. Potential by lifestyle modification in obese polycystic ovary syndrome: role of insulin sensitivity and luteinizing hormone. J Clin Endocrinol Metab 1999;84: 1470–4.

87. Moran LJ, Noakes M, Clifton PM, et al. Short term energy restriction (using meal replacements) improves reproductive parameters in polycystic ovary syndrome. Asia Pac J Clin Nutr 2004;13(Suppl):S88.

88. Hoeger KM, Kochman L, Wixom N, et al. A randomized 48 week, placebo controlled trial of intensive lifestyle modification and/or metformin therapy in overweight women with polycystic ovary syndrome: a pilot study. Fertil Steril 2004;82:421–9.

89. Sheiner E, Levy A, Silverberg D, et al. Pregnancy after bariatric surgery is not associated with adverse perinatal outcome. Am J Obstet Gynecol 2004;190: 1335–40.

90. The effect of intensive treatment of diabetes on the development and progression of long-term complications in insulin-dependent diabetes mellitus. The Diabetes Control and Complications Trial Research Group. N Engl J Med 1993;329: 977–86.

91. Robertson RP, Davis C, Larsen J, et al. Pancreas and islet transplantation for patients with diabetes mellitus [technical review]. Diabetes Care 2000;23:112–6.

92. Tice JA, Karliner L, Walsh J, et al. Gastric banding or bypass? A systematic review comparing the two most popular bariatric procedures. Am J Med 2008;121(10):885–93.

93. Hoerger TJ, Zhang P, Segel JE, et al. Cost-effectiveness of bariatric surgery for severely obese adults with diabetes. Diabetes Care 2010;33(39):1933–9.

94. Mason ME, Jalagani H, Vinik AI. Metabolic complications of bariatric surgery: diagnosis and management issues. Gastroenterol Clin North Am 2005;34(1): 25–33.

95. Buchwald H, Oien D. Metabolic/Bariatric surgery worldwide 2008. Obes Surg 2009;19:1605–11.

96. Scavini M, Pontiroli A, Folli F. Asymptomatic hyperinsulinemic hypoglycemia after gastric banding. N Engl J Med 2005;353:2822–3.

97. Service GT, Thompson GF, Service FJ, et al. Hyperinsulinemic hypoglycemia with nesidioblastosis after gastric-bypass surgery. N Engl J Med 2005;353: 249–54.

98. Patti ME, McMahon G, Mun EC, et al. Severe hypoglycaemia post-gastric bypass requiring partial pancreatectomy: evidence for inappropriate insulin secretion and pancreatic islet hyperplasia. Diabetologia 2005;48:2236–40.

99. Goldfine AB, Mun EC, Devine E, et al. Patients with neuroglycopenia after gastric bypass surgery have exaggerated incretin and insulin secretory responses to a mixed meal. J Clin Endocrinol Metab 2007;92:4678–85.

100. Service FJ, Natt N, Thompson GB, et al. Noninsulinoma pancreatogenous hypoglycemica: a novel syndrome of hyperinsulinemic hypoglycemia in adults independent of mutations in Kir6.2 and SUR1 genes. J Clin Endocrinol Metab 1999; 84:1582–9.

101. Deitel M. The change in the dumping syndrome concept. Obes Surg 2008;18: 1622–4.

102. Z'graggen K, Guweidhi A, Steffen R, et al. Severe recurrent hypoglycemia after gastric bypass surgery. Obes Surg 2008;18:981–8.

103. Clancy TE, Moore FD, Zinner MJ. Post-gastric bypass hyperinsulinism with ne-sidioblastosis: subtotal or total pancreatectomy may be needed to prevent recurrent hypoglycemia. J Gastrointestinal Surgery 2006;10:1116–9.
104. Meier JJ, Butler AE, Galasso R, et al. Hyperinsulinemic hypoglycemia after gastric bypass surgery is not accompanied by islet hyperplasia or increased beta cell turnover. Diabetes Care 2006;29:1554–9.
105. Rumilla KM, Erickson LA, Service FJ, et al. Hyperinsulinemic hypoglycemia with nesidioblastosis: histologic features and growth factor expression. Modern Pathology 2009;22:239–45.
106. Todd JF, Stanley SA, Roufosse CA, et al. A tumour that secretes glucagon-like peptide-1 and somatostatin in a patient with reactive hypoglycaemia and dia-betes. Lancet 2003;361:228–30.
107. McLaughlin T, Peck M, Holst J, et al. Reversible hyperinsulinemic hypoglycemia after gastric bypass: a consequence of altered nutrient delivery. J Clin Endocri-nol Metab 2010;95:1851–5.
108. Abellan P, Camara R, Merino-Torres JF, et al. Severe hypoglycemia after gastric bypass surgery for morbid obesity. Diabetes Res and Clin Practice 2008;79: e7–e9.
109. Kellogg TA, Bantle JP, Leslie DB, et al. Postgastric bypass hyperinsulinemic hypoglycemia syndrome: characterization and response to a modified diet. Surg Obes Relat Dis 2008;4:492–9.
110. Moreira RO, Moreira RB, Machado N, et al. Post-prandial hypoglycemia after bariatric surgery: pharmacological treatment with verapamil and acarbose. Obes Surg 2008;18:1618–21.
111. D'Cruz DP, Reynard J, Tatman AJ, et al. Long-term symptomatic relief of post-prandial hypoglycaemia following gastric surgery with a somatostatin analogue. Postgrad Med J 1989;65:116–7.
112. Spanakis E, Gragnoli C. Successful medical management of status post-roux-en-y-gastric-bypass hyperinsulinemic hypoglycemia. Obes Surg 2009;19: 1333–4.
113. Pories WJ, Swanson MS, MacDonald KG, et al. Who would have thought it? An operation proves to be the most effective therapy for adult-onset diabetes mellitus. Ann Surg 1995;222:339–52.

Measuring the Relationship of Quality of Life and Health Status, Including Tumor Burden, Symptoms, and Biochemical Measures in Patients with Neuroendocrine Tumors

Etta Vinik, MA(Ed)[a],*, Maria P. Silva, MD[a],
Aaron I. Vinik, MD, PhD, FCP, MACP[b]

KEYWORDS

- Neuroendocrine tumors • Health-related quality of life
- QOL-NET questionnaire

Concern for quality of life (QOL) and respect for the sanctity of life were both concepts expressed by the earliest medical and philosophic writings of ancient Greece. In the Christian world, the sanctity of life was extolled as paramount. For the ancient Greeks and Romans, and in many post-Renaissance philosophies, quality of life assumed greater importance. These two opposing themes are woven into western history, and opponents for each philosophy exist today.[1]

The term, quality of life was first mentioned in modern times by Arthur C. Pigou (1920) in his book, "The Economics of Welfare," wherein he proposed, "the surroundings of work react on the quality of life of workers."[2]

After the Second World War, the World Health Organization (WHO) revived the social concept of QOL in 1948 and broadened the definition to include health, defining it as, "a state of complete physical, mental, and social well being and not merely the

[a] Neuroendocrine Unit, Strelitz Diabetes Center for Endocrine and Metabolic Disorders, Eastern Virginia Medical School, 855 West Brambleton Avenue, Norfolk, VA 23510, USA
[b] Eastern Virginia Medical School, Strelitz Diabetes Center, 855 West Brambleton Avenue, Norfolk, VA 23510, USA
* Corresponding author.
E-mail address: vinikai@evms.edu

Endocrinol Metab Clin N Am 40 (2011) 97–109
doi:10.1016/j.ecl.2010.12.008
0889-8529/11/$ – see front matter © 2011 Elsevier Inc. All rights reserved.

absence of disease or infirmity." This new definition of health-related QOL (HQOL) led to conjecture on whether HQOL could be measured.

Although the concept of HQOL was generally accepted in theory, it retained an ephemeral quality that provoked concern reflected in this statement from Fallowfield,

> "Hundreds of generic and specific tests purporting to measure different aspects of quality of life (QOL) have been developed. Acknowledgment that QOL is a valid outcome measure in clinical trials has been hampered by a variety of factors, including the conceptual vagueness of QOL, the use of assessment tools of dubious validity and reliability, the inappropriateness of methods, and the weakness of statistical analysis of the resulting data.... Consequently we have a responsibility to ensure that the tests employed to measure QOL are psychometrically sound, and that they are administered thoughtfully and analyzed correctly."[3]

In "Assessing quality of life in clinical research: from where have we come and where are we going?" Wood Dauphine describes the history of HRQOL assessment, discusses its current status, and suggests challenges for the future.[4] She wrote,

> "The development of generic measures began in the early 1970s and continues today. Disease-specific measures have also proliferated. The 1980s and 1990s saw an increase in methodological rigor, and additional emphasis on analytic approaches, interpretation of scale scores, cultural and language issues, as well as on the development of shorter measures. Future challenges include conceptualization and testing of theoretical models, further refinement of individualized measures for use in routine clinical practice, the use of computer adapted testing in quality of life assessment, and the inclusion of quality of life information in health databases."[4]

INTRODUCTION

Neuroendocrine tumors have always been regarded as a Cinderella condition. Yet it is estimated that there are now more than 100,000 patients with gastroenteropancreatic neuroendocrine tumors (NETs) in the United States. NETs are more prevalent than stomach and gastric cancer combined. While the incidence of all neoplasms in the surveillance, epidemiology, and end results registry shows a small increase up to and until 2004, NETs (which include neuroendocrine tumors of the gastroenteropancreatic axis) have risen from 1 case per 100,000 population in 1973 to 5 cases per 100,000 in 2004, and this increase appears to be rising. Patients with well-differentiated NETs have a survival probability of 35% compared with patients with poorly differentiated tumors, predicted to have a survival rate of 4% for 5 years. The survival of patients with well-differentiated tumors can be improved markedly if diagnosed before the advent of metastases, increasing from 30 to 120 months if localized, showing the importance of early recognition. Early studies bear testimony to the fact that time from the first appearance of symptoms to the diagnosis is usually 9.2 years. It is clear that both patients and practitioners need a heightened awareness of the symptoms of the condition, which often masquerade as other disease states. Early recognition, together with the advent of new approaches to therapy—the use of somatostatin analogs alone and in combinations with other chemotherapeutic, surgical, and advanced technological procedures—has had a very significant impact on the course of the disease, which now may be regarded as chronic rather than a rapidly progressive and fatal condition. In this milieu, the need for developing a questionnaire to capture patients' responses may have been predicated by the notion that the instrument would be able to help define those patients who have the condition, while excluding those without it.

With regard to therapy, a fundamental objective of any health care intervention is enhancement of the patient's QOL and overall well being. A patient's HRQOL encompasses his or her experience as a result of the underlying condition and his or her response to medical treatment, and consequently how his or her illness impacts his or her overall well being.[5] Consideration of a patient's QOL has become increasingly important in evaluating the adverse health effects resulting from chronic illnesses such as NETs. Knox and colleagues[6] found that advanced therapy like resection surgery for NETs is associated with significantly improved and sustained functional QOL. On the contrary, QOL may be severely impaired by the devastating effects of many chemotherapeutic agents causing nausea, vomiting, and fatigue. The effects of radiation, too, can compromise QOL.

PATIENT-REPORTED OUTCOMES IN CLINICAL TRIALS

In the current patient-centered environment, there has been an increasing interest in incorporating patients' assessments of their health status, giving rise to questionnaires designed to collect and analyze patient-reported outcomes (PROs).

The abbreviation QOL used in this article will denote HQOL. Thus subjective, self-reported patient assessments of their health status as it affects their QOL reflects health outcomes related to QOL. Although QOL as a marker for health outcomes is a recently recognized value, the importance of QOL for evaluating results of clinical research is now indisputable. No clinical trial for a new therapy will pass muster with the US Food and Drug Administration (FDA) without the use of a suitable validated QOL instrument to assess patient-reported outcomes. QOL measures also are used to discriminate the presence or absence of a condition, discriminate the different levels of severity within a condition, correlate subjective and objective measures, and most importantly, to monitor patients' progress. QOL questionnaires administered to patients may help to bridge the gap between patient and physician interaction and touch on issues too sensitive for the patient to address personally. As reported by Clauser and colleagues,[7] PROs are used in various cancer clinical trials to better understand the burden of cancer and the adverse effects of cancer therapy such as pain, fatigue, and nausea. Also mentioned in this article is the fact that the evolution of PROs in cancer trials has been documented by the National Cancer Institutes (NCI)-supported Cancer Outcomes measurement Working Group. In their endeavor to measure QOL across a range of cancers and other diseases, the NCI created the Patient Reported Outcomes Measurement Information System (PROMIS).[8]

In Europe, the European Organization for Research and Treatment of Cancer (EORTC) developed the first generation of a core questionnaire in 1987 for measuring PROs in cancer clinical trials, EORTC-QLQ-C-36.[9] Subsequently, EORTC-QLQ-C-36 was modified to EORTC-QLQ-C-30, and after further iteration the EORTC-QLQ-C-30 (version 3.0) now in use since December 1997 is the recommended version for new studies. Although there was a concerted effort in Europe and later in the United States toward the development of cancer-related questionnaires, no specific tool was available for assessing subjective QOL outcomes in patients with NETs. In fact it was recognized that although the EORTC-QLQ-C-30 was an important tool to measure generic aspects of cancer, it had limitations for capturing specific aspects of cancer-related diseases. This realization of the lack of disease-specific self-reported QOL measures motivated the development of disease-specific modules.

DEVELOPMENT OF TWO DISEASE-SPECIFIC QUESTIONNAIRES

Until recently, only a limited body of research literature on carcinoid tumors and NETS existed, and, as previously mentioned, there was no disease-specific tool to measure HLQOL in patients with this disease. To fill this need, two questionnaires were simultaneously but independently developed, on two different continents, to measure the subjective, self-reported effects of NETs on QOL. Although there are some distinct similarities, there are also notable differences in the perspectives of each and their paths to the common goal of measuring QOL.

The Norfolk QOL-NET, a 72-item all-inclusive single questionnaire, was developed in 2004 at the Neuroendocrine Unit, a department within Eastern Virginia Medical School (EVMS), located in Norfolk, Virginia. The development process, which extended over 3 years in different patient populations in the United States ,has been described and published.[10]

In the interim, the European group working in the field of NETs also found a need for a tool to capture the responses from patients with NETs of the gut.[11] They developed a 21-item disease-specific QOL questionnaire to supplement the EORTC QLQ-C30, (their generic cancer measure updated in 1995). They named the new, disease-specific tool EORTC QLQ-C30 GI.NET-21.[9]

DESCRIPTION OF TWO DISEASE-SPECIFIC QUESTIONNAIRES

The measurements in the Norfolk QOL-NET relate to a 4-week time frame as opposed to the single week reports in the EORTC QLQ-C30 GI.NET-21, with the exception of the question on sexual activity in the European tool, which later was changed to a 4-week time frame.

Norfolk QOL-NET captures 11 symptoms and it measures both frequency and severity of symptoms: flushing, joint/bone pain, other pain, peripheral edema, wheezing, diarrhea/constipation, rash, cyanosis, telangiectasia, fatigue, and coughing. It also assesses in detail severity of dysfunction in daily activities, impaired work performance, family life, and psycho/social activities. The authors have shown that the burden of disease plays a major role on physical functioning and consequently on QOL. Twenty questions in the Norfolk QOL-NET were designed to capture activities of daily living and physical functioning. EORTC QLQ-C30 GI.NET-21 does not measure frequency and severity of symptoms, nor does it cover physical functioning as one of its scales. It has three defined multi-item symptom scales: endocrine, gastrointestinal (GI), and treatment-related side effects. It has two single-item symptoms (bone/muscle pain and worry about weight loss), two psychosocial scales (social function and disease-related worries), and two other single items (sexuality and communication). Certain symptoms in the QLQ-GI.NET-21, such as headaches, night sweats, and abdominal bloating are not included in the Norfolk QOL-NET. However, these are generic cancer questions and not specific to this condition. Also featured in the QLQ-GI.NET-21 are items that deal with worry about general cancer issues, but an important NET-specific question related to coughing is not included, nor are items related to diarrhea and constipation.

Norfolk QOL-NET does include diarrhea and constipation, specific to NETS, and addresses these symptoms in depth:

> *"Have you had diarrhea even if you did not eat?"*
> *"Have you had continuous diarrhea even if you did not eat?"*
> *"Have you had a cough, not related to a cold or allergies?"*

During the psychometric validation process of the Norfolk QOL-NET, factor analysis confirmed the subscales/factors and items. Several factors emerged from the analyses

Principal components showing a scree plot
Forced 7-factor analysis with varimax rotation
Physical functioning
Flushing
GI disturbances
Respiratory
Cardiovascular
Depression
Attitude.

Cronbach α values ranged from 0.86 to 0.97, showing excellent internal consistency of the items in each factor. This analysis has not been shown to date in the European version.

In the course of the development process of Norfolk QOL-NET,[10] the authors related measures of QOL to tumor burden, biochemical values, and symptoms, using the results of both questionnaires to demonstrate criterion validity. In this article, they compare the structure of both questionnaires in more detail and discuss the ability of each to capture the salient features of the disease and each questionnaire's capacity to correlate patient-related QOL scores with objective health measures.

STUDY METHODS FOR COMPLETING BOTH QUESTIONNAIRES

During clinic visits to the Neuroendocrine Unit at the Eastern Virginia Medical School, patients with a diagnosed NET (from August through November 2008) were informed about the study and asked to participate. Those in agreement signed the consent form and completed the Norfolk QOL-NET and the EORTC QLQ-C30 GI.NET 21 questionnaires. At the end of that period, 29 patients were enrolled; information about the status of the disease in terms of the tumor burden, biochemistry, and carcinoid symptoms was extracted from their files matching the date they completed the questionnaires.

For the evaluation of the tumor burden, a scale was developed, from 1 to 6, "1" representing status post tumor resection, "2" no evident tumor, "3" single tumor without metastasis, "4" tumor with metastasis to liver or elsewhere but not to bone, "5" tumor with metastasis to bone, and "6" tumor with metastasis to bone and liver or elsewhere. Most of the blood samples for biochemical values were assayed and analyzed at the Norfolk Sentara Laboratory System. The markers for this study were: chromogranin A (CgA), urinary 5-hydroxyindoleacetic acid (5-HIAA) and serotonin, with normal values as follows: chromogranin A in the range of 0 to 5 nmol/L, 5-HIAA 2 to 8 mg/d, and serotonin 12 to 44 pg/mL.

The Norfolk Carcinoid Symptom Score is another tool developed in the Endocrine Unit at Eastern Virginia Medical School to address the usual symptoms present in individuals with neuroendocrine tumors (see Appendix). It has a total of 18 scored questions. Included in the total number of questions, are three questions related to flushing, four to respiratory symptoms, three to gastro-intestinal symptoms, two to cardiovascular, three to physical functioning and two to diabetes. There are also questions about family history and personal medical history. Each question is scored from 0 to 1, "0" denoting absence of the symptom, and "1" denoting that the symptom is present. The total possible score (worst scenario) is 18 points.

Statistical Analysis

From the data on the condition of these 29 patients, the means and SE were calculated for the total scores of both questionnaires, for biochemical values and for symptom scores; the median was calculated for tumor burden. Because these data were not a Gaussian distribution, nonparametric correlations were used to explore the relationship between total QOL scores from both questionnaires, each individual domain of the Norfolk QOL-NET, tumor burden, biochemical markers, and symptom scores. P values <.05 were accepted as statistically significant.

Missing data were handled in the following way: for CgA values, the mean of the results for each variable was used, on condition that more than two-thirds of the values were available. For the analysis of the other biochemical markers, 5-HIAA and serotonin, only the patients who had these measures were included.

Regression analysis was used to determine the predictability of whether the scores of each domain of the Norfolk QOL-NET correlated with the total scores of the Norfolk QOL-NET and the EORTC QLQ C30 GI.NET-21 questionnaires.

Results

Twenty-nine patients completed both the Norfolk QOL-NET and the EORTC QLQ C30 QLQ-GI.NET21, and the results were compared using Spearman's nonparametric correlations. The results showed a strong correlation between the total scores of the two questionnaires ($r= 0.93$, $P<.0001$); all the domains of the Norfolk QOL-NET correlated positively with the EORTC QLQ C30 QLQ-GI.NET-21 total score, except for the cardiovascular domain, which did not correlate at all (**Table 1**).

Both questionnaires correlated strongly with the Norfolk Carcinoid Symptom Score and also with tumor burden. No correlation was found between the QOL scores and CgA values.

The analysis of the data from the serotonin values that matched the date the patients completed the questionnaires showed a positive strong correlation between serotonin and QOL, either assessed by the Norfolk QOL-NET or by the EORTC QLQ C30 GI.NET-21 questionnaires. This marker also correlated positively with three of the Norfolk QOL-NET domains. **Table 2** shows the r and P values of these correlations.

When comparing the Norfolk QOL-NET with the QLQ C30GI NET-21, certain differences emerged. Although there was a good correlation between the total scores with the two tools, a clear distinction emerged when the correlations between the different domains of the Norfolk QOLNET and the total scores of the two tools were examined.

All the domains of Norfolk QOL-NET—physical functioning, depression, GI, flushing, respiratory, positive attitude, and cardiovascular—correlated strongly with the total QOL Norfolk NET score, with P values <.05. In contrast, only three domains of the Norfolk QOL-NET predicted the total QOL score of the EORTC QLQ C30 GI.NET-21. These were: physical functioning, GI, and respiratory, which reached significance. The remaining four domains—flushing, depression, cardiovascular, and positive attitude—failed to reach significance (**Figs. 1** and **2**).

However, correlation of the domains of the Norfolk QOL-NET—physical functioning, GI, depression, flushing, respiratory, and positive attitude—was stronger with the total Norfolk QOL-NET score than it was with the total scores of the EORTC QLQ C30 QLQ-GI.NET-21. Similarly, there was a stronger correlation of QOL-NET domains with tumor burden and the Norfolk Carcinoid Symptom Score.

Table 1

Comparison of the Norfolk quality of life–neuroendocrine tumor (QOL-NET) total scores, Norfolk QOL-NET domains, tumor burden, biochemical markers, and the Norfolk carcinoid symptom scores with the European Organization for Research and Treatment of Cancer QLQ-C30 GI.NET-21 scores

	Total Norfolk QOL		Total European QOL		Domain 1 Depression		Domain 2 Flushing		Domain 3 Respiratory		Domain 4 Gastrointestinal		Domain 5 Cardiovascular		Domain 6 Physical Functioning		Domain 7 Positive Attitude	
	r	P	r	P	r	P	r	P	r	P	r	P	r	P	r	P	r	P
Total Norfolk QOL			0.94	<.001	0.73	<.0001	0.62	.0003	0.65	.0002	0.78	<.0001	0.46	.012	0.96	<.0001	0.52	.004
Tumor Burden	0.52	.004	0.5	.005	0.42	.023	0.24	.216	0.02	.935	0.58	.001	0.18	.343	0.56	.002	0.18	.346
Serotonin	0.62	.013	0.71	.003	0.56	.03	0.08	.78	0.32	.25	0.62	.013	0.29	.3	0.62	.013	0.12	.67
CgA	0.06	.764	0.06	.765	−0.15	.433	0.26	.176	0.08	.663	0.03	.891	0.34	.07	0.07	.735	0.12	.55
Carcinoid Symptom Score	0.67	<.0001	0.67	<.0001	0.37	.051	0.58	.001	0.53	.003	0.6	.0006	0.55	.0018	0.7	<.0001	0.59	.0009

Table 2
Correlations between serotonin, total QOL scores, and domains of the Norfolk QOL-NET in patients with NETs

Total QOL and Domain Scores	Serotonin	
	r	P
Total Scores Norfolk QOL NET	0.62	.013
Total Scores EORTC C-30 GI.NET 21	0.71	.003
Domain 1: Depression	0.56	.03
Domain 2: Flushing	0.08	.78
Domain 3: Respiratory	0.32	.25
Domain 4: Gastrointestinal	0.62	.013
Domain 5: Cardiovascular	0.29	.3
Domain 6: Physical Functioning	0.62	.013
Domain 7: Positive Attitude	0.12	.67

SUMMARY

In the United States and in Europe the need arose to evaluate the impairment of QOL in patients with NETs as more patients were diagnosed (or misdiagnosed) with this disease. Because of the lack of specific questionnaires to assess the spectrum of symptoms present in this disease, two disease-specific QOL, the Norfolk QOL-NET and the combination EORTC QLQ C30 GI.NET-21, were developed.

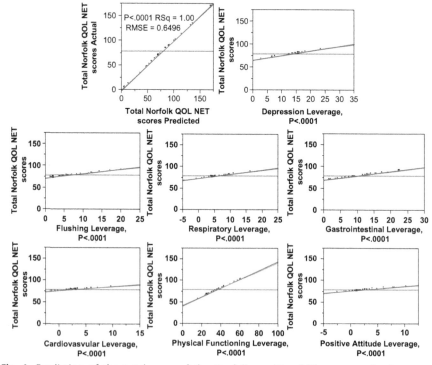

Fig. 1. Prediction of the total score of the Norfolk quality of life–neuroendocrine tumor (QOL- NET) by the scores of each of the Norfolk QOL-NET domains. Logistic regression analysis shows how each domain predicts the total scores of the Norfolk QOL-NET. All the domains have significant values. The order in which they predict the scores is: physical functioning, depression, gastrointestinal symptoms, flushing, respiratory symptoms, positive attitude and cardiovascular symptoms.

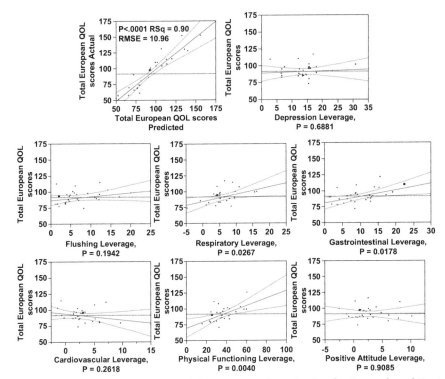

Fig. 2. Prediction of the total score of the European Organization for Research and Treatment of Cancer (EORTC) QLQ C30 GI.NET-21 by the scores of each of the Norfolk QOL-NET domains. Logistic regression analysis to show how each domain of the Norfolk QOL-NET predicts the total score of the EORTC QLQ C-30 GI.NET-21. Only physical functioning, gastrointestinal, and respiratory domains correlated significantly with the total score.

The Norfolk QOL-NET questionnaire is an all-inclusive single tool of 72 questions for measuring subjective, self-reported effects of neuroendocrine on QOL. It measures both frequency and severity of symptoms; the measurements relate to a 4-week time frame as opposed to the single-week reports in the EORTC QLQ C30 GI.NET-21, with the exception of the question on sexual activity, which was later changed to a 4-week time frame. The Norfolk QOL-NET captures clinical symptoms related to NETS that have been classified by factor analysis into domains. There are 10 questions in the depression domain and eight in the flushing domain that include actual flushing, rash, and teleangiectasia, while the European tool has only two questions related to flushing. In the respiratory domain, there are eight questions related to shortness of breath, wheezing, and coughing compared with only one question related to shortness of breath present in the European questionnaire. In contrast to the lack of cardiovascular questions in the European questionnaire, the Norfolk QOL-NET has six questions assessing the presence of edema and cyanosis. The physical functioning domain in the Norfolk QOL-NET is comprised of 26 questions. Additionally, there are three questions related to positive attitude and four related to the impact of treatment with somatostatin on the QOL of these patients.

The psychometric analysis performed on the Norfolk QOL-NET tool resulted in seven domains, providing a structure for entering, analyzing, and interpreting patient data for proposed interventions, directed to specific problems. As yet, there is no publication to show that psychometric analysis has been performed on EORTC QLQ C30 GI.NET-21.

The Norfolk QOL-NET assesses the impact of treatment with Somatostatin on the QOL of patients with NETS. Since new treatment options are being developed that may affect the QOL of patients in different ways, this issue should be addressed. The European tool has no questions addressing this concern.

There is a strong positive correlation between the Norfolk QOL-NET and the European questionnaires. All the domains of the Norfolk QOL-NET, except for the cardiovascular domain, correlated with the EORTC QLQ C30 GI.NET-21 total score. This might be because the European questionnaire has no questions related to cardiovascular symptoms, while there are six questions addressing this issue in the Norfolk tool.

The strongest correlation found between the total scores of both questionnaires and the Norfolk QOL-NET domains was with the physical functioning domain. This domain also was found to be the biggest predictor of total scores for both questionnaires after logistic regression analysis.

Both questionnaires and each domain correlate positively with the Carcinoid Symptom Score, except for depression; this might be because there are no questions about depression in the Carcinoid Symptom Score tool.

Tumor burden correlates with both questionnaires and with the depression, GI, and physical functioning domains. The authors recommend the use of the tumor burden scale, proposed in this study, for future studies, since it gives an easy and reproducible way to assess and classify this variable and compare it with others.

Of the biochemical markers investigated in this study, only serotonin was found to have a significant positive and strong correlation with the total QOL scores assessed with either questionnaire; it also correlated with three domains: depression, GI, and physical functioning. Serotonin regulates numerous biologic processes including cardiovascular function, bowel motility, ejaculatory latency, and bladder control, as well as other processes including platelet aggregation.[12] Serotonin may be incriminated in several symptoms of carcinoid, particularly diarrhea and cardiomyopathy. While the relationship between serotonin and total QOL, and in particular the depression domain, appears counterintuitive, there may be a plausible explanation. Serotonin does not cross the blood–brain barrier, but 5-HTP (the precursor to serotonin) is able to, and is required for brain synthesis of 5-HT (serotonin). Since the tumor deviates 5-HTP into tumor production of 5-HT, which is released into the circulation, high levels of blood 5-HT reflect a deficiency of 5-HT in the brain. The authors are continuing to study this fascinating phenomenon to ascertain whether the proposed hypothesis on the inverse relationship between high blood serotonin levels and depression can be confirmed in a larger population of patients with NETs.[13]

Finally, the authors demonstrated a strong correlation between Norfolk QOL-NET and the EORTC QLQ-C30 GI.NET-21, indicating that either tool can be considered for use in a clinical trial. However, the Norfolk QOL-NET captures additional features: a larger number of questions covering aspects of the flushing and respiratory domains, and, in particular, the cardiovascular impact, which has been found in 37% of patients with carcinoid tumors.[14] Nevertheless, it should be mentioned that the prevalence of these cardiovascular complications of carcinoid tumors may be falling for reasons that are not obvious.[15] The authors believe that the Norfolk QOL-NET is an important tool for measuring patients' perception of the burden of their disease and impact of treatment modalities on their QOL and may be a useful guide in deciding changes in therapy to alter apparent health status. Norfolk QOL-NET should be particularly sensitive to symptom change, physical functioning, respiratory and cardiovascular disease progression, or remission, and in this respect it may have advantages over the EORTC QLQ-C30 GI.NET-21. This remains to be seen when longitudinal studies have been completed.

It has been reported that there has been very little change in the natural history of carcinoid tumors.[16] However, with the recent advent of new drugs for treating NETS,[17,18] there are new inroads into the rapid pace of nonprogress[16,19] or the odyssey in the land of slow-growing tumors.[20] To this end, tools that can identify the selective impact of these agents on the different domains determining health status and QOL should be welcome, particularly if they pave the way for new therapeutic options that derive their logic from HRQOL measures.

APPENDIX

TO BE COMPLETED BY HEALTH PROESSIONAL

Patient Name:_____Date:_____

CARCINOID SYMPTOM SCORE
(0=NO SYMPTOM, 1=SYMPTOM IS PRESENT)

SCORE: 0 or 1

1.	Have you experienced any flushing?	_____
	Does the flush last minutes or hours? __ minutes __hours	no score
	Is the flush a hot flush or wet flush? __ hot ___wet	no score
2.	Have you been experiencing any joint pain?	_____
3.	Have you noticed any	
	a) Wheezing?	_____
	b) Shortness of breath with or without activity?	_____
	c) Shortness of breath when lying flat?	_____
	d) Cough?	_____
4.	Have you been having any diarrhea?	_____
5.	If you do have diarrhea, is it persistent if you do not eat?	_____
6.	Are you having any abdominal colicky pain?	_____
7.	Are you able to get out of a chair without pushing on the arms of the chair?	_____
8.	Can you do your own hair?	_____
9.	Have you noticed any skin color changes or changes in your pigmentation?	_____
10.	Do you have a family history of any endocrine tumors (pituitary, parathyroid, thyroid, adrenal)?	_____
11.	Do you have an endocrine tumor (pituitary, parathyroid, thyroid, adrenal)?	_____
12.	Do you have a history of high blood pressure?	_____
13.	Do you have diabetes?	_____
14.	Are your ankles swelling?	_____
15.	Do you have numbness or tingling or pain in your feet or hands?	_____

TOTAL SCORE_____

How have you been feeling in general?_____
_____

Revised 9/14/09

REFERENCES

1. Vinik E, Vinik AI. Transcending tradition: quality of life as the inextricable link between activities of daily living and specific organ and disease states. In: Farquhar I, Summers K, Sorkin A, editors. Research in human capital and development. The value of innovation: impact on health, life quality, safety and regulatory research, vol. 1. Bingley (UK): Emerald Group Publishing Limited; 2008. p. 29–52.
2. Pigou AC. The economics of welfare. 1st edition. London: Macmillan and Company; 1920.
3. Fallowfield L. Quality of quality-of-life data. Lancet 1996;348:421–2.
4. Wood-Dauphinee S. Assessing quality of life in clinical research: from where have we come and where are we going? J Clin Epidemiol 1999;52:355–63.
5. Berzon RA. Understanding and using health-related quality of life instruments within clinical research studies. In: Staquet MJ, Hays RD, Fayers PM, editors. Quality of life assessment in clinical trials. Methods and practice. New York: Oxford University Press; 1998.
6. Knox CD, Feurer ID, Wise PE, et al. Survival and functional quality of life after resection for hepatic carcinoid metastasis. J Gastrointest Surg 2004;8:653–9.
7. Clauser SB, Ganz PA, Lipscomb J, et al. Patient-reported outcomes assessment in cancer trials: evaluating and enhancing the payoff to decision making. J Clin Oncol 2007;25:5049–50.
8. Garcia SF, Cella D, Clauser SB, et al. Standardizing patient-reported outcomes assessment in cancer clinical trials: a patient-reported outcomes measurement information system initiative. J Clin Oncol 2007;25:5106–12.
9. Aaronson NK, Cull A, Kaasa S. The EORTC modular approach to quality-of-life assessment in oncology. Int J Ment Health 1994;23:75–96.
10. Vinik E, Carlton CA, Silva MP, et al. Development of the Norfolk quality-of-life tool for assessing patients with neuroendocrine tumors. Pancreas 2009;38:e87–95.
11. Davies AH, Larsson G, Ardill J, et al. Development of a disease-specific quality-of-life questionnaire module for patients with gastrointestinal neuroendocrine tumours. Eur J Cancer 2006;42:477–84.
12. Berger M, Gray JA, Roth BL. The expanded biology of serotonin. Annu Rev Med 2009;60:355–66.
13. Vinik E, Silva M, Vinik A. Relationship between quality of life and health-related measures including symptoms, biochemical markers and tumor burden. International Society for Pharmacoeconomics and Outcomes Research (ISPOR), May 2009; National Association of Neuroendocrine Tumors (NANETS), October 2009. Abstract and poster presentation.
14. Vinik AI, Feliberti E, Perry RR, et al. Carcinoid tumors. Updated January 28, 2008. In: de Groot LC, editor. Diffuse hormonal systems and endocrine tumor syndromes. 2008. Chapter 2. Available at: Endotext.com. Accessed December 17, 2010.
15. Vinik AI, Anthony L, Boudreaux JP, et al. Neuroendocrine tumors: a critical appraisal of management strategies pancreas. Conference report: NETs summit 2010;39(6):801–18.
16. Modlin IM, Moss SF, Chung DC, et al. Priorities for improving the management of gastroenteropancreatic neuroendocrine tumors. J Natl Cancer Inst 2008;100: 1282–9.
17. Kulke MH, Lenz HJ, Meropol NJ, et al. Activity of sunitinib in patients with advanced neuroendocrine tumors. J Clin Oncol 2008;26:3403–10.
18. Yao JC, Phan A, Hoff PM, et al. Targeting vascular endothelial growth factor in advanced carcinoid tumor: a random assignment phase II study of depot

octreotide with bevacizumab and pegylated interferon alpha-2b. J Clin Oncol 2008;26:1316–23.

19. Modlin IM, Champaneria MC, Chan AK, et al. A three-decade analysis of 3911 small intestinal neuroendocrine tumors: the rapid pace of no progress. Am J Gastroenterol 2007;102:1464–73.

20. Moertel CG. Karnofsky memorial lecture. An odyssey in the land of small tumors. J Clin Oncol 1987;5:1502–22.

The Clinical Relevance of Chromogranin A as a Biomarker for Gastroenteropancreatic Neuroendocrine Tumors

Ben Lawrence, MBChB, MSc[a], Bjorn I. Gustafsson, MD, PhD[b,c],
Mark Kidd, PhD[a], Marianne Pavel, MD[d], Bernhard Svejda, MD[a],
Irvin M. Modlin, MD, PhD, DSc, FRCS(Eng & Ed)[a,*]

KEYWORDS

- Chromogranin • Granin family • Neuroendocrine tumor
- Carcinoid • Enterochromaffin cell • Tumor marker

THE BIOCHEMICAL DIAGNOSIS OF NEUROENDOCRINE TUMORS

An accurate tumor marker is a critical tool in tumor management because it establishes an uncertain diagnosis, offers a basis for individual prognostication, signals response to therapy, and identifies relapse. In classical terms, a high-quality tumor marker should represent a biologic attribute unique to the tumor cell or its local environment. Although this has proved manageable in a homogenous tumor population, the goal has been difficult to attain in gastroenteropancreatic neuroendocrine tumors (GEP-NETs) because they comprise an extremely heterogeneous group of cancers. Thus, the conundrum of identifying a global marker for NETs has remained a considerable technical challenge.

The identification of chromogranin A (CgA) in secretory vesicles in the adrenal medulla,[1] the development of a specific antibody,[2] and localization to extra-adrenal neuroendocrine cells[3,4] provided a partial solution. The clinical utility of this tool is blunted, however, by the ubiquity of CgA in normal tissue, the variable methodology

[a] Gastrointestinal Pathobiology Research Group, Department of Surgery, Yale University School of Medicine, 310 Cedar Street, PO Box 208602, New Haven, CT 06520-8062, USA
[b] Department of Gastroenterology, St Olavs Hospital, 7006 Trondheim, Norway
[c] Department of Cancer Research and Molecular Medicine, Norwegian University of Science and Technology, Prinsesse Kristinas Gate 1, 7006 Trondheim, Norway
[d] Med. Klinik m.S. Hepatologie und Gastroenterologie, Charité - Campus Virchow Klinikum, Universitätsmedizin Berlin, Augustenburger Platz 1, 13353 Berlin, Germany
* Corresponding author. Department of Gastroenterological Surgery, Yale University School of Medicine, 333 Cedar Street, PO Box 208062, New Haven, CT 06520-8062.
E-mail address: imodlin@optonline.net

Endocrinol Metab Clin N Am 40 (2011) 111–134
doi:10.1016/j.ecl.2010.12.001
0889-8529/11/$ – see front matter © 2011 Elsevier Inc. All rights reserved.

of its measurement, and the diverse disease processes and physiologic events that perturb the granin family of peptides. To assess the utility of CgA measurement for clinical application, a basic understanding of essential CgA biology is necessary. This article provides an overview of the strengths and limitations of CgA as a tumor marker. It encompasses the physiologic role of CgA and evaluates the causes of CgA elevation in non-NET disease states and assesses the test platform variations and the impact on clinical care of NETs.

THE BIOLOGY OF CHROMOGRANIN A IN NORMAL CELLS
The Neuroendocrine Cell

Neuroendocrine cells aggregate in classical endocrine glands (eg, adrenal, pituitary, and parathyroid) but also in the diffuse neuroendocrine system (DNES)—the diaphanous, ill-defined, and poorly understood neuroendocrine syncytium integrated throughout the bronchopulmonary and gastrointestinal (GI) systems.[5] Although the overarching role of the DNES as a wide-ranging regulator of secretion, absorption, and motility is broadly understood, the precise mechanistic basis of its function and its cell lineage remains, for the most part, opaque.

The cellular origins of GEP-NETs are diverse and reflect the numerous neuroendocrine cell types of the DNES in the GI tract.[6] Certain neuroendocrine cells are localized to a single organ (eg, gastric enterochromaffin-like [ECL] cells) whereas others (eg, the enterochromaffin [EC] cells), are ubiquitous throughout the GI tract (**Table 1**). Neuroendocrine cells share several common features, including production of secretory granules, maturation, and exocytosis as well as the synthesis of specific proteins and the presence of electron-dense or translucent secretory granules that are prototypical of the neuroendocrine cell type.[6] Of particular interest is the synthesis and biologic role of the granin family of proteins and peptides, especially that of CgA.[7]

The Granin Family

Granins are found as major, or principal, components of the soluble core of dense-core secretory granules in neuroendocrine cells and are secreted in a physiologically regulated manner.[8–11] There are 8 members in granin family, including CgA, CgB, CgC (secretogranin [Sg] II), SgIII, SgIV, SgV (7B2), Sg VI (NESP55), and VGF nerve growth factor–inducible (VGF) (**Fig. 1**). Granins have been proposed as playing important roles in secretory granule formation, processing, and development. The precise function, however, of individual granins is dependent on the presence of other granins and hormones produced by a specific neuroendocrine cell, the presence of proteolytic processing enzymes, and their inhibitors and activators as well as the density and localization of calcium pumps and exchangers. Of critical relevance to their clinical utility is the observation that irrespective of the cellular type, processing milieu, or expression of other granins, all are cosecreted with a variety of peptide and amine hormones depending on the neuroendocrine cell type.

Neuroendocrine Cell Types and CgA Secretion

Each neuroendocrine cell type in the DNES produces different amines, peptides, and proteins with a variety of biologic functions. At the same time, neuroendocrine cells cosecrete CgA during the secretory granule exocytotic process. Based on this biologic event, CgA has come to represent a common denominator peptide with the putative ability to be a marker of neuroendocrine cell activity (see **Table 1**). CgA was the initial member of the granin family identified, and its name represents the

Table 1
GEP-NET cell types and CgA secretion

Organ	Cell Type	Active Peptide	Related Tumor	Positive CgA Immunohistochemistry
Stomach—fundus	ECL cell	Histamine	ECLoma (types I, II, III)	Yes[63]
Antrum	X cell	Amylin	—	—
Antrum (and duodenum)	G cell	Gastrin	Gastrinoma	Yes[63]
Duodenum	I cell	CCK	CCKoma	Yes[145]
	S cell	Secretin	—	Yes[145]
	M cell	Motilin	—	No[145,146]
Duodenum/jejunum	K cell	GIP	GIPoma	Yes[145]
Small intestine	L cell	GLP1, PYY, NPY	—	Yes[145]
	N cell	Neurotensin	—	Yes[145]
Pancreas	β cell	Insulin	Insulinoma	Yes[63]
	α cell	Glucagon	Glucagonoma	Yes[63]
	F cell	Pancreatic PP	PPoma	Yes[63]
Entire GI tract	EC cell	Serotonin, substance P, guanylin, melatonin	Carcinoid, SI-NET	Yes[63]
	D cell	Somatostatin	Somatostatinoma	Yes[104,145]
	VIP cell	Vasoactive intestinal peptide	VIPoma	Yes[147]

Abbreviations: CCK, cholecystokinin; SI-NET, small intestinal neuroendocrine tumor.

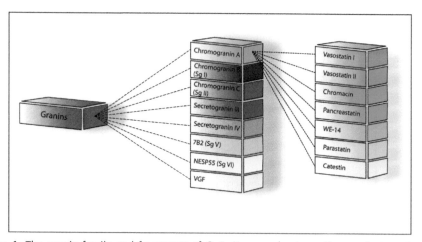

Fig. 1. The granin family and fragments of CgA. Neuroendocrine cells manufacture the 8 granin proteins in large dense-core secretory vesicles, including chromogranin (Cg) A, CgB, SgII (CgC), SgIII, SgIV, 7B2 (SgV), neuroendocrine secretory protein 55 (NESP55 or SgVI), and VGF nerve growth factor–inducible (VGF). CgA may be present in the blood as a major constituent, or as a series of smaller biologically active peptides created by postsecretory processing (right-hand box stack). These peptides include pancreastatin, catestin, vasostatin I and II, and others.

original detection in the catecholamine-containing chromaffin granules of the adrenal medulla.[1,12] It is encoded by the *CHGA/CgA* gene located on chromosome 14.

CgA mRNA and protein are pan-neuronally expressed,[13] which reflects the extent of dense-core granule formation in diverse cell types throughout the DNES. CgA expression generally correlates with dense-core granule number within a neuroendocrine cell. In PC12 and 6T3 neuroendocrine cells (rat pheochromocytoma and pituitary corticotroph cell lines, respectively), CgA is considered to function as on/off switch for the formation of large dense-core granules.[11] Sequence comparisons of CgA from various mammalian (eg, man, monkey, equine, pig, cattle, rat, and mouse), avian (ostrich *Struthio camelus*), and teleostean species have revealed considerable interspecies homology,[14–17] underlining the fundamental importance of CgA in cellular function.

Cleavage of CgA to Other Peptides

Granins serve as precursor proteins that can be proteolytically processed by prohormone or proprotein convertases at multiple cleavage sites to produce a large number of small bioactive peptides, with a wide range of proposed biologic activity.[8] CgA is a 439 amino acid protein[18] produced as a component of a complex processing mechanism; it may be present in the blood as a major constituent or as a series of smaller biologically active peptides, such as vasostatin I and II, chromacin, pancreastatin, WE14, parastatin, and catestin (see **Fig. 1**). Evidence for biologic activity in granin-derived peptides has accumulated since pancreastatin was first demonstrated to inhibit insulin secretion in 1986.[19]

Physiologic Role of CgA and Peptide Fragments

Although a definitive function for the complete CgA protein remains to be determined, a range of biologic functions is mediated by CgA-derived peptides (**Figs. 2** and **3**). CgA can exist in a variety of molecular forms and has been proposed as subsuming

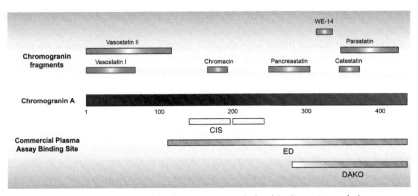

Fig. 2. The CgA protein, its peptide fragments, and the binding sites of the commercial p-CgA assays (CIS, ED, and DAKO). CgA is an approximately 460 amino acid protein that undergoes postsecretion processing into fragments, including pancreastatin (corresponding to human CgA residues 250–301), catestatin (residues 352–372), vasostatin I (residues 1–76), and vasostatin II (residues 1–113). The different sensitivities of 3 commercial CgA assays reflect the different binding epitopes of the antibody used in each test and the differential ability to bind to peptide fragments. The binding region of the DAKO antibody is not stated in product information, but because is standardized against a 23-kDa CgA fragment at the C- terminal, it will include at least some portion of the fragment indicated.

a diverse array of biofunctions ranging from neuroendocrine secretory regulation to cardiac function, vasomotor activity, and antimicrobial and antifungicidal activity to influences on intestinal smooth muscle contraction and modulatory roles in cell adhesion and homeostasis.[19–34] Possible additional roles include regulation of glomerular

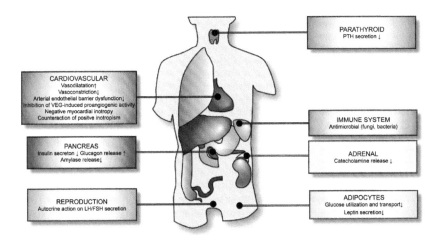

Fig. 3. Physiologic role of CgA. Although the definitive function for CgA itself remains unclear, CgA-derived peptides mediate a diverse array of biologic functions. These include regulation of parathyroid hormone secretion, carbohydrate metabolism, lipid metabolism, catecholamine secretion, several cardiovascular processes, immune properties, and reproduction. Variations in P-CgA may, therefore, reflect numerous functional alterations in a wide variety of biologic systems. In addition, CgA levels fluctuate on average by approximately 30% on repeated testing of normal individual and increase after food intake or physiologic stress.

filtration,[35] inflammation,[36–40] and microglial activation in the central nervous system.[41]

The physiologic role of many CgA peptide fragments is more certain. Vasostatins inhibit arterial vasoconstriction, including small and medium resistance vessels[22,23,25] as well as coronary and cerebral arteries,[30,42,43] and protect the heart against positive inotropism caused by β-adrenergic stimulation. Vasostatins also have antimicrobial properties by encouraging macrophage migration in inflammatory response,[27,29] inhibit PTH secretion,[25] and might regulate gonadotrophins.[44] Vasostatin I further inhibits tumor necrosis factor α–induced disruption of endothelial cells[45] and vascular endothelial growth factor.[46] Pancreastatin inhibits glucose-induced insulin release,[47] inhibits insulin-evoked glucose transport,[48] inhibits leptin secretion,[49] inhibits acid secretion from parietal cells,[50] and suppresses cholecystokinin-induced amylase secretion.[51] WE14 secretion might regulate gonadotrophins.[44] Parastatin inhibits PTH secretion,[24] inhibits pancreatic β-cells insulin release, and stimulates histamine release from ECL cells. Catestatin inhibits catecholamine release from adrenal chromaffin cells,[52] is coreleased with atrial natriuretic peptide,[53,54] has been proposed as protecting the heart against sympathetic overactivation,[54] and has antimicrobial activity against bacteria, fungi, and yeast.[55,56]

CGA MEASUREMENT

Based on post-translational processing (cleavage), CgA circulates as a highly heterogeneous antigen composition—comprising complete protein or constituent fragments. The efficacies of antibodies used in a particular CgA immunoassay therefore are of considerable relevance (see **Fig. 2**). CgA processing varies between different neuroendocrine organs, such that there is more extensive cleavage of CgA in pancreatic islets than in the adrenals, and different fragment profiles exist for each of the pancreatic α, β, D, and PP cells.[57]

CgA Testing Platforms for Blood

There are several commercially available and laboratory-developed assays for the measurement of circulating CgA concentrations. Three examples of commercial CgA assay kits are CgA-RIA CT (CIS bio international, Gif-sur-Yvette Cedex, France), DAKO Chromogranin A ELISA Kit (DAKO A/S, Glostrup, Denmark), and CgA EuroDiagnostica (Malmö, Sweden). These kits differ in methodologic techniques, such as radioimmunoassay and enzyme-linked immunosorbent assay (ELISA), have different standardization, and use different antibodies and binding epitopes (see **Fig. 2**). The calculated CgA level subsequently varies broadly between test platforms, with varying sensitivity and specificity.[58] Coefficients of variation also differ between testing kits.[59] At present, no universally accepted CgA assay exists and caution should be exhibited in the comparison of CgA concentration undertaken in different sites using different assay techniques.

CgA can be measured in plasma CgA (P-CgA) or serum CgA (S-CgA) without significantly changing the CgA level. A comparison of P-CgA to S-CgA concentration identified a strong positive linear relationship between these two measures ($r = 0.9858$, $P<.0001$), indicating CgA measurement can be undertaken in either sample type.[60] Although CgA measurement in saliva has been analyzed as a measure of stress response, this compartment has not, however, been investigated in NET patients.[61,62]

CgA Testing Platforms for Tissue

Immunohistochemical staining for CgA and synaptophysin is regarded as standard for a histopathologic diagnosis of NETs. CgA staining can be achieved in many neuroendocrine cell types, including pancreatic α, β, and polypeptide (PP) cells; gut EC, ECL, and G cells; thyroid C cells; parathyroid cells; adrenal medullary cells; and pituitary thyroid-stimulating hormone, follicle-stimulating hormone, and luteinizing hormone cells as well as some axons of visceral nerves.[63] An increased sensitivity in CgA-positive tumor detection by immunohistochemistry can be achieved by tyramide signal amplification, which is of value in diagnosing dedifferentiated neuroendocrine carcinomas.[64,65] Immunohistochemical staining for the NESP55 fragment (as well as CDX-2, PDX-1, and TTF-1) can help distinguish GI-NETs from pancreatic endocrine and pulmonary NETs.[66]

Several different CgA antibodies are commercially available for histopathologic use. Each antibody has variable sensitivity for different neuroendocrine cell types, for example, in the different pancreatic neuroendocrine cells. The monoclonal antibodies clone, LK2H10 (eg, Roche Molecular Biochemicals, Mannheim, Germany), is widely used for routine histopathology, has binding epitopes located in the CgA residues 250–284 (the N-terminal part of pancreastatin), and stains normal islet α cells well and β cells weakly but is nonreactive for D and PP cells.[57] The DAKO polyclonal antibody (A-0430) binds to the C-terminal part of the CgA molecule, has a broader range of epitopes, and may provide positive immunoreactivity in tumors where the monoclonal antibody is negative. The CgA 176–195 antibody[67] against the CgA midportion, however, displays strong immunoreactivity in all islet cell types except D cells and was the only CgA antibody expressed in all NETs, making it a superior pancreas endocrine cell and tumor marker compared with the other CgA antibodies.[68] Similar variability should be expected when staining neuroendocrine cells outside the pancreas.

A systematic immunocytochemical investigation of CgA fragments demonstrated expression of a more extensive variety of CgA fragments in NETs than normal neuroendocrine cells.[68] The CgA fragment pattern may thus be of value in evaluating the biologic behavior of NETs and region-specific antibodies of potential use when differentiating between benign and malignant NET types.[68] Staining variation is also exhibited by NETs of different histologic grade. The staining intensity of CgA antibodies is high in well-differentiated NETs and is comparable to staining in a normal neuroendocrine cell. Conversely, poorly differentiated neuroendocrine carcinomas (PDECs) are often nonimmunoreactive for CgA because of the rarity of large, dense-core granules.[69] The loss of CgA expression in PDECs indicates their incomplete or partial endocrine differentiation, in keeping with the on/off switch function of the *CHGA/CgA* gene for endocrine differentiation in mammalian cells.[11] Thus, P-CgA, which is related to the hormone's expression in the granules, may be within the reference interval or only slightly elevated in PDECs.[69]

PATHOLOGIC ELEVATION OF CGA
Nonmalignant but Pathologic Causes of Elevated CgA

As a consequence of the ubiquitous cosecretion of CgA with other regulatory peptides (see **Table 1**), there are multiple causes of CgA elevation that are unrelated to NETs. CgA elevation is associated with diverse GI, cardiovascular, pulmonary, rheumatologic, and endocrine diseases (**Fig. 4**).[36,38,70–72] CgA elevation in GI disease occurs in chronic atrophic gastritis,[73] liver cirrhosis, chronic hepatitis,[71] pancreatitis,[74] inflammatory bowel disease,[75] *Helicobacter pylori* infection,[76] and even irritable bowel syndrome (**Table 2**).[77,78] The elevated levels of CgA in inflammatory bowel disease

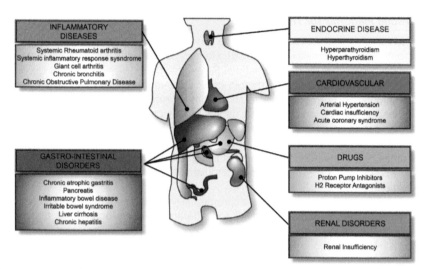

Fig. 4. Non-neoplastic causes of CgA elevation. CgA is elevated in endocrine diseases, chronic and acute inflammation, and cardiac insufficiency. Acid-suppressive medications result in hypergastrinemia (G-cell and ECL-cell hyperplasia) and a concomitant increase in cosecreted CgA. Renal failure increases detectable p-CgA by reducing glomerular filtration of CgA-related peptides. P-CgA alone cannot discriminate between GEP-NETs, pancreatitis, inflammatory bowel disease, irritable bowel syndrome, or hepatitis.

are of particular interest because the incidence of GI-NETs is significantly elevated in inflammatory bowel disease, possibly reflecting increased neuroendocrine cell proliferation in an inflammatory milieu.[79]

Elevated levels of circulating CgA as a consequence of non-GI disease occur in patients with hypertension,[80–82] heart failure,[37,83] renal failure,[84,85] systemic inflammatory response syndrome,[86] hyperthyroidism,[87] pulmonary obstructive disease,[62,88]

Table 2
Sensitivity of elevated P-CgA levels in detection of non-neuroendocrine GEP disease

Disease/Disorder		Detection Sensitivity (%)
Non-neoplastic	Chronic atrophic gastritis[73]	78–100
	Pancreatitis[74]	23
	Inflammatory bowel disease[71,75]	28–55[a]
	Irritable bowel syndrome[77]	20–31[b]
	Liver cirrhosis[71]	19–48
	Chronic hepatitis[71]	20
Neoplastic	Colon cancer[148]	1–20
	HCC[40]	70–83
	Pancreatic adenocarcinoma[74]	43–83
Drugs	PPIs[58,149]	100[c]
	H$_2$ blockers[92,150,151]	0–8

[a] In active disease using a cutoff value of >20 μ/L.
[b] Normal range 0–20 μ/L.
[c] Medium (6 weeks–1 year) and long-term treatment (1–8 years).

and exercise-induced physical stress.[89] Furthermore, giant cell arteritis,[38] rheumatoid arthritis, and systemic lupus erythematosus have been associated with increased circulating concentrations of CgA.[88]

Iatrogenic Causes of CgA Elevation

The widespread use of the proton pump inhibitor (PPI) class of drugs and other acid-suppressive medications is a substantial cause of CgA elevation.[76,90,91] In the setting of PPI medication, the lack of gastric acid engenders hypergastrinemia, G-cell hyperplasia, and ECL cell hyperplasia, with both neuroendocrine cell types cosecreting CgA with their respective products (gastrin and histamine). Omeprazole therapy may engender CgA elevations that are in excess of 690 μg/L (mean 45 ± 18 μg/L [normal range: 16–97 μg/L]) and can occur as early as 6 days after first intake of PPI.[91] Higher CgA levels are noted after long-term treatment (1–8 years) compared with midterm treatment (<1 year).[92] CgA concentration is higher with PPI usage compared with histamine type-2 receptor antagonist (H2RA).[92] Withdrawal of PPI leads to normalization of CgA within 1 to 2 weeks,[91] so elevated CgA concentration consequent on the use of acid-suppressive pharmacotherapy can be confirmed by withdrawal of the PPI for a period of 2 weeks followed by review of the CgA levels.

Malignant but Non-neuroendocrine Causes of CgA Elevation

Although increased circulating CgA concentrations are moderately sensitive markers of GI-NETs, they are not specific for a neuroendocrine malignancy.[93] CgA elevation in non-NET tumors usually reflects an underlying pattern of neuroendocrine differentiation (eg, pancreatic, colorectal, gastric, or prostate adenocarcinoma), although in HCC or breast cancer, the cause is unclear.[94–96]

Underlying neuroendocrine differentiation has been postulated to occur in several cancers, although CgA is only expressed in cell nests within these cancers and is not considered an adequate humoral tumor marker when compared with standard tumor markers for these cancers. Neuroendocrine differentiation is not an uncommon event in primary colorectal cancer (34%) and these patients exhibit a worse prognosis after routine surgical therapy.[97] This suggests that neuroendocrine differentiation correlates with a more aggressive disease course and reflects the observation that neuroendocrine differentiation is often identifiable in small cell undifferentiated colorectal cancer.[98] Prostatic and pancreatic adenocarcinomas also exhibit a neuroendocrine component, with the incidence of these cells in prostatic adenocarcinomas ranging from 10% to 100%. There is a positive correlation between the proportion of prostate cancer cells that stain for CgA and the serum levels of CgA,[95] and elevated CgA has been reported as indicative of a poor prognosis in localized[99] and metastatic[100] prostate carcinomas. In patients with pancreatic adenocarcinoma, mean CgA levels were significantly higher (192.9 ± 66.5 ng/mL) as compared with a group of healthy subjects (36.0 ± 22.0 ng/mL) and those with chronic pancreatitis (96.0 ± 31.0 ng/mL).[74] As with prostate cancer, individuals with high CgA levels and pancreatic cancer exhibited a poorer prognosis and survival.

Elevation of CgA has been identified in hepatocellular cancer (HCC) but its pathophysiologic basis is unknown. Elevated CgA above normal values occurred in 83% of patients with HCC, well in excess of the rates in liver cirrhosis, chronic hepatitis, and inflammatory bowel disease (48%, 20%, and 33%, respectively).[71] Diagnostic accuracy is, however, inferior to α-fetoprotein,[40] which remains the tumor marker of choice for HCC.

The relationship between CgA expression and breast cancer is also uncertain. P-CgA elevation can occur in breast adenocarcinoma, even in the absence of immunostaining for neuroendocrine markers (including CgA) in the tumor.[101] On the contrary, P-CgA was elevated in only 2 of 8 pathologically confirmed neuroendocrine carcinomas of the breast,[101] suggesting a limited role for circulating CgA in this cancer.

THE CLINICAL UTILITY OF CGA IN NEUROENDOCRINE TUMORS
Rationale for CgA as a Tumor Marker

CgA is used as an important and reliable broad-spectrum marker for immunohisto-chemical identification of normal and neoplastic neuroendocrine cells (**Fig. 5**). The major advantage of CgA is co-secretion by multiple different neuroendocrine cell types. The major difficulty that limits the accuracy of CgA as a tumor marker is extensive postsecretion processing into several fragments; the fragment pattern varies between tumor primary sites and individuals, and the commercially available tests have differing abilities to detect the fragments.

A reasonable approach to developing a tumor marker for NETs might be to measure a specific peptide or amine produced by the tumor; however, many of these tumor products are obscure, difficult to measure, and unreliable due to diurnal fluctuation that exceeds the variation caused by the tumor itself. The original neuroendocrine cell type is also not immediately obvious on routine pathologic testing, and therefore the peptide of interest is not always initially apparent. By comparison, CgA is present in most NETs and is relatively stable, and commercially available assays are available.

CgA concentrations have, therefore, become regarded as moderately sensitive but nonspecific markers of individual NETs. Increased CgA concentrations can be detected in GEP-NETs, bronchopulmonary NETs (including small cell lung cancer), pheochromocytomas, neuroblastomas, medullary thyroid carcinoma, and Merkel

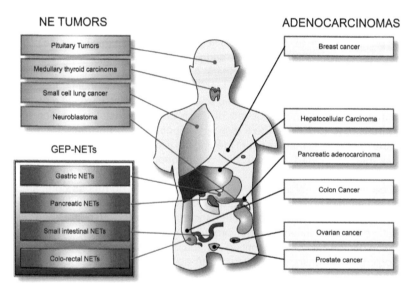

Fig. 5. Neoplastic causes of elevated CgA. CgA elevations occur in diverse NETs but are usually more pronounced in GEP-NETs (small intestinal, gastric, and pancreatic NETs). CgA elevations may occur in carcinomas with a complete or a partial neuroendocrine phenotype (left and right box stacks, respectively). In HCC, the cause of CgA elevation In HCC, the CgA elevation may reflect impaired metabolism of CgA fragments due to concurrent liver failure.

cell carcinoma of the skin.[58,69,93,102–118] CgA has limited use in diagnosis of pituitary adenomas where more specific biochemical markers (eg, prolactin, throid-stimulating hormone, luteinizing hormone, follicle-stimulating hormone, adrenocorticotrophic hormone, and insulinlike growth factor 1) are available.[107,119] Small cell lung carcinomas exhibit higher levels of CgA than any other type of lung cancer or healthy controls,[102] and the level is higher in extensive stage disease. CgB is a major granin of the human adrenal medulla,[120] plays a role in regulating secretion,[121] and may be a more sensitive marker for pheochromocytoma and related endocrine tumors than CgA or SgII.[122]

Sensitivity and Specificity of Elevated CgA

Diagnosis
Fluctuations in CgA concentration P-CgA levels vary in healthy control participants and patients with NETs; both eating and exercise lead to increases in CgA concentration. Levels are increased after eating in healthy controls and in multiple endocrine neoplasia type 1 (MEN-1) patients with or without a pancreatic NET (by 16%, 20%, and 31%, respectively).[70] The mean day-to-day variation of CgA in NET patients is 29.3% (range 0–113.5%), irrespective of a normal or elevated CgA or type of NET, and healthy subjects showed similar variability (21%, range 0%–47%). The maximum CgA values occur 30 to 60 minutes after eating and increase between 2- and 3-fold after meals.[90] Exercise-induced CgA elevation is evident as early as 2 minutes after high-intensity exercise and at 15 minutes postexercise and rises from a baseline value of 41 ± 10 µg/L to a peak of 56 ± 4 µg/L ($P<.005$).[123,124] To facilitate comparison and increase accuracy, CgA should, therefore, be measured in fasting patients and exercise should be avoided before the testing.

Comparison to alternative tumor markers for NETs Alternative NET tumor markers quantify the primary secretory product of the malignant neuroendocrine cell (see **Table 1**). The most widely used tumor marker for serotonin secreting NETs has previously been 24-hour urine measurement of the serotonin metabolite, urinary 5-hydroxyindoleacetic acid (u5-HIAA). Elevation of u5-HIAA correlates with the intensity of radiolabeled somatostatin uptake (tumor:background ratio) on somatostatin receptor scintigraphy (SRS), and the same relationship is observed between SRS and CgA.[111] CgA, however, demonstrates higher diagnostic accuracy than either u5-HIAA or other markers, including neuron-specific enolase (NSE) and carcinoembryonic antigen, in distinguishing NETs from controls (**Table 3**).[125] CgA correlates better than u5-HIAA in regard to physical functioning and quality of life[126] and is more convenient than u5-HIAA measurement. The latter requires a 24-hour urine collection and a complex dietary regime abstention from tryptophan/serotonin-rich foods (eg, bananas, avocados, plums, eggplant, tomatoes, plantain, pineapples, and walnuts) for 3 days before the collection period. Both markers may be considered complementary, however. Many other neuroendocrine cell–specific biochemical markers, including insulin, gastrin, glucagon, vasoactive intestinal peptide, serotonin, bradykinin, substance P, neurotensin, human chorionic gonadotropin, neuropeptide K, and neuropeptide L and pancreatic PP, have been identified in association with GI-NETs; for the most part, few have the specificity or predictive value of CgA (or even u5-HIAA) and their measurement is often complex and usually expensive.

Tumor markers of more generic cellular processes have also been examined and CgA identifies NETs from other forms of cancer more effectively than NSE and the alpha subunit of glycoprotein hormones.[107] In a group of patients with GEP-NETs, immunoassays identified elevated CgA in 99% of patients and elevated CgB levels

Table 3
Sensitivity and specificity of CgA in the detection of NETs

Study	NET Group	Comparison Group	Test	Sensitivity (%)	Specificity (%)
Bajetta et al[125]	n = 127 GEP NETs	N = 103 Blood donors	CgA[a]	68	86
			NSE	33	100
			Urine 5HIAA	35	100
			CEA	15	91
Campana et al[152]	n = 238 GEP-NETs	N = 42 CAG N = 48 disease-free patients	CgA vs disease free	85	96
			CgA vs CAG and disease free	75	84
Nobels et al[107]	n = 211 NETs	n = 180 non-NET cancers	CgA[b]	53	93
			NSE	46	65
			α-SU	26	85
Cimitan et al[69]	N = 63 Lung and GEP-NETs	No control	CgA[a]	55	94
			SRS[c]	77	94
Namwongprom et al[106]	N = 125 NET	No control	CgA[d]	62	84
			SRS[e]	83	98
			CgA and SRS	93	81
Nehar et al[112]	N = 124 GEP-NETs	N = 34 MEN-1 N = 127 controls	CgA[f]	63	98

Abbreviations: α-SU, alpha subunit of glycoprotein hormones; CAG, with chronic atrophic gastritis; CEA, carcinoembryonic antigen.
[a] ELISA (Dako A/S, Glostrup, Denmark).
[b] Polyclonal radioimmunoassay (UCB, Brussels, Belgium).
[c] 111In-pentetreotide SRS.
[d] Enzyme immunoassay.
[e] Indium-111-DTPA-Phel-octreotide including whole-body images as well as single-photon emission CT and CT.
[f] CgA-RIA CT kit (Cis bio international, Gif-sur-Yvette Cedex, France).

in 86% of patients.[127] Overall, CgA (despite its limitations) seems a better tumor marker than u5-HIAA, NSE, CEA, and alpha subunit of glycoprotein.

It has been proposed that improvement in diagnostic sensitivity can be achieved by combining CgA with a second diagnostic test. Thus, CgA and SRS detect NETs with approximately 60% and approximately 80% sensitivity, respectively,[69,106] which can be increased, by combining both tests, to 93% diagnostic sensitivity (see **Table 3**).[106] Combining CgA and pancreatic PP concentrations enhances the sensitivity in diagnosis of overall GEP-NETs, as well as in both functioning and nonfunctioning endocrine pancreatic tumors, to greater than 95%.[128]

Surveillance for pancreatic NETs is an important clinical issue in MEN-1. Identification of substantially elevated CgA levels strongly suggests the presence of an occult GEP-NET (especially concomitant gastrinoma in Zollinger-Ellison syndrome) because primary hyperparathyroidism or pituitary adenomas rarely are associated with marked CgA increases.[119,129,130] Thus, CgA not only is an important tool not only for the diagnosis of sporadic NETs but also is of value in MEN-1.

Prognosis and tumor burden

There is a substantial but indirect rationale for a prognostic role of CgA because it has some correlation to tumor stage, and advanced staging predicts diminished survival.[131] CgA levels are higher with extensive metastases than with localized disease or even limited hepatic involvement.[114,116,132] An investigation of 124 patients with sporadic GEP-NETs indicated that the degree of elevation of CgA levels reflected disease extent, with higher CgA levels occurring in metastatic compared with localized disease.[112] This relationship altered the sensitivity of CgA as a diagnostic tool with CgA apparently more sensitive in metastatic (73%) as opposed to localized disease (26%; $P<.01$).[112] Thus, CgA exhibits a relationship with the extent of hepatic tumor burden.[133]

An association between CgA and survival has been observed retrospectively in patients with metastatic GEP-NETs,[133] pancreatic NETs,[110] and nonfunctioning pancreatic NETs.[132] A CgA concentration 3 times above the upper normal limit at diagnosis is a significant predictor of shorter survival (hazard ratio 2.6) in patients with GEP-NETs.[110] In midgut carcinoid patients, an increase of CgA (>5000 µg/L) was an independent predictor of shorter survival,[116] and those with CgA less than 5000 µg/L had a significantly longer median survival (57 months) as compared with those with higher values (33 months). Elevated CgA levels were associated with a significantly poorer survival in 39 patients with midgut tumors with liver metastases treated with long-acting octreotide,[126] whereas no significant association was observed between 5-HIAA levels and survival time.

The relationship between CgA elevation and extent of disease is, however, not evident in all NET phenotypes. Gastrinomas are associated with high circulating CgA values even in the absence of liver metastasis, most likely representing the dual impact of tumor gastrin-associated CgA secretion and gastrin-driven ECL-cell histamine release. Also, some studies have noted an association between CgA and tumor location that is not always correlated with survival.[134] The highest maximum CgA values have been reported in ileal NETs (200 times the normal upper limit) and GEP-NETs associated with MEN-1 (150 times the normal upper limit). Types II and III gastric ECLomas (80–100 times normal) and pancreatic NETs and Zollinger-Ellison syndrome (in MEN-1) had intermediate values (60–80 times the upper limit of normal). In a variety of NETs (n = 211), CgA was found most frequently increased in gastrinomas (100%), followed by pheochromocytomas (90%), NETs (80%), nonfunctioning pancreatic NETs (70%), and medullary thyroid carcinomas (50%).[107] These findings directly contradict the proposal that CgA concentration correlates positively with diminished survival.

An additional problem with CgA as a prognostic indicator occurs in the relationship with tumor grade. Because higher tumor grade is related to poorer survival,[131] it might be predicted that CgA should be higher in high-grade tumors if it was accurately prognostic. CgA is more frequently elevated in well-differentiated tumors, however, as compared with poorly differentiated tumors. This may reflect the functional integrity of the neuroendocrine secretory system in individual tumors or the individual secretory profile of the small bowel EC cell per se. In a study of 63 NETs, the diagnostic accuracy of CgA was 76% for well-differentiated NETs, 68% for well-differentiated neuroendocrine carcinomas, and 50% for PDECs.[69] None of the poorly differentiated NETs in this study occurred in the GI system. Nonetheless, it is apparent that overall, CgA provides only limited prognostic information, because, although it generally correlates with tumor burden, it does not consistently correspond to tumor grade. Thus, CgA is a useful tumor marker in well-differentiated NEC but is of less reliability in PDEC.

Response to treatment

Theoretically, it might be considered that a correlation between CgA and tumor burden should culminate in a reduction in CgA after successful therapeutic intervention. Simplistic validation of the relationship between CgA concentration and tumor bulk is confirmed by a reduction in CgA after surgical resection.[112] This provides the rationale for monitoring more speculative pharmacotherapeutic intervention. Clinical response to medical therapy has been reported with stable or reduced CgA in GEP-NETs[93,125,135,136] and in gastric carcinoids.[137–141] Reduction in CgA is observed after successful peptide receptor radionuclide therapy[142] and liver transplantation.[143] Overall, it seems that CgA has some degree of utility in monitoring therapeutic response with the proviso that an elevation must be detectable before intervention.

Relapse

A critical role of a tumor marker is to identify disease recurrence after definitive or palliative therapeutic intervention, especially when further therapeutic options may need to be initiated. CgA is well correlated to the tumor burden and, therefore, may be considered a moderately useful tool in NET treatment surveillance.[137] In patients followed up for radically operated midgut carcinoids, CgA was reported to represent the first indication of recurrence, ahead of u5-HIAA and traditional radiologic examinations (transabdominal ultrasound, CT, or MRI).[144] Specifically, CgA became pathologically elevated in 85% of patients who ultimately relapsed (in 33 of 56 patients after a median of 32 months).[144] The authors of this study concluded that in asymptomatic patients who underwent resection of a midgut NET primary, follow-up should only comprise measurement of CgA twice a year and annual transabdominal ultrasonography.[144] Further support for the value of CgA in detecting recurrence was reported in a heterogeneous group of NETs, where an elevation of CgA was identified in 83% undergoing clinical progression and in 100% of patients with progressive liver metastases.[125] Similarly, concordance with tumor progression was 81% in a large group of GEP-NETs and concordance was higher for CgA than levels of serotonin (54%).[112] It seems that CgA is a useful tool in the detection of disease relapse in selected patient groups, although further characterization of subgroups is required to delineate NET specific follow-up protocols.

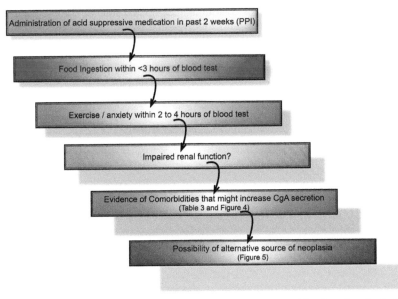

Fig. 6. A clinical checklist effective in ascertaining that detectable elevation in CgA identifies a neuroendocrine cancer. Although not exhaustive, this aide memoire summarizes the key issues clinically relevant to a clinician seeking to determine that an elevated CgA represents NET disease. The most common cause of CgA elevation is administration of PPIs, or the presence of either chronic atrophic gastritis or renal failure.

SUMMARY

CgA, although it exhibits limitations, is currently the most useful general tumor biomarker available for use in the diagnosis and management of GEP-NETs. The value of the CgA lies in its universal cosecretion by the majority of neuroendocrine cells that persists after malignant transformation. The added utility provided by the measurement of specific primary tumor–type biomarkers is rarely of prognostic value. The limitations of CgA measurement include a modest sensitivity of 50% to 60% when all stages and grades are considered and perturbation of the analysis by numerous physiologic and pathologic events unrelated to neuroendocrine cancer (**Fig. 6**). CgA also has mild to modest prognostic value in GEP-NETs, although some NET subtypes produce higher overall levels irrespective of prognosis. Circulating CgA is not useful as a prognostic tool in poorly differentiated tumors. Alteration of CgA levels has some utility in monitoring tumor relapse or progression. Clinicians aware of the physiologic role of CgA and its diverse implications in a variety of non-NET related pathologic conditions can adequately use this protein as a moderately effective tumor biomarker in the management of GEP-NETs.

REFERENCES

1. Banks P, Helle K. The release of protein from the stimulated adrenal medulla. Biochem J 1965;97(3):40C–1C.
2. Helle K. Antibody formation against soluble protein from bovine adrenal chromaffin granules. Biochim Biophys Acta 1966;117(1):107–10.

3. Geffen LB, Livett BG, Rush RA. Immunological localization of chromogranins in sheep sympathetic neurones, and their release by nerve impulses. J Physiol 1969;204(2):58P–9P.

4. O'Connor DT. Chromogranin: widespread immunoreactivity in polypeptide hormone producing tissues and in serum. Regul Pept 1983;6(3):263–80.

5. Modlin IM, Champaneria MC, Bornschein J, et al. Evolution of the diffuse neuroendocrine system—clear cells and cloudy origins. Neuroendocrinology 2006; 84(2):69–82.

6. Barakat MT, Meeran K, Bloom SR. Neuroendocrine tumours. Endocr Relat Cancer 2004;11(1):1–18.

7. Taupenot L, Harper KL, O'Connor DT. The chromogranin-secretogranin family. N Engl J Med 2003;348(12):1134–49.

8. Natori S, Huttner WB. Chromogranin B (secretogranin I) promotes sorting to the regulated secretory pathway of processing intermediates derived from a peptide hormone precursor. Proc Natl Acad Sci U S A 1996;93(9):4431–6.

9. Jain RK, Joyce PB, Gorr SU. Aggregation chaperones enhance aggregation and storage of secretory proteins in endocrine cells. J Biol Chem 2000; 275(35):27032–6.

10. Gorr SU, Jain RK, Kuehn U, et al. Comparative sorting of neuroendocrine secretory proteins: a search for common ground in a mosaic of sorting models and mechanisms. Mol Cell Endocrinol 2001;172(1–2):1–6.

11. Kim T, Tao-Cheng JH, Eiden LE, et al. Chromogranin A, an "on/off" switch controlling dense-core secretory granule biogenesis. Cell 2001;106(4):499–509.

12. Blaschko H, Comline RS, Schneider FH, et al. Secretion of a chromaffin granule protein, chromogranin, from the adrenal gland after splanchnic stimulation. Nature 1967;215(5096):58–9.

13. Woulfe J, Deng D, Munoz D. Chromogranin A in the central nervous system of the rat: pan-neuronal expression of its mRNA and selective expression of the protein. Neuropeptides 1999;33(4):285–300.

14. Lazure C, Paquet L, Litthauer D, et al. The ostrich pituitary contains a major peptide homologous to mammalian chromogranin A(1–76). Peptides 1990;11(1):79–87.

15. Winkler H, Fischer-Colbrie R. The chromogranins A and B: the first 25 years and future perspectives. Neuroscience 1992;49(3):497–528.

16. Turquier V, Vaudry H, Jegou S, et al. Frog chromogranin A messenger ribonucleic acid encodes three highly conserved peptides. Coordinate regulation of proopiomelanocortin and chromogranin A gene expression in the pars intermedia of the pituitary during background color adaptation. Endocrinology 1999; 140(9):4104–12.

17. Yang HW, Kutok JL, Lee NH, et al. Targeted expression of human MYCN selectively causes pancreatic neuroendocrine tumors in transgenic zebrafish. Cancer Res 2004;64(20):7256–62.

18. Konecki DS, Benedum UM, Gerdes HH, et al. The primary structure of human chromogranin A and pancreastatin. J Biol Chem 1987;262(35):17026–30.

19. Tatemoto K, Efendic S, Mutt V, et al. Pancreastatin, a novel pancreatic peptide that inhibits insulin secretion. Nature 1986;324(6096):476–8.

20. Ishizuka J, Asada I, Poston GJ, et al. Effect of pancreastatin on pancreatic endocrine and exocrine secretion. Pancreas 1989;4(3):277–81.

21. Fasciotto BH, Gorr SU, DeFranco DJ, et al. Pancreastatin, a presumed product of chromogranin-A (secretory protein-I) processing, inhibits secretion from porcine parathyroid cells in culture. Endocrinology 1989;125(3):1617–22.

22. Aardal S, Helle KB. The vasoinhibitory activity of bovine chromogranin A fragment (vasostatin) and its independence of extracellular calcium in isolated segments of human blood vessels. Regul Pept 1992;41(1):9–18.

23. Aardal S, Helle KB, Elsayed S, et al. Vasostatins, comprising the N-terminal domain of chromogranin A, suppress tension in isolated human blood vessel segments. J Neuroendocrinol 1993;5(4):405–12.

24. Fasciotto BH, Trauss CA, Greeley GH, et al. Parastatin (porcine chromogranin A347–419), a novel chromogranin A-derived peptide, inhibits parathyroid cell secretion. Endocrinology 1993;133(2):461–6.

25. Ronchi CL, Boschetti M, Uberti EC, et al. Efficacy of a slow-release formulation of lanreotide (Autogel 120 mg) in patients with acromegaly previously treated with octreotide long acting release (LAR): an open, multicentre longitudinal study. Clin Endocrinol (Oxf) 2007;67(4):512–9.

26. Russell J, Gee P, Liu SM, et al. Inhibition of parathyroid hormone secretion by amino-terminal chromogranin peptides. Endocrinology 1994;135(1):337–42.

27. Lamberts R, Creutzfeldt W, Struber HG, et al. Long-term omeprazole therapy in peptic ulcer disease: gastrin, endocrine cell growth, and gastritis. Gastroenterology 1993;104(5):1356–70.

28. Gasparri A, Sidoli A, Sanchez LP, et al. Chromogranin A fragments modulate cell adhesion. Identification and characterization of a pro-adhesive domain. J Biol Chem 1997;272(33):20835–43.

29. Lugardon K, Raffner R, Goumon Y, et al. Antibacterial and antifungal activities of vasostatin-1, the N-terminal fragment of chromogranin A. J Biol Chem 2000; 275(15):10745–53.

30. Feng D, Nagy JA, Brekken RA, et al. Ultrastructural localization of the vascular permeability factor/vascular endothelial growth factor (VPF/VEGF) receptor-2 (FLK-1, KDR) in normal mouse kidney and in the hyperpermeable vessels induced by VPF/VEGF-expressing tumors and adenoviral vectors. J Histochem Cytochem 2000;48(4):545–56.

31. Ghia JE, Crenner F, Rohr S, et al. A role for chromogranin A (4–16), a vasostatin-derived peptide, on human colonic motility. An in vitro study. Regul Pept 2004; 121(1–3):31–9.

32. Nishida A, Miyata K, Tsutsumi R, et al. Pharmacological profile of (R)-1-[2,3-dihydro-1-(2'-methylphenacyl)-2-oxo-5-phenyl-1H-1,4-benzodiazepin-3-yl]-3-(3-methylphenyl)urea (YM022), a new potent and selective gastrin/cholecystokinin-B receptor antagonist, in vitro and in vivo. J Pharmacol Exp Ther 1994;269(2):725–31.

33. Agarwal SK, Lee Burns A, Sukhodolets KE, et al. Molecular pathology of the MEN1 gene. Ann N Y Acad Sci 2004;1014:189–98.

34. Mazza R, Mannarino C, Imbrogno S, et al. Crucial role of cytoskeleton reorganization in the negative inotropic effect of chromogranin A-derived peptides in eel and frog hearts. Regul Pept 2007;138(2–3):145–51.

35. Jackson LN, Chen LA, Larson SD, et al. Development and characterization of a novel in vivo model of carcinoid syndrome. Clin Cancer Res 2009;15(8):2747–55.

36. Sorhaug S, Langhammer A, Waldum HL, et al. Increased serum levels of chromogranin A in male smokers with airway obstruction. Eur Respir J 2006;28(3): 542–8.

37. Ceconi C, Ferrari R, Bachetti T, et al. Chromogranin A in heart failure; a novel neurohumoral factor and a predictor for mortality. Eur Heart J 2002;23(12): 967–74.

38. Di Comite G, Previtali P, Rossi CM, et al. High blood levels of chromogranin A in giant cell arteritis identify patients refractory to corticosteroid treatment. Ann Rheum Dis 2009;68(2):293–5.

39. Capellino S, Lowin T, Angele P, et al. Increased chromogranin A levels indicate sympathetic hyperactivity in patients with rheumatoid arthritis and systemic lupus erythematosus. J Rheumatol 2008;35(1):91–9.

40. Massironi S, Fraquelli M, Paggi S, et al. Chromogranin A levels in chronic liver disease and hepatocellular carcinoma. Dig Liver Dis 2009;41(1):31–5.

41. Ciesielski-Treska J, Ulrich G, Taupenot L, et al. Chromogranin A induces a neurotoxic phenotype in brain microglial cells. J Biol Chem 1998;273(23): 14339–46.

42. Mandala M, Brekke JF, Serck-Hanssen G, et al. Chromogranin A-derived peptides: interaction with the rat posterior cerebral artery. Regul Pept 2005; 124(1–3):73–80.

43. Helle KB, Corti A, Metz-Boutigue MH, et al. The endocrine role for chromogranin A: a prohormone for peptides with regulatory properties. Cell Mol Life Sci 2007; 64(22):2863–86.

44. Zhao E, Zhang D, Basak A, et al. New insights into granin-derived peptides: evolution and endocrine roles. Gen Comp Endocrinol 2009;164(2–3):161–74.

45. Blois A, Srebro B, Mandala M, et al. The chromogranin A peptide vasostatin-I inhibits gap formation and signal transduction mediated by inflammatory agents in cultured bovine pulmonary and coronary arterial endothelial cells. Regul Pept 2006;135(1–2):78–84.

46. Belloni D, Scabini S, Foglieni C, et al. The vasostatin-I fragment of chromogranin A inhibits VEGF-induced endothelial cell proliferation and migration. FASEB J 2007;21(12):3052–62.

47. O'Connor DT, Cadman PE, Smiley C, et al. Pancreastatin: multiple actions on human intermediary metabolism in vivo, variation in disease, and naturally occurring functional genetic polymorphism. J Clin Endocrinol Metab 2005; 90(9):5414–25.

48. Sanchez-Margalet V, Gonzalez-Yanes C, Santos-Alvarez J, et al. Pancreastatin. Biological effects and mechanisms of action. Adv Exp Med Biol 2000;482: 247–62.

49. Gonzalez-Yanes C, Sanchez-Margalet V. Pancreastatin, a chromogranin A-derived peptide, inhibits leptin and enhances UCP-2 expression in isolated rat adipocytes. Cell Mol Life Sci 2003;60(12):2749–56.

50. Lewis JJ, Zdon MJ, Adrian TE, et al. Pancreastatin: a novel peptide inhibitor of parietal cell secretion. Surgery 1988;104(6):1031–6.

51. Funakoshi A, Miyasaka K, Nakamura R, et al. Bioactivity of synthetic human pancreastatin on exocrine pancreas. Biochem Biophys Res Commun 1988;156(3): 1237–42.

52. Mahata SK, O'Connor DT, Mahata M, et al. Novel autocrine feedback control of catecholamine release. A discrete chromogranin a fragment is a noncompetitive nicotinic cholinergic antagonist. J Clin Invest 1997;100(6):1623–33.

53. Ontsouka EC, Reist M, Graber H, et al. Expression of messenger RNA coding for 5-HT receptor, alpha and beta adrenoreceptor (subtypes) during oestrus and dioestrus in the bovine uterus. J Vet Med A Physiol Pathol Clin Med 2004;51(9–10):385–93.

54. Pieroni M, Corti A, Tota B, et al. Myocardial production of chromogranin A in human heart: a new regulatory peptide of cardiac function. Eur Heart J 2007; 28(9):1117–27.

55. Pawlikowski M, Gruszka A, Radek M, et al. Chromogranin A in pituitary adenomas: immunohistochemical detection and plasma concentrations. Folia Histochem Cytobiol 2004;42(4):245–7.
56. Briolat J, Wu SD, Mahata SK, et al. New antimicrobial activity for the catecholamine release-inhibitory peptide from chromogranin A. Cell Mol Life Sci 2005; 62(3):377–85.
57. Portela-Gomes GM, Stridsberg M. Selective processing of chromogranin A in the different islet cells in human pancreas. J Histochem Cytochem 2001; 49(4):483–90.
58. Stridsberg M, Eriksson B, Oberg K, et al. A comparison between three commercial kits for chromogranin A measurements. J Endocrinol 2003;177(2):337–41.
59. Verderio P, Dittadi R, Marubini E, et al. An Italian program of External Quality Control for chromogranin A (CgA) assay: performance evaluation of CgA determination. Clin Chem Lab Med 2007;45(9):1244–50.
60. Woltering EA, Hilton RS, Zolfoghary CM, et al. Validation of serum versus plasma measurements of chromogranin a levels in patients with carcinoid tumors: lack of correlation between absolute chromogranin a levels and symptom frequency. Pancreas 2006;33(3):250–4.
61. Miyakawa M, Matsui T, Kishikawa H, et al. Salivary chromogranin A as a measure of stress response to noise. Noise Health 2006;8(32):108–13.
62. Hoshino K, Suzuki J, Yamauchi K, et al. Psychological stress evaluation of patients with bronchial asthma based on the chromogranin a level in saliva. J Asthma 2008;45(7):596–9.
63. Rindi G, Buffa R, Sessa F, et al. Chromogranin A, B and C immunoreactivities of mammalian endocrine cells. Distribution, distinction from costored hormones/prohormones and relationship with the argyrophil component of secretory granules. Histochemistry 1986;85(1):19–28.
64. Bofin AM, Qvigstad G, Waldum C, et al. Neuroendocrine differentiation in carcinoma of the breast. Tyramide signal amplification discloses chromogranin A-positive tumour cells in more breast tumours than previously realized. APMIS 2002;110(9):658–64.
65. Qvigstad G, Sandvik AK, Brenna E, et al. Detection of chromogranin A in human gastric adenocarcinomas using a sensitive immunohistochemical technique. Histochem J 2000;32(9):551–6.
66. Srivastava A, Padilla O, Fischer-Colbrie R, et al. Neuroendocrine secretory protein-55 (NESP-55) expression discriminates pancreatic endocrine tumors and pheochromocytomas from gastrointestinal and pulmonary carcinoids. Am J Surg Pathol 2004;28(10):1371–8.
67. Portela-Gomes GM, Stridsberg M. Chromogranin A in the human gastrointestinal tract: an immunocytochemical study with region-specific antibodies. J Histochem Cytochem 2002;50(11):1487–92.
68. Portel-Gomes GM, Grimelius L, Johansson H, et al. Chromogranin A in human neuroendocrine tumors: an immunohistochemical study with region-specific antibodies. Am J Surg Pathol 2001;25(10):1261–7.
69. Cimitan M, Buonadonna A, Cannizzaro R, et al. Somatostatin receptor scintigraphy versus chromogranin A assay in the management of patients with neuroendocrine tumors of different types: clinical role. Ann Oncol 2003;14(7): 1135–41.
70. Granberg D, Stridsberg M, Seensalu R, et al. Plasma chromogranin A in patients with multiple endocrine neoplasia type 1. J Clin Endocrinol Metab 1999;84(8): 2712–7.

71. Spadaro A, Ajello A, Morace C, et al. Serum chromogranin-A in hepatocellular carcinoma: diagnostic utility and limits. World J Gastroenterol 2005;11(13): 1987–90.

72. Sidhu R, Drew K, McAlindon ME, et al. Elevated serum chromogranin A in irritable bowel syndrome (IBS) and inflammatory bowel disease (IBD): a shared model for pathogenesis? Inflamm Bowel Dis 2010;16(3):361.

73. Peracchi M, Gebbia C, Basilisco G, et al. Plasma chromogranin A in patients with autoimmune chronic atrophic gastritis, enterochromaffin-like cell lesions and gastric carcinoids. Eur J Endocrinol 2005;152(3):443–8.

74. Malaguarnera M, Cristaldi E, Cammalleri L, et al. Elevated chromogranin A (CgA) serum levels in the patients with advanced pancreatic cancer. Arch Gerontol Geriatr 2009;48(2):213–7.

75. Sciola V, Massironi S, Conte D, et al. Plasma chromogranin a in patients with inflammatory bowel disease. Inflamm Bowel Dis 2009;15(6):867–71.

76. Waldum HL, Arnestad JS, Brenna E, et al. Marked increase in gastric acid secretory capacity after omeprazole treatment. Gut 1996;39(5):649–53.

77. Sidhu R, McAlindon ME, Leeds JS, et al. The role of serum chromogranin A in diarrhoea predominant irritable bowel syndrome. J Gastrointestin Liver Dis 2009;18(1):23–6.

78. Valeur J, Milde AM, Helle KB, et al. Low serum chromogranin A in patients with self-reported food hypersensitivity. Scand J Gastroenterol 2008;43(11):1403–4.

79. West NE, Wise PE, Herline AJ, et al. Carcinoid tumors are 15 times more common in patients with Crohn's disease. Inflamm Bowel Dis 2007;13(9):1129–34.

80. O'Connor DT. Plasma chromogranin A. Initial studies in human hypertension. Hypertension 1985;7(3 Pt 2):I76–9.

81. Hsiao RJ, Parmer RJ, Takiyyuddin MA, et al. Chromogranin A storage and secretion: sensitivity and specificity for the diagnosis of pheochromocytoma. Medicine (Baltimore) 1991;70(1):33–45.

82. Takiyyuddin MA, Parmer RJ, Kailasam MT, et al. Chromogranin A in human hypertension. Influence of heredity. Hypertension 1995;26(1):213–20.

83. Larsen AI, Helle KB, Christensen M, et al. Effect of exercise training on chromogranin A and relationship to N-ANP and inflammatory cytokines in patients with chronic heart failure. Int J Cardiol 2008;127(1):117–20.

84. O'Connor DT, Pandlan MR, Carlton E, et al. Rapid radioimmunoassay of circulating chromogranin A: in vitro stability, exploration of the neuroendocrine character of neoplasia, and assessment of the effects of organ failure. Clin Chem 1989;35(8):1631–7.

85. Hsiao RJ, Mezger MS, O'Connor DT. Chromogranin A in uremia: progressive retention of immunoreactive fragments. Kidney Int 1990;37(3):955–64.

86. Zhang D, Lavaux T, Sapin R, et al. Serum concentration of chromogranin A at admission: an early biomarker of severity in critically ill patients. Ann Med 2009;41(1):38–44.

87. Al-Shoumer KA, Vasanthy BA. Serum chromogranin A concentration in hyperthyroidism before and after medical treatment. J Clin Endocrinol Metab 2009; 94(7):2321–4.

88. Di Comite G, Rossi CM, Marinosci A, et al. Circulating chromogranin A reveals extra-articular involvement in patients with rheumatoid arthritis and curbs TNF-alpha-elicited endothelial activation. J Leukoc Biol 2009;85(1):81–7.

89. Allgrove JE, Gomes E, Hough J, et al. Effects of exercise intensity on salivary antimicrobial proteins and markers of stress in active men. J Sports Sci 2008; 26(6):653–61.

90. Fossmark R, Jianu CS, Martinsen TC, et al. Serum gastrin and chromogranin A levels in patients with fundic gland polyps caused by long-term proton-pump inhibition. Scand J Gastroenterol 2008;43(1):20–4.
91. Giusti M, Sidoti M, Augeri C, et al. Effect of short-term treatment with low dosages of the proton-pump inhibitor omeprazole on serum chromogranin A levels in man. Eur J Endocrinol 2004;150(3):299–303.
92. Sanduleanu S, Stridsberg M, Jonkers D, et al. Serum gastrin and chromogranin A during medium- and long-term acid suppressive therapy: a case-control study. Aliment Pharmacol Ther 1999;13(2):145–53.
93. Stivanello M, Berruti A, Torta M, et al. Circulating chromogranin A in the assessment of patients with neuroendocrine tumours. A single institution experience. Ann Oncol 2001;12(Suppl 2):S73–7.
94. Pinkus GS, Etheridge CL, O'Connor EM. Are keratin proteins a better tumor marker than epithelial membrane antigen? A comparative immunohistochemical study of various paraffin-embedded neoplasms using monoclonal and polyclonal antibodies. Am J Clin Pathol 1986;85(3):269–77.
95. Angelsen A, Syversen U, Haugen OA, et al. Neuroendocrine differentiation in carcinomas of the prostate: do neuroendocrine serum markers reflect immunohistochemical findings? Prostate 1997;30(1):1–6.
96. Syversen U, Ramstad H, Gamme K, et al. Clinical significance of elevated serum chromogranin A levels. Scand J Gastroenterol 2004;39(10):969–73.
97. Gulubova M, Vlaykova T. Chromogranin A-, serotonin-, synaptophysin- and vascular endothelial growth factor-positive endocrine cells and the prognosis of colorectal cancer: an immunohistochemical and ultrastructural study. J Gastroenterol Hepatol 2008;23(10):1574–85.
98. Grabowski P, Schonfelder J, Ahnert-Hilger G, et al. Heterogeneous expression of neuroendocrine marker proteins in human undifferentiated carcinoma of the colon and rectum. Ann N Y Acad Sci 2004;1014:270–4.
99. Alessandro S, Vincenzo G, Maria AG, et al. Chromogranin A and biochemical progression-free survival in prostate adenocarcinomas submitted to radical prostatectomy. Endocr Relat Cancer 2007;14(3):625–32.
100. Sciarra A, Di Silverio F, Autran AM, et al. Distribution of high chromogranin A serum levels in patients with nonmetastatic and metastatic prostate adenocarcinoma. Urol Int 2009;82(2):147–51.
101. Giovanella L, Marelli M, Ceriani L, et al. Evaluation of chromogranin A expression in serum and tissues of breast cancer patients. Int J Biol Markers 2001;16(4):268–72.
102. Sobol RE, O'Connor DT, Addison J, et al. Elevated serum chromogranin A concentrations in small-cell lung carcinoma. Ann Intern Med 1986;105(5):698–700.
103. Stridsberg M, Eriksson B, Oberg K, et al. A panel of 11 region-specific radioimmunoassays for measurements of human chromogranin A. Regul Pept 2004;117(3):219–27.
104. Vinik AI, Strodel WE, Eckhauser FE, et al. Somatostatinomas, PPomas, neurotensinomas. Semin Oncol 1987;14(3):263–81.
105. Aparicio T, Ducreux M, Baudin E, et al. Antitumour activity of somatostatin analogues in progressive metastatic neuroendocrine tumours. Eur J Cancer 2001;37(8):1014–9.
106. Namwongprom S, Wong FC, Tateishi U, et al. Correlation of chromogranin A levels and somatostatin receptor scintigraphy findings in the evaluation of metastases in carcinoid tumors. Ann Nucl Med 2008;22(4):237–43.

107. Nobels F, Kwekkeboom D, Coopmans W, et al. Chromogranin A as serum marker for neuroendocrine neoplasia: comparison with neuron-specific enolase and the alphasubunit of glycoprotein hormones. J Clin Endocrinol Metab 1997; 82:2622–8.
108. Oberg K, Eriksson B. The role of interferons in the management of carcinoid tumours. Br J Haematol 1991;79(Suppl 1):74–7.
109. Blind E, Schmidt-Gayk H, Sinn HP, et al. Chromogranin A as tumor marker in medullary thyroid carcinoma. Thyroid 1992;2(1):5–10.
110. Ekeblad S, Skogseid B, Dunder K, et al. Prognostic factors and survival in 324 patients with pancreatic endocrine tumor treated at a single institution. Clin Cancer Res 2008;14(23):7798–803.
111. Kalkner KM, Janson ET, Nilsson S, et al. Somatostatin receptor scintigraphy in patients with carcinoid tumors: comparison between radioligand uptake and tumor markers. Cancer Res 1995;55(Suppl 23):5801s–4s.
112. Nehar D, Lombard-Bohas C, Olivieri S, et al. Interest of Chromogranin A for diagnosis and follow-up of endocrine tumours. Clin Endocrinol (Oxf) 2004; 60(5):644–52.
113. Schurmann G, Raeth U, Wiedenmann B, et al. Serum chromogranin A in the diagnosis and follow-up of neuroendocrine tumors of the gastroenteropancreatic tract. World J Surg 1992;16(4):697–701 [discussion: 701–2].
114. Tomassetti P, Migliori M, Lalli S, et al. Epidemiology, clinical features and diagnosis of gastroenteropancreatic endocrine tumours. Ann Oncol 2001;12(Suppl 2): S95–9.
115. Boomsma F, Bhaggoe UM, Man in 't Veld AJ, et al. Sensitivity and specificity of a new ELISA method for determination of chromogranin A in the diagnosis of pheochromocytoma and neuroblastoma. Clin Chim Acta 1995;239(1):57–63.
116. Janson ET, Holmberg L, Stridsberg M, et al. Carcinoid tumors: analysis of prognostic factors and survival in 301 patients from a referral center. Ann Oncol 1997;8(7):685–90.
117. Seregni E, Ferrari L, Bajetta E, et al. Clinical significance of blood chromogranin A measurement in neuroendocrine tumours. Ann Oncol 2001;12(Suppl 2):S69–72.
118. Wassberg E, Stridsberg M, Christofferson R. Plasma levels of chromogranin A are directly proportional to tumour burden in neuroblastoma. J Endocrinol 1996;151(2):225–30.
119. Nobels FR, Kwekkeboom DJ, Coopmans W, et al. A comparison between the diagnostic value of gonadotropins, alpha-subunit, and chromogranin-A and their response to thyrotropin-releasing hormone in clinically nonfunctioning, alpha-subunit-secreting, and gonadotroph pituitary adenomas. J Clin Endocrinol Metab 1993;77(3):784–9.
120. Schober M, Fischer-Colbrie R, Schmid KW, et al. Comparison of chromogranins A, B, and secretogranin II in human adrenal medulla and pheochromocytoma. Lab Invest 1987;57(4):385–91.
121. Eiden LE, Huttner WB, Mallet J, et al. A nomenclature proposal for the chromogranin/secretogranin proteins. Neuroscience 1987;21(3):1019–21.
122. Eriksson B, Arnberg H, Oberg K, et al. Chromogranins–new sensitive markers for neuroendocrine tumors. Acta Oncol 1989;28(3):325–9.
123. Elias AN, Wilson AF, Pandian MR, et al. Chromogranin A concentrations in plasma of physically active men after acute exercise. Clin Chem 1992;38(11): 2348–9.
124. Takiyyuddin MA, Cervenka JH, Sullivan PA, et al. Is physiologic sympathoadrenal catecholamine release exocytotic in humans? Circulation 1990;81(1):185–95.

125. Bajetta E, Ferrari L, Martinetti A, et al. Chromogranin A, neuron specific enolase, carcinoembryonic antigen, and hydroxyindole acetic acid evaluation in patients with neuroendocrine tumors. Cancer 1999;86(5):858–65.

126. Korse CM, Bonfrer JM, Aaronson NK, et al. Chromogranin A as an alternative to 5-hydroxyindoleacetic acid in the evaluation of symptoms during treatment of patients with neuroendocrine Tumors. Neuroendocrinology 2009;89(3):296–301.

127. Stridsberg M, Oberg K, Li Q, et al. Measurements of chromogranin A, chromogranin B (secretogranin I), chromogranin C (secretogranin II) and pancreastatin in plasma and urine from patients with carcinoid tumours and endocrine pancreatic tumours. J Endocrinol 1995;144(1):49–59.

128. Panzuto F, Severi C, Cannizzaro R, et al. Utility of combined use of plasma levels of chromogranin A and pancreatic polypeptide in the diagnosis of gastrointestinal and pancreatic endocrine tumors. J Endocrinol Invest 2004;27(1):6–11.

129. Gussi IL, Young J, Baudin E, et al. Chromogranin A as serum marker of pituitary adenomas. Clin Endocrinol (Oxf) 2003;59(5):644–8.

130. Nanes MS, O'Connor DT, Marx SJ. Plasma chromogranin-A in primary hyperparathyroidism. J Clin Endocrinol Metab 1989;69(5):950–5.

131. Ahmed A, Turner G, King B, et al. Midgut neuroendocrine tumours with liver metastases: results of the UKINETS study. Endocr Relat Cancer 2009;16(3):885–94.

132. Nikou GC, Marinou K, Thomakos P, et al. Chromogranin a levels in diagnosis, treatment and follow-up of 42 patients with non-functioning pancreatic endocrine tumours. Pancreatology 2008;8(4–5):510–9.

133. Arnold R, Wilke A, Rinke A, et al. Plasma chromogranin A as marker for survival in patients with metastatic endocrine gastroenteropancreatic tumors. Clin Gastroenterol Hepatol 2008;6(7):820–7.

134. Modlin IM, Moss SF, Oberg K, et al. Gastrointestinal neuroendocrine (carcinoid) tumours: current diagnosis and management. Med J Aust 2010; 193(1):46–52.

135. Yao JC, Phan AT, Chang DZ, et al. Efficacy of RAD001 (everolimus) and octreotide LAR in advanced low- to intermediate-grade neuroendocrine tumors: results of a phase II study. J Clin Oncol 2008;26(26):4311–8.

136. Arnold R, Muller H, Schade-Brittinger C, et al. Placebo-controlled, double-blind, prospective, randomized study of the effect of octreotide LAR in the control of tumor growth in patients with metastatic neuroendocrine midgut tumors: a report from the PROMID study group [abstract #121]. ASCO 2009, Gastrointestinal Cancers Symposium. San Francisco, January 15, 2009.

137. Granberg D, Wilander E, Stridsberg M, et al. Clinical symptoms, hormone profiles, treatment, and prognosis in patients with gastric carcinoids. Gut 1998;43(2):223–8.

138. Tomassetti P, Migliori M, Caletti GC, et al. Treatment of type II gastric carcinoid tumors with somatostatin analogues. N Engl J Med 2000;343(8):551–4.

139. Kouraklis G, Misiakos E, Glinavou A, et al. Management of enterochromaffin-like gastric carcinoid tumour metastasized to the liver. Scand J Gastroenterol 2002; 37(2):246–8.

140. Shojamanesh H, Gibril F, Louie A, et al. Prospective study of the antitumor efficacy of long-term octreotide treatment in patients with progressive metastatic gastrinoma. Cancer 2002;94(2):331–43.

141. Fykse V, Sandvik AK, Waldum HL. One-year follow-up study of patients with enterochromaffin-like cell carcinoids after treatment with octreotide long-acting release. Scand J Gastroenterol 2005;40(11):1269–74.

142. Kwekkeboom DJ, Teunissen JJ, Bakker WH, et al. Radiolabeled somatostatin analog [177Lu-DOTA0, Tyr3]octreotate in patients with endocrine gastroentero-pancreatic tumors. J Clin Oncol 2005;23(12):2754–62.

143. Olausson M, Friman S, Herlenius G, et al. Orthotopic liver or multivisceral transplantation as treatment of metastatic neuroendocrine tumors. Liver Transpl 2007;13(3):327–33.

144. Welin S, Stridsberg M, Cunningham J, et al. Elevated plasma chromogranin A is the first indication of recurrence in radically operated midgut carcinoid tumors. Neuroendocrinology 2009;89(3):302–7.

145. Cetin Y, Muller-Koppel L, Aunis D, et al. Chromogranin A (CgA) in the gastro-entero-pancreatic (GEP) endocrine system. II. CgA in mammalian entero-endocrine cells. Histochemistry 1989;92(4):265–75.

146. Weynand B, Guiot Y, Doriaux M, et al. Motilin-producing liver and bone metastases evidenced 14 years after resection of a rectal polyp. Am J Surg Pathol 1999;23(7):838–43.

147. Song S, Shi R, Li B, et al. Diagnosis and treatment of pancreatic vasoactive intestinal peptide endocrine tumors. Pancreas 2009;38(7):811–4.

148. Tsao KC, Wu TL, Chang PY, et al. Detection of carcinomas in an asymptomatic Chinese population: advantage of screening with multiple tumor markers. J Clin Lab Anal 2006;20(2):42–6.

149. Hirschowitz BI, Worthington J, Mohnen J, et al. Chromogranin A in patients with acid hypersecretion and/or hypergastrinaemia. Aliment Pharmacol Ther 2007; 26(6):869–78.

150. Kim BW, Lee BI, Kim HK, et al. [Influence of long-term gastric acid suppression therapy on the expression of serum gastrin, chromogranin A, and ghrelin]. Korean J Gastroenterol 2009;53(2):84–9 [in Korean].

151. Sanduleanu S, De Bruine A, Stridsberg M, et al. Serum chromogranin A as a screening test for gastric enterochromaffin-like cell hyperplasia during acid-suppressive therapy. Eur J Clin Invest 2001;31(9):802–11.

152. Campana D, Nori F, Piscitelli L, et al. Chromogranin A: is it a useful marker of neuroendocrine tumors? J Clin Oncol 2007;25(15):1967–73.

Modern Laboratory Evaluation of Peptide and Amines: A Continuing Role for Radioimmunoassay?

Gregg Mamikunian, MS

KEYWORDS

• Biogenic amines • Serotonin • Radioimmunoassay • Carcinoid

PROLOGUE

Since the early 1900s, the clinical confirmational diagnosis for the presence of neuro-endocrine tumors of the pancreas and gut relied on the search for and identification of circulating markers. However, the challenge in accurately measuring these circulating amines and peptides proved elusive if not impossible. Thus, an analytical journey commenced, which began in 1901 to the most resent publication in 2010. This quest presented difficulties, not only in identification of the specific biogenic amines and the neuroendocrine peptides but also even in use of the most advanced bioanalytical techniques and instrumentation to achieve valid and reproducible data that correlate with manifestations of the symptoms and disease (Appendix 1).

Modern medicine, and specifically clinical diagnosis, relies, among other diagnostic procedures, on the measurements of the biogenic analytes for elucidation and correlation of specific neuroendocrine markers. Tremendous advances have been made in imaging and radioactive uptake procedures to elucidate tumor presence and characterization. However, such advances only partially provide the fundamental degree of tumor activity and clinical confirmational validity.

The current review of more than 100 published articles in peer review journals with respect to the topic at hand presents an amorphous and disjointed view of the data. Moreover, in a critical compilation of the reported levels, it became apparent that a 10- to 1000-fold difference in results of various peptides and amines is the norm rather than the exception. These measured analyte numbers that resulted from the use of various laboratory procedures, lacked critical data review for justification of methodological acceptance.

Financial disclosure: No financial interest associated with this article.
Inter Science Institute, 944 West Hyde Park Boulevard, Inglewood, CA 90302, USA
E-mail address: gmisi@earthlink.net

Endocrinol Metab Clin N Am 40 (2011) 135–151
doi:10.1016/j.ecl.2010.08.005
0889-8529/11/$ – see front matter
© 2011 Elsevier Inc. All rights reserved.

Absence of standardization from different laboratories was almost always a factor in evaluating the validity of the generated numbers. To this end, the literature does not point to any specific approach that may be used to duplicate the numbers in another laboratory. Variances are exaggerated from procedure to procedure and from laboratory to laboratory, both in academic settings and specialized reference laboratories.

In the following pages of this article, the author points out in some detail the problems that may arise when the methodological differences presented by each investigational study and investigators are not standardized. This variation causes a concern with the specific objectives of the investigator and the specific aims of the research project at hand, and ultimately for the validity of the published results.

Numerous methods have been established for the measurement of serotonin, its precursors and metabolites, and other biogenic amines. The earliest methods for the quantitation of the serotonin precursor tryptophan were based on the isolation of this compound from other protein cleavage products[1] and fraught with problems caused by gross loss of product. Levene and Rouiller[2] attempted to obviate the need for total isolation of tryptophan by titrating solutions of the digests with bromine water, which nevertheless necessitated precipitation with mercuric sulfate reagent to account for the many other compounds that also combine with bromine water.[1] Even with this cleanup step measures had to be taken to account for the presence of any tyrosine and cystine, steps which involved the estimation of nitrogen and sulfur, respectively, in the solution.

Colorimetric techniques were put in place fairly early although not without considerable debate regarding possible interference in the determination of compounds, such as tryptophan, hydroxytryptophan, hydroxyproline, and tyrosine,[3,4] and suffering from low sensitivity and narrow dynamic ranges. Later colorimetric methods were able to overcome most of the selectivity issues[5] and sensitivity issues continue to be improved.[6]

For serotonin (5-hydroxytryptamine, enteramine), the first quantitative measurements involved biologic semiquantitative assays on perfused rabbit ear,[7,8] first created to aid in the isolation and identification of serotonin,[9] with serotonin finally being synthesized in 1951 by Hamlin and Fisher.[10] Measurements of serotonin levels were also reported using carotid artery contraction[11] able to measure down to about 0.02 μg/mL, rat uterus[12] with high selectivity, rat colon,[13] or the heart of the Quahog (*Venus mercenaria*) with sensitivity down to 0.18 ng/mL of the 10-mL bath water used in the assay and that used 1 mL or less of biologic fluid.[14] For a review of work done on serotonin before 1954, refer to Page, 1954.[15]

High levels of serotonin (2.5 mg per gram of tumor) in carcinoid tumors were reported by Lembeck and others as determined through bioassay and chromatographic and colorimetric estimations.[16–18] Shortly afterwards, Udenfriend and others published several colorimetric and ultraviolet absorption and fluorescence methods for the estimation of serotonin as well as a colorimetric method for the determination of the serotonin metabolite 5-hydroxyindoleacetic acid (5-HIAA).[19,20] It is to be noted that in all these methods, the specificity was directly related to their ability to physically isolate the analyte of interest from significant amounts of any interfering substances and that this was performed through the use of multiple extractions and washing schemes. Sensitivities for serotonin were a low of 0.04 μmol of serotonin in as much as 500 mg of tissue for the ultraviolet absorption method (upper limit was 0.4 μmol). An equal sensitivity was obtained with the colorimetric method that used a reaction with 1-nitroso-2-naphthol to generate a violet color; the fluorometric method allowed the measurement of 0.1 to 0.3 μg of serotonin in 10 mL of blood.

In 1956, Sjoerdsma and colleagues[21] used Udenfriend's method to establish greatly elevated levels of serotonin in the blood (0.5–2.7 μg/mL vs 0.1–0.3 μg/mL in controls) and in the urine of patients with carcinoids, but lack of sensitivity (0.02 μg per ml) precluded them from being able to observe any serotonin in plasma or in cerebrospinal fluid (CSF). The nitrosonaphthol reagent was also used in the generation of a colorimetric derivative of 5-hydroxyindoleacetic acid,[20] which allowed them to easily distinguish endogenous levels in the urine of controls (2.0–8.2 mg per 24 hours) from that of subjects diagnosed with intestinal carcinoid (142–384 mg per 24 hours), a fact corroborated by Sjoerdsma and colleagues[21] who reported 2 to 9 mg per 24 hours for controls versus 76 to 580 mg per 24 hours in subjects with carcinoids. Sjoerdsma and colleagues[21] also reported that they were unable to find any (logarithm of odds of 0.5 μg/mL) 5-HIAA in plasma, CSF, or feces in their study. The following year, Sjoerdsma and colleagues[22] reexamined serotonin and 5-HIAA levels in blood, plasma, urine, and CSF. They again found elevated levels of 5-HIAA in the urine and elevated serotonin in the blood platelets of subjects with carcinoids when compared with normal controls. Despite a report by Snow and colleagues[23] using a rat uterus bioassay detailing the presence of 0.5 μg/mL serotonin in CSF (obtained 9 days after death and heavily infected), Sjoerdsma and colleagues[22] again failed to find any serotonin (<0.03 μg/mL) in the CSF of their subjects. Sjoerdsma and colleagues were able to measure 5-HIAA in the blood of subjects with carcinoids (0.2–0.8 μg 5-HIAA per mL of plasma), and although they also reported measuring serotonin (0.05 μg to 0.3 μg/mL) in platelet-poor plasma, as did Snow and colleagues,[23] Sjoerdsma and colleagues questioned whether this is a true reflection of levels in plasma or an artifact of the platelet separation step in the process of obtaining plasma. Young and Anderson,[24] Mohler[25] also provided a thorough and recent critique of this old problem.

The usefulness of urinary 5-HIAA by the method of Udenfriend and colleagues[19] was demonstrated by reports showing no false positives among 1023 subjects and no elevated values (<12 mg per 24 hours) among subjects without carcinoids.[26] On the other hand, Kabakow and colleagues[27] reported the usefulness of the method of Udenfriend and colleagues for the measurement of 5-hydroxyindoles while noting many compounds (most notably many phenothiazines and elemental iodine) can mask the developing color in the test and lead to underestimations of 5-hydroxyindoles. For urine containing these compounds, Kabakow and colleagues[27] used the qualitative paper-chromatography method developed by Curzon[28] that appears not to be affected by these interferences but which suffers from sensitivity problems (urine requiring a minimum of 20 mg/L of 5-HIAA or 2 mg/L of serotonin for detection).

The following years brought about continued use of spectrofluorometric techniques to investigate serotonin, 5-HIAA, and other biogenic amines from biologic tissues with emphasis on automation[29] and expanding the range of analytes that could be investigated from fractionated extracts of the same tissue[30,31] which could then be measured by separate spectral analysis. Issues regarding sensitivity, however, remained, problematic when trying to measure the small amounts present in platelet-free or platelet-poor plasma and in CSF. As late as 1981, Vatassery and colleagues[32] reported that most spectrophotofluorometric methods for serotonin used to that date continued to be based on the method first developed by Udenfriend and colleagues, although the use of acidic solutions had been found to increase specificity; whereas, ethanol increased the fluorescence of serotonin. Vatassery and colleagues[32] also reported that other 5-hydroxyindole compounds interfered with the assay, contributing up to almost 6% of the apparent serotonin content under normal physiologic conditions and that measurements of the individual components in such mixtures had to be separated first by chromatography and then assayed individually. This chromatographic separation before fluorescence detection was ideally resolved through the use of high-performance liquid chromatography (HPLC). Mais and colleagues[33] used HPLC with fluorescence detection to measure, in a single injection, levels of serotonin, 5-HIAA, 5-hydroxytrptophan, 5-hydroxyindoleacetic acid O-sulfate, 5-hydroxytryptophol, tyramine, N-acetylserotonin, and indole-3-acetic acid in mouse lung and plasma. Although Mais and colleagues[33] did not report limits of detection for these compounds in their matrix, they provided limits for on-column values of 30 to 70 pg and rough assumptions on their methodology would suggest limits of detection of about 12 ng/mL for serotonin and 37 ng/mL for 5-HIAA. Actual plasma values in mice were found to be 1.7 µg/mL for serotonin; whereas, no HIAA could be routinely detected in plasma.

The use of the fluorescence detector, coupled to HPLC, continued to be a preferred method for the measurements of biogenic amines, especially as the continued advances in HPLC, now ultra high-performance liquid chromatography (UHPLC), push the limits of the ability to separate and detect metabolites in ever decreasing amounts of matrix. Developments in sampling technology, as well as the use of derivatives to aid in the fluorescence of these analytes, have also contributed to the continued usefulness of this technique. Wu and colleagues[34] used polymer monolith microextraction to extract derivatized urinary serotonin, 5-HIAA, 5-hydroxytryptophan, N-acetyl-5-hydroxytryptamine, and 6 catechol amines and subject them to HPLC with fluorescence detection. Wu and colleagues[34] reported limits of quantitation, calculated from regression equations rather than actual measurements, with ranges as low as 0.36 nM for epinephrine or as high as 71 nM for l-dopa and of about 5 nM for serotonin and 2.5 nM for 5-HIAA; linear working ranges appear to be excellent: 10 to 3000 nM for both serotonin and 5-HIAA. Wu and colleagues[34] argued that the initial derivatization and cleanup steps were necessary because of a combination of the comparatively low sensitivity of fluorescence detectors, the low concentration of the analytes, and multitude of interferences present in the matrix. Wu and colleagues[34] also found that in HPLC-electron chemical detector (EC), an often used alternative to HPLC-fluorescence, the electrochemical detector suffered from high noise and instrument instability. In the same vein, Muñoz and colleagues[35] reported that electrochemical detection of melatonin, although postulated to have higher sensitivity than native fluorescence for indole compounds, was problematic because oxidation/reduction of melatonin required high electric potentials that gave rise to elevated background currents, resulting in a lack of stability of baseline and lower reproducibility. Their LC-fluorescence for measuring melatonin in fish plasma and bile appeared to be sensitive (80 pg/mL).[35] HPLC-fluorescence continued to be used in the determination of biogenic amines in a recent article by Kolevzon and colleagues,[36] studying the behavioral symptoms of autism and giving a range of 78 to 471 ng/mL serotonin in whole blood.

Use of electrochemical detection for the quantitation of biologic amines also began at an early date and benefited just as much as fluorescence detection from the coupling with HPLC technologies.[37] A recent article by Lechin and colleagues[38] reported the use of an HPLC fitted with a regular C18 column and sodium octyl sulfate as ion-pair for chromatography. Sensitivity with the electrochemical detector was said to be 0.1 ng/mL for serotonin, 6.4 pg/mL for noradrenaline, 5.8 pg/mL for adrenaline, and 2.0 pg/mL for dopamine. Serotonin was measured in one assay; whereas, adrenaline, noradrenaline, and catechol amine were measured in a second assay. Lechin and colleagues[38] developed the method to measure adrenaline, noradrenaline, and dopamine in plasma, and to measure platelet-serotonin and free-serotonin in platelet-rich and platelet-poor plasma, respectively, using 1 mL each for free and platelet serotonin.

The question of appropriate sampling methodology and associated issues of detection sensitivity were recently discussed by Young and Anderson[24] in an editorial on bioanalytical inaccuracy. Young and Anderson wrote that a large number of articles reported serotonin human lumbar CSF mean values ranging from 0.02 ng/mL to 10.0 ng/mL. With fairly selective and highly sensitive methods using an HPLC fitted with a hypersil column and electrochemical detection, or with an HPLC fitted with a C18 column and a fluorometric detector using a 350-nm peak transmission to isolate the "indolic fluorescence," Anderson and colleagues[39] claimed to have obtained limits of detection of 7 to 8 pg/mL with the EC detector and 7 to 15 pg/mL CSF with the fluorometric detector. From their studies, these investigators were able to establish a high limit for serotonin in normal human lumbar CSF of 0.01 ng/mL, which is in contrast with the many literature reports they cited in their editorial.[5–13,24] Young and Anderson stated that several papers reported erroneously elevated levels (1–100 ng/mL) for serotonin in platelet-poor plasma in contrast to their HPLC fluorometric method[40] establishing mean values less than 0.5 ng/mL. Their method used ion-pairing HPLC with fluorometric detection, which afforded limits of detection of 2 to 4 pg on column from a 50-µl injection. This method also used anticoagulant (ethylenediaminetetraacetic acid sorbate, acid-citrate-dextrose, or sodium citrate) in the syringe used to collect blood before immediate platelet removal (centrifugation or ultrafiltration); if no anticoagulant was present in the syringe, higher serotonin levels (1–3 ng/mL) were obtained; on the other hand, lower amounts were obtained the longer the time period between collection and platelet removal.[40] These values (<0.5 ng/mL) agreed with the gas chromatography/mass spectrometry (GC/MS) values reported by Beck and colleagues[41] who found a range of 0.048 to 0.262 ng/mL serotonin in normal human plasma. The method of Anderson and colleagues[40] also permitted the measurement of indolepropionic acid and indole acetic acid but not of tryptophan, and provided mean values for whole blood serotonin of 140 ng/mL, confirming existing literature; tryptophan was measured through a similar technique by Anderson and colleagues.[42]

GC coupled to MS, as well as to ionization and electrochemical detectors, is another powerful technique that has sometimes been used to measure biogenic amines. Among the first articles to appear detailing GC of biologic amines was that of Fales and Pisano[43] reporting GC of biologically important amines, including histamine, serotonin, 5-methoxytryptamine, N-acetyltryptamine, melatonin, benzylamine, N-methylbenzylamine, β-phenylethylamine, amphetamine, β-phenylethanolamine, norephedrine, ephedrine, tyramine, octopamine, synephrine, normetanephrine, metanephrine, tryptamine, and dimethyltryptamine; and although limits of detection were not investigated, the investigators used a 1-µl injection of 1% solutions (approximately 10 µg on column). Sen and McGeer's work[44] soon followed, detailing analysis of mixtures of trimethylsilyl derivatives of epinephrine, norepinephrine, dopamine, metanephrine, normetanephrine, and 3-methoxytyramine, as did work reported by Brooks and Horning[45] detailing the analysis of mixtures of 0.1 µg on column of more than 30 biologic amines, including catecholamines, melatonin, 5-methoxytryptamine, serotonin, and tryptamine after acetylation. Derivatization of biogenic amines to be measured by GC coupled to any type of detector, whether by acetylation, silylation, or other techniques, is almost universally necessary to afford the necessary volatility and chromatographic separations. These derivatizations must be performed with care because they might give rise to artifacts, as was the case for the reported presence of 5-methoxytryptamine in hypothalamus tissue[46] identified by GC/MS and that was later found, also by GC/MS, to be an artifact of the deacetylation of the hypothalamus's melatonin in the derivatization step.[47]

Sensitive and specific methods by GC/MS for serotonin in tissues have been reported by Cattabenni and colleagues,[48] Abramson,[49] and Beck and colleagues.[50] Although Markey and colleagues[51] found these methods to be effective for tissues, they were not readily applicable to aqueous biologic fluids (CSF, blood, urine). Markey and colleagues were, however, able to use the method developed by Welsh[52] to quantitatively separate biogenic amines from aqueous solutions, a method that involved acetylation by acetic anhydride, or by propionic or deuteroacetic anhydride in cases where endogenous N-acetylated serotonin, such as the pineal gland, might be found. This step was followed by extraction into a nonpolar solvent and a second derivatization step with pentafluoropropionic anhydride was performed.[51] Their method required GC/MS on a quadrupole mass spectrometer allowing single ion monitoring (SIM) and using negative chemical ionization (NCI) with methane as reagent gas for analysis of CSF while using electron impact ionization (EI) for the higher concentrations found in platelets. The authors[51] reported serotonin values in CSF to be less than 1 ng/mL, confirming previously reported measurements by a bioassay method[53] but in contrast to the much higher levels reported in other bioassay and fluorometric studies.[54,55] Beck and colleagues[41] also commented that most previous studies reported values for plasma serotonin greater than 10 nmol/L (1.76 ng/mL); whereas, actual values, as shown by their work, should be much lower (0.27–1.49 nmol/L; 0.048–0.262 ng/mL). Their method[41] called for GC/MS on a quadrupole mass spectrometer, permitting SIM and NCI with methane as reagent gas, to afford the desired sensitivity. A sample, 1 mL of plasma, was extracted through a C-18 solid phase extraction cartridge and serotonin derivatized, first with acetic anhydride and then with pentafluoropropionic anhydride, to afford a volatile analyte giving sharp peaks. Tetradeuterated serotonin was used as an internal standard. The final product was reconstituted into 15 μL and 1 to 2 μL were injected. The investigators reported a limit of detection, based on a signal-to-noise ratio (S/N) of 3, of 0.03 nmol/L (5.3 pg/mL). Assuming a typical S/N of 10 for the limit of quantitation (LOQ), this leads to a LOQ of approximately 0.017 ng/mL. Beck and colleagues also stated that their method was based on that of Markey and colleagues[51] and that problems encountered when applying it to plasma, namely the loss of serotonin in the protein precipitation step with perchloric acid, were resolved through the use of the initial C-18 solid phase extraction and that previous overestimations of serotonin in plasma were avoided through appropriate blood collection and processing techniques.[41]

Many of the GC-MS (and LC-MS) methodologies use a combination of SIM and NCI. Mass spectrometry, in full scan, is one of the most information-rich detectors as well as being highly selective when the contribution of individual ions of different masses can be quantitated separately, and is rivaled in selectivity perhaps only by the best designed antibodies used in immunoassays. In practice this means that one can use the unique combination of retention times and individual mass ions to insure the analyte being measured is the desired one and, at full scan, the presence of potential interferences, whether previously examined or not, can readily be ascertained. The author uses this type of full-scan GC/MS with quantitation based on extracted ions for the analysis of many biologic, clinical, and research studies. The author's preferred instrument is an ion trap because, in his experience, it provides much lower levels of detection than comparable quadrupoles set at full-scan information-rich settings. The author can examine analytes down to the 20 pg on-column level and routinely develop validated methods for quantitation with LOQs as low as 60 pg on column from a 1-μl injection (3 ng/50 μL of derivatized extract; 1 ng/mL of original biologic fluid). Nevertheless, this sensitivity, although good, falls far short of that needed for work on many other analytes found in biologic fluids and tissues. Much of the published work uses quadrupoles in the SIM mode for this reason. In the SIM mode, the quadrupole is set to isolate only 1 or a few individual mass ions all of the time. This selectivity leads, in the author's experience, to at least a 2-orders-of-magnitude improvement in sensitivity, although at the cost of losing the information-rich full scan and therefore the degree of certainty that the analyte being measured is in fact the right one. To regain at least some of this selectivity, most assays using SIM use at least 2 ions for each analyte, one to quantitate and the other as a confirmatory ion. Newer technology, on the other hand, allows an increasing number of measurements to be obtained across a peak so that, in some cases, quadrupoles are now able to acquire at least 1 full scan within a peak while acquiring the rest of the peak in SIM mode, thus providing a combination of the scan's full range of information and the sensitivity of the SIM. The other technique used by many researchers to increase MS sensitivity is through the use of NCI, which can afford another 1- to 2-orders of magnitude better sensitivity, depending on the nature of the background and of appropriately derivatized analytes.

Like GC, HPLC is another chromatographic technique well suited for use with MS detectors. Monaghan and colleagues[56] used a micro-UHPLC fitted with a strong cation exchange guard column on line with a monolithic C-18 column coupled to a tandem mass spectrometer run in the positive electrospray ionization (ESI) mode to measure plasma serotonin; tetradeuterated serotonin was used as an internal standard and lowest limits of quantitation were established at 5 nmol/L (0.880 ng/mL) based on calibrators made from standards. The method uses 50 μL of platelet-depleted plasma, the retention time of serotonin was 2.79 minutes, and total analysis time was 6 minutes. Miller and colleagues[57] also used an UHPLC fitted with a C-18 guard column online with a mixed-mode reverse/anion exchange column and coupled to a tandem MS running in the positive ESI mode to measure 5-HIAA; bis-deuterated 5-HIAA was used as an internal standard and the lowest limit of quantitation established at 15 nmol/L (2.9 ng/mL) based on coefficient of variation of dilutions of 5-HIAA. The method uses 50 μL plasma and the retention time of 5-HIAA was 2.1 minutes with a total analysis time of 7 minutes. Miller and colleagues[57] at the Leeds Teaching Hospital also routinely measured 5-HIAA with an HPLC fitted with a C-18 column and coupled to a fluorescence detector using the 280-nm wavelength for excitation and with the 345-nm wavelength for emission but confirmed that this method was longer (17 minutes), used more sample (500 μL), and had a smaller linear range (to 1000 nmol/L vs to 10,000 nmol/L). Other recent relevant reports using this technique included that of Minami and colleagues,[58] who used fluorometric HPLC and LC-MS/MS to facilitate the study of diverse urinary serotonin and melatonin metabolites and which led them to report new tryptamine-related compounds in urine, and an LC-ESI-MS/MS method[59] requiring no derivatization for the detection of histamine from basophilic cells and with a limit of quantitation of 1.1 ng/mL.

So where do immunoassays, and more specifically radioimmunoassay, fit against this background? Paralleling the previously mentioned methods, many radioimmunoassays profit from derivatization or extraction steps to improve selectivity or sensitivity. Nevertheless, the author routinely performs direct unextracted radioimmunoassays, on 100 μL or less of sample, with limits of detection in the femtograms per test tube range, meaning 1 pg/mL or less in the original biologic fluid. Use of these assays presents huge advantages over chromatographic techniques, especially when these must be coupled to high-maintenance, high-sensitivity detectors. In the author's experience, direct radioimmunoassays are much preferred over the more complex methods mentioned previously with the exception, perhaps, of assays for the diagnosis of conditions that require the quantitation of multiple analytes. Many other researchers also continue to develop these types of radioimmunoassays to provide the specific and sensitive quantitative results that they cannot obtain with alternative methods. A recent article by Welp and colleagues,[60] for instance, detailed the development of a direct radioimmunoassay method for the quantitation of as low as 3 pg of melatonin from 50 to 200 μL of serum or plasma and with a large working range (up to thousands of pg/ml). The method uses activated-charcoal-stripped plasma or serum to make the standards (calibrators) and to dilute the samples, and protease is used to reduce nonspecific binding in samples and standards. Welp and colleagues cited Chegini and colleagues[61] in pointing out several of the shortcomings in the measurements of melatonin for their high-volume purposes by GC-MS or by HPLC methods, which they found to be limited by low throughput, the need for extensive sample preparation, and a need for technical expertise by the analyst in using and maintaining sophisticated equipment.[61] Engbaek and Voldby[62] also reported the development and use of a 1-hour direct tritium-based radioimmunoassay for the measurement of serotonin in CSF, platelet-poor plasma, and serum with limits of detection of 2 nmol/L (0.352 ng/mL) in a 200-μl sample. Engbaek and Voldby's method was free of cross reaction from tryptophan, 5-hydroxytryptophan, 5HIAA, and 5-hydroxytryptophol; however, it cross reacted with tryptamine and 5-methoxytryptamine but at levels that were satisfactory for their studies. Engbaek and Voldby reported normal serotonin ranges of 5 to 14 nmol/L (0.880–2.464 ng/mL) in plasma and 380 to 900 nmol/L (67–158 ng/mL) in serum. Two-thirds of their subjects had CSF levels less than their limits of detection and one-third were in the 2 to 4 nmol/L range.[62]

Many times measurements by radioimmunoassay require extraction or derivatization steps to improve either the selectivity, sensitivity, or both. Several such assays have been developed in the study of biogenic amines. Geffard and colleagues[63] used a single I-125-based radioimmunological assay to measure serotonin, N-acetylserotonin, 5-methoxytryptamine, and melatonin with high sensitivity (0.01 pmol; 2 pg). Their method involved the chemical conversion of serotonin, N-acetylserotonin, or 5-methoxytryptamine in serum to melatonin, effectively allowing them to use the same highly sensitive melatonin method for the measurements of the other analytes. In 1987, Gow and colleagues[64] developed a 125-I-based radioimmunoassay to measure serotonin, after acetylation, in platelet-rich plasma. They were able to measure 100 samples per day. Their limit of detection was 2.0 nmol/L (70 pg per tube), which corresponds to 40 nmol/L (7 ng/mL) in platelet-rich-plasma. Their working range, stated as that corresponding to 80% to 15% binding/binding of traser in the absence of the analyte (B/Bo), was 17 to 1144 ng/mL platelet-rich plasma.[64] Gow and colleagues found that the results obtained with their method compared well in sensitivity with a highly sensitive HPLC-EC method, although precision was poorer when the HPLC results were corrected by the use of an internal standard. Radioimmunoassays of many analytes involving derivatization are now readily available commercially. Ericson and colleagues,[65] for instance, reported on the measurements of serotonin with such a commercially available radioimmunoassay to measure variations in serotonin on isolated human antral glands treated with capsaicin. That particular manufacturer provides 3 different kits, 1 radioimmunoassay-based kit and 2 enzyme-linked immunosorbent assay-(ELISA) based kits, for serotonin measurements. The manufacturer claims that its radioimmunoassay method provides a limit of quantitation of 6.7 ng/mL serum, urine, or platelets and of 0.3 ng/mL of CSF or platelet-free plasma. A volume of 25 μL urine, serum, or platelets and 100 μL CSF or platelet-free plasma is needed and total assay time is 2.5 hours with each sample, control, and calibrator being counted for 1 minute. Their 2 ELISAs provide sensitivity of 5 ng/mL with an assay time of 1 hour and 15 minutes and a sensitivity of 5 pg/mL with a 24-hour assay, respectively. In 1995, Chegini and colleagues[61] compared the use of a radioimmunoassay based on extracted samples with a commercial ELISA geared to the direct measurement of melatonin in serum. Direct ELISA was found to be simpler and to require less sample (100 μL). The ELISA method, however, appeared to suffer from matrix (serum) effect, and the detection limits of the ELISA failed to cover the physiologic daytime melatonin concentrations in humans.[61] An extraction and concentration step of 1.5 mL of sample was determined to be necessary with the ELISA, to lower its sensitivity and to eliminate matrix effects, before it could compare with results obtained with radioimmunoassay.[61]

One last method of note in the measurement of biogenic amines involves the use of radioenzymatic methods. These methods are based in the enzymatic conversion of a precursor into a radiolabelled metabolite. As such it can provide high specificity, because particularly selective enzymes are available for many of these conversions, coupled with the high sensitivity of radioactive labels. Feldman[66] has advocated for the use of urinary serotonin measurements in the diagnosis of carcinoid tumors based on results he obtained after separately measuring platelet and urinary serotonin and urinary 5-hydoxytrptophan (5-HTP) and 5-HIAA. Feldman's radioenzymatic method for 5-HTP quantitation involved removal of serotonin through a cation exchange column and conversion of 5-HTP to serotonin with aromatic-L-amino acid decarboxylase. Assaying for serotonin involved acetylation to N-acetylserotonin with acetic anhydride and methylation, to tritium-labeled melatonin, with S-adenosyl-L-[3H] methylmethionine and hydroxyindole-O-methyl transferase, followed by solvent extractions and TLC.[66] Some subjects with carcinoids had normal platelet serotonin and normal urine 5-HIAA (the usual markers for carcinoid) but elevated urine serotonin. No limits of detection are given by Feldman, but the normal range for urine serotonin is given as 53 to 229 μg/24 hours.[66] Hussain and Sole[67] used an almost identical method for tissue and plasma (low-speed, platelet-poor, and platelet-rich) and reported their assay to be sensitive to about 50 pg of serotonin, although their reports of 3.98 ng/mL serotonin in platelet-poor plasma might constitute an overestimation.[24] Hindberg and Naesh[68] also used a radioenzymatic method involving acetylation with acetic anhydride and methylation with S-adenosyl-L-[3H] methylmethionine and hydroxyindole-O-methyl transferase, followed by a toluene extraction, wash, and re-extraction of the resulting tritiated melatonin. The limit of detection was 0.9 nmol/L (158 pg/mL) and they reported a platelet-poor plasma median level of 0.495 ng/mL.

The author finds that methods for the estimation of biogenic amines have evolved. Methods providing superb detection limits, such as HPLC-EC, or specificity, such as LC-MS of GC-MS, have been developed to satisfy many of the rigorous requirements needed in this field. An additional advantage of these methods, in many cases, is that they permit the analysis of many metabolites in one run. Nevertheless, proven methods based on immunoassays, including radioimmunoassay, continue to provide invaluable contributions because of their high sensitivity, specificity, and throughput coupled to analytical instrumentation that, in contrast to LC- or GC-hyphenated methods, are stable and require minimum expertise and maintenance.

EPILOGUE

The analytical methods (**Table 1**) employed for quantitative and qualitative analysis of biogenic amines (**Fig. 1**) play a focal role in the understanding and diagnosis of human disease. The early, impractical, imprecise, and laborious bioassay procedures[69] were too insensitive to detect the low levels of hormones, enzymes, and other bioactive substances involved in the regulation of vital cellular and metabolic function.

The finding of insulin-binding antibodies in the blood of patients with diabetes treated with bovine insulin laid the groundwork for the development of competitive

Table 1
History of analytical methods for the measurement of biogenic amines

Analytical Technique	Sensitivity	Benefits	Drawbacks	Reference
Bioassays	1.8 ng/mL	Directly measures biologic activity and directs isolation efforts Good sensitivity	Not specific Methods are hard to replicate and to maintain	Woolley & Shaw[11] Erspamer[12] Dalgliesh et al[13] Twarog & Page[14] Snow et al[23]
Colorimetric	500 ng/mL	Simple protocols and detector Can be used for cases where highly elevated values are to be expected	Specificity and sensitivity relies on prior isolation of analyte Small dynamic range Spurious interferences not recognized	Udenfriend et al[19] Kabakow et al[27]
Fluorometric	20 ng/mL	Simple protocols and detector Can be used for cases were moderately elevated values are to be expected	Specificity relies on prior isolation of analyte May need derivatization for sensitivity Spurious interferences not recognized	Udenfriend et al[19] Sjoerdsma et al[22] Hardeman et al[29] Welch & Welch[30] Crawford & Rudd[31] Vatassery et al[32]
LC-fluorescence	7–15 pg/mL	Can measure many analytes in one run Superb sensitivity Detector may provide some degree of specificity	Specificity relies on chromatographic performance and extraction conditions Spurious interferences not likely to be recognized May need derivatization LC operation and maintenance requires technical expertise	Wu et al[34] Muñoz et al[35] Anderson et al[39] Anderson et al[40]
LC-ECD	7–8 pg/mL	Can measure many analytes in one run Superb sensitivity Detector may provide some degree of specificity	Specificity relies on chromatographic performance and extraction conditions Spurious interferences not likely to be recognized May need derivatization Both LC and detector operation and maintenance require technical expertise	Wightman et al[37] Lechin et al[38] Anderson et al[39]

Method	Detection limit	Features	Limitations/Comments	References
LC-MS	880 pg/mL	Can measure many analytes in one run; Good sensitivity (SIM) Detector provides a good degree of specificity Spurious interferences might be recognized if confirmation ions are used Tandem MS may improve sensitivity and specificity Derivatization not needed in many cases	Spurious interferences not likely be recognized unless confirmation ions or tandem MS is used Both LC and detector operation and maintenance require high technical expertise	Miller et al[57] Minami et al[58] Koyama et al[59] Welp et al[60]
GC-MS	Full scan: 1 ng/mL SIM/NCI: 5 pg/mL	Can measure many analytes in one run Good sensitivity and specificity with SIM/NCI where spurious interferences might be recognized if confirmation ions are used Use of tandem MS may improve sensitivity/ specificity Good sensitivity and superb specificity in full-scan mode where spurious interferences will likely be recognized	Limited to volatile analytes Almost always needs derivatization May need preliminary cleanup Both GC and detector operation and maintenance require high technical expertise	Cattabeni et al[48] Abramson[49] Beck et al[50] Markey et al[51] Monaghan et al[56]
Radioimmunoassay	1 pg/mL	Superb sensitivity and good specificity Unextracted, underivatized protocols provide high throughput and minimal operator error Detectors are rugged/easy to use	May need derivatization Specificity directly related to ability of antibodies to select analyte over interferences Spurious interferences not likely to be recognized	Chegini et al[61] Engbaek & Voldby[62] Geffard et al[63] Gow et al[64] Ericson et al[65] Feldman[66] Hussain & Sole[67]
ELISA	5 pg/mL	Superb sensitivity and good specificity 96-well plate formats provide high throughput and minimal operator error Detectors are rugged and easy to use	May need derivatization Specificity directly related to ability of antibodies to select analyte over interferences Spurious interferences not likely to be recognized	Hussain & Sole[67]
Radio-enzymatic	150 pg/mL	Good sensitivity and good specificity Unextracted, underivatized protocols provide high throughput and minimal operator error Detectors are rugged and easy to use	Involves derivatization Specificity directly related to ability of enzymes to react with analyte over interferences Spurious interferences not likely to be recognized	Hindberg & Naesh[68] Odell & Daughaday[69] Yalow & Berson[70]

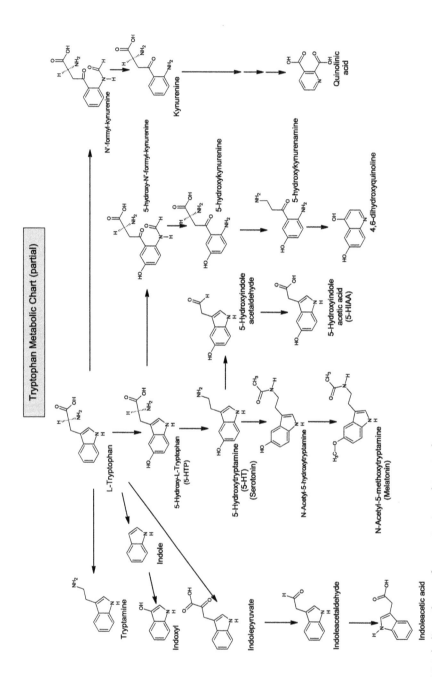

Fig. 1. Metabolic pathways for serotonin and tryptophan.

binding assays. The discovery by Yalow and Berson[70–72] in 1958 unleashed a proliferation of this new technique of radioimmunoassay for endocrinology, clinical chemistry, and other fields of biochemical research.

This novel methodological technique of radioimmunoassay provided the catalyst for the advancement of the field of clinical endocrinology and metabolism to unparalleled advantage in diagnosis and treatment of endocrine gland disorders. Within a decade of Yalow and Berson's discovery, radioimmunoassay for gastrin, glucagon, aldosterone, adrenocorticotropin, prolactin, parathyroid, and a great number of hormones had become measurable entities in many laboratories throughout the world.

As in any scientific field, there is a period whereby such discovery is overshadowed by newer, unique, or advanced technologies that may be superior or not. Consequently, radioimmunoassay techniques and procedures are not immune from this syndrome. Nevertheless, to banish the analytical techniques of radioimmunoassay to *analytical exile* would be a disadvantage to the field of clinical endocrinology in particular and science in general. The simple eloquent radioimmunoassay procedures still commands praise because it has served science well for the past 50 years and it should not find itself on the marquee at the Smithsonian Museum of Science and Industry…yet.

APPENDIX 1: GLOSSARY

5-HIAA: 5-hydroxyindoleacetic acid
5-HT: 5-hydroxytryptamine; 3-(2-aminoethyl)-1H-indol-5-ol; serotonin; enteramine
5-HTP: 5-hydroxytrptophan; 2-amino-3-(5-hydroxy-1H-indol-3-yl) propanoic acid
HPLC: high pressure liquid chromatography; high performance liquid chromatography
UHPLC: ultra high performance liquid chromatography
EC: ECD; electrochemical detector
LC-MS: liquid chromatography coupled to mass spectrometry
GC/MS: gas chromatography coupled to mass spectrometry
SIM: single ion monitoring; monitoring for only one ion at a time
ESI: electrospray ionization
EI: electron impact ionization
NCI: Negative chemical ionization
C18: octadecyl phase
SPE: Solid phase extraction
LOD: limit of detection
LOQ: Limit of quantitation
S/N: signal-to-noise ratio
CSF: cerebrospinal fluid
PDP: Platelet depleted plasma; akin to PPP, platelet poor plasma
PFP: platelet free plasma
ELISA: enzyme linked immunosorbent assay

REFERENCES

1. Hopkins FG, Cole SW. A contribution to the chemistry of proteids. Part I. A preliminary study of a hitherto undescribed product of tryptic digestion. J Physiol 1901; 27(4&5):418–28.
2. Levene PA, Rouiller CA. On the quantitative estimation of tryptophan in protein cleavage products. J Biol Chem 1907;2:481–4.

3. Folin O, Denis W. Tyrosine in proteins as determined by a new colorimetric method. J Biol Chem 1912;12:245–51.

4. Abderhalden EJ. Comments on the communications of Folin and Denis. J Biol Chem 1913;15:357–8.

5. Folin O, Ciocalteu V. On tyrosine and tryptophan determinations in proteins. J Biol Chem 1927;73:627–50.

6. Acharya MM, Katyare SS. An improved method for tyrosine estimation. Z Naturforsch 2004;59:897–900.

7. Page IH. A method for perfusion of rabbit's ears, and its application to study of the reninangiotonin vasopressor system, with a note on angiotonin tachyphylaxis. Am Heart J 1942;23:336–48.

8. Page IH, Green AA. Perfusion of rabbit's ear for study of vasoconstrictor substances. In: Potter VR, editor. Methods in medical research. Chicago: Year Book Publishing; 1948. p. 123–9.

9. Rapport MM, Green AA, Page IH. Serum vasoconstrictor (serotonin) IV. Isolation and characterization. J Biol Chem 1948;176:1243–51.

10. Hamlin KE, Fisher FE. Synthesis of 5-hydroxytryptamine. J Am Chem Soc 1951; 73:5007–8.

11. Woolley DW, Shaw E. Some antimetabolites of serotonin and their possible application to treatment of hypertension. J Am Chem Soc 1952;74:2948–9.

12. Erspamer V. Pharmacological studies on enteramine (5-hydroxytryptamine). IX. Influence of sympathomimetic and sympatholytic drugs on the physiological and pharmacological actions of enteramine. Arch Int Pharmacodyn 1953;93: 293–316.

13. Dalgliesh CE, Toh CC, Work TS. Fractionation of the smooth muscle stimulants present in extracts of gastro-intestinal tract. Identification of 5-hydroxytryptamine and its distinction from substance P. J Physiol 1953;120:298–310.

14. Twarog BM, Page IH. Serotonin content of some mammalian tissues and urine and a method for its determination. Am J Physiol 1953;175:157–61.

15. Page IH. Serotonin (5-hydroxytryptamine). Physiol Rev 1954;34:563–88.

16. Lembeck F. 5-Hydroxytryptamine in carcinoid tumor. Nature 1953;172:910–1.

17. Lembeck F. Uber den nachweis von 5-oxytryptamin (enteramin, serotonin) in carcinoidemetastasen. Arch Exp Path u Pharmakol 1954;221:50–66 [in German].

18. Ratzenhofez M, Lembeck F. Uber den gehalt an 5-oxytryptamin in carcinoiden des darmtraktes. Zeitschrift fur Krebsforschung 1954;60:169–95 [in German].

19. Udenfriend S, Weissbach H, Clark T. The estimation of 5-hydroxytryptamine (serotonin) in biological tissues. J Biol Chem 1955;215:337–44.

20. Udenfriend S, Titus E, Weissbach H. The identification of 5-hydroxyindoleacetic acid in normal urine and a method for its assay. J Biol Chem 1955;216: 499–505.

21. Sjoerdsma A, Weissbach H, Udenfriend S. A clinical, physiologic and biochemical study of patients with malignant carcinoid (argentaffinoma). Am J Med 1956;20:520–32.

22. Sjoerdsma A, Weissbach H, Terry LL. Further observations on patients with malignant carcinoid. Am J Med 1957;23:5–15.

23. Snow PJD, Lennard-Jones JE, Curzon G, et al. Humoral effects of metastasing carcinoid tumors. Lancet 1955;269:1004–9.

24. Young SN, Anderson GM. Bioanalytical inaccuracy: a threat to the integrity and efficiency of research. J Psychiatry Neurosci 2010;35:3–6.

25. Mohler DN. Evaluation of the urine test for serotonin metabolites. JAMA 1957; 163(13):1138.

26. Haverback BJ, Sjoerdsma A, Terry LL. Urinary excretion of the serotonin metabolite, 5-hydroxyindoleacetic acid, in various clinical conditions. N Engl J Med 1956;255(6):270–2.
27. Kabakow B, Weinstein B, Ross G, et al. A clinical and metabolic study of metastatic carcinoid. Am J Med 1959;26(4):636–45.
28. Curzon G. A rapid chromatographic test for high urinary excretion of 5-hydroxyindole-acetic acid and 5-hydroxytryptamine. Lancet 1955;266:1361–2.
29. Hardeman MR, Den Uyl A, Prins HK. A semi-mechanized method for the fluorometric determination of 5-hydroxytryptamine (serotonin) in blood plasma and platelets. Clin Chim Acta 1972;37:71–9.
30. Welch AS, Welch BL. Solvent extraction method for simultaneous determination of norepinephrine, dopamine, serotonin, and 5-hydroxyindoleacetic acid in a single mouse brain. Anal Biochem 1969;30:161–79.
31. Crawford N, Rudd BT. A spectrofluorometric method for the determination of serotonin (5-hydroxytryptamine) in plasma. Clin Chim Acta 1962;7:114–21.
32. Vatassery GT, Sheridan MA, Krezowski AM. Spectrofluorometry of serotonin in blood platelets. Clin Chem 1981;27:328–30.
33. Mais DE, Lahr PD, Bosin TR. Determination of serotonin, its precursors, metabolites and [3H]serotonin in lung by high-performance liquid chromatography with fluorescence detection. J Chromatogr Biomed App 1981;225:27–35.
34. Wu YB, Wu JH, Shi ZG, et al. Simultaneous determination of 5-hydroxyindoles and catechols from urine using polymer monolith microextraction coupled to high-performance liquid chromatography with fluorescence detection. J Chromatogr B 2009;77:1847–55.
35. Muñoz JLP, Ceinos RM, Soengas JL, et al. A simple and sensitive method for determination of melatonin in plasma, bile and intestinal tissues by high performance liquid chromatography with fluorescence detection. J Chromatogr B 2009;877:2173–7.
36. Kolevzon A, Newcorn JH, Kryzak L, et al. Relationship between whole blood serotonin and repetitive behaviors in autism. Psy Res 2010;175:274–6.
37. Wightman MR, Plotsky PM, Strope E, et al. Liquid chromatographic monitoring of CSF metabolites. Brain Res 1977;131:345–9.
38. Lechin F, van der Dijs B, Pardey-Maldonado B. Effects of amantadine on circulating neurotransmitters in healthy subjects. J Neural Transm 2010;117: 293–9.
39. Anderson GM, Mefford IN, Tolliver TJ, et al. Serotonin in human lumbar cerebrospinal fluid: A reassessment. Life Sci 1990;46:247–55.
40. Anderson GM, Feibel FC, Cohen DJ. Determination of serotonin in whole blood, platelet-rich plasma, platelet-poor plasma and plasma ultrafiltrate. Life Sci 1987;40:1063–70.
41. Beck O, Wallen NH, Broijersen A, et al. On the accurate determination of serotonin in human plasma. Biochem Biophys Res Commun 1993;196:260–6.
42. Anderson GM, Young JG, Cohen DJ, et al. Liquid-chromatographic determination of serotonin and tryptophan in whole blood and plasma. Clin Chem 1981;27: 775–6.
43. Fales HM, Pisano JJ. Gas chromatography of biologically important amines. Anal Biochem 1962;3:337–42.
44. Sen NP, McGeer PL. Gas chromatography of phenolic and catecholic amines as the trimethylsilyl ethers. Biochem Biophys Res Comm 1963;13:390–4.
45. Brooks CJW, Horning EC. Gas chromatographic studies of catecholamines, tryptamines, and other biological amines. Anal Chem 1964;36:1540–5.

46. Green AR, Koslow SH, Costa E. Identification and quantitation of a new indoleal-kylamine in rat hypothalamus. Brain Res 1973;51:371–4.
47. Narasimhachari N, Kempster E, Anbar M. 5-Methoxytryptamine in rat hypothal-amus and human CSF. A fact or artifact? Biomed Mass Spectrom 1980;7:231–5.
48. Cattabeni F, Koslow SH, Costa E. Gas chromatographic-mass spectrometric assay of four indole alkylamines of rat pineal. Science 1972;178:166–8.
49. Abramson FP. Femtomole level of analysis of biogenic amines and amino acids using functional group mass spectrometry. Anal Biochem 1974;51:482–99.
50. Beck O, Wiesel FA, Sedvall G. Mass fragmentographic determination of 5-hydroxytryptamine and 5-hydroxyindole-3-acetic acid in brain tissue using deuterated internal standards. J Chromatogr 1977;134:407–14.
51. Markey SP, Colburn RW, Johannessen JN. Efficient extraction and mass spectro-metric assay of serotonin in biological fluids. Biomed Mass Spec 1981;8:301–4.
52. Welsh LH. The analysis of solutions of epinephrine and norepinephrine. J Am Pharm Assoc 1955;44:507–14.
53. Turner WJ, Mauss EA. Serotonin (5-hydroxytryptamine) and acetylcholine in human ventricular and spinal fluids. Arch Gen Psychiatry 1959;1:646–50.
54. Singh KS, Mira SS, Bhargava KP. 5-Hydroxytryptamine (5-Ht) content of cerebro-spinal fluid in infective conditions of the central nervous system. J Lab Clin Med 1964;64:802–7.
55. Kriek JA, Bester AJ, Rossouw JJ. A new method of measuring serotonin in plasma and cerebrospinal fluid. S Afr Med J 1979;55:260–2.
56. Monaghan PJ, Brown HA, Houghton LA, et al. Measurement of serotonin in platelet depleted plasma by liquid chromatography tandem mass spectrometry. J Chrom B 2009;877:2163–7.
57. Miller AG, Brown H, Degg T, et al. Measurement of plasma 5-hydroxyindole acetic acid by liquid chromatography tandem mass spectrometry–Comparison with HPLC methodology. J Chrom B 2010;878(7–8):695–9.
58. Minami M, Takahashi H, Inagaki H, et al. Novel tryptamine-related substances, 5-sulphatoxydiacetyltryptamine, 5-hydroxydiacetyltryptamine, and reduced melatonin in human urine and the determination of those compounds, 6-sul-phatoxymelatonin, and melatonin with fluorometric HPLC. J Chrom B 2009; 877(8–9):814–22.
59. Koyama J, Takeuchi A, Tode C, et al. Development of fan LC-ESI-MS/MS method for the determination of histamine: application to the quantitative measurement of histamine degranulation by KU812 cells. J Chrom B 2009;877(3):207–12.
60. Welp A, Manz B, Peschke E. Development and validation of a high throughput direct radioimmunoassay for the quantitative determination of serum and plasma melatonin (N-acetyl-5-methoxytryptamine) in mice. J Immunol Methods 2010; 358(1–2):1–8.
61. Chegini S, Ehrhart-Hofmann B, Kaider A, et al. Direct enzyme-linked immunosor-bent assay and a radioimmunoassay for melatonin compared. Clin Chem 1995; 41:381–6.
62. Engbaek F, Voldby B. Radioimmunoassay of serotonin (5-hydroxytryptamine) in cerebrospinal fluid, plasma, and serum. Clin Chem 1982;28:624–8.
63. Geffard MR, Puizillout JJ, Delaage MA. A single radioimmunological assay for sero-tonin, N-acetylserotonin, 5-methoxytryptamine, and melatonin. J Neurochem 1982; 39:1271–7.
64. Gow IF, Corrie JE, Williams BC, et al. Development and validation of an improved radioimmunoassay for serotonin in platelet-rich plasma. Clin Chim Acta 1987;162: 175–88.

65. Ericson A, Mohammed Nur E, Petersson F, et al. The effects of capsaicin on gastrin secretion in isolated human antral glands: before and after ingestion of red chili. Dig Dis Sci 2009;54:491–8.
66. Feldman JM. Urinary serotonin in the diagnosis of carcinoid tumors. Clin Chem 1986;32:840–4.
67. Hussain MN, Sole MJ. A simple, specific, radioenzymatic assay for picogram quantities of serotonin or acetylserotonin in biological fluids and tissues. Anal Biochem 1981;111:105–10.
68. Hindberg I, Naesh O. Serotonin concentrations in plasma variations during the menstrual cycle. Clin Chem 1992;38:2087–9.
69. Odell WD, Daughaday WH, editors. Principles of competitive protein-binding assays, eds. Philadelphia: J.B. Lippincott Company; 1971.
70. Yalow RS, Berson SA. Immunoassay of endogenous plasma insulin in man. J Clin Invest 1960;39:1157–75.
71. Berson SA, Yalow RS. Isotopic tracers in the study of diabetes. Adv Biol Mol Phys 1958;6:349–430.
72. Yalow RS, Berson SA. Assay of plasma insulin in human subjects by immunological methods. Nature (London) 1959;184(Suppl 21):1648–9.

Standard Imaging Techniques for Neuroendocrine Tumors

David L. Bushnell, MD[a,b,*], Richard P. Baum, MD[c]

KEYWORDS

- Computed tomography • Magnetic resonance imaging
- Positron emission tomography • Neuroendocrine tumors

Several diagnostic imaging techniques including computed tomography (CT), magnetic resonance imaging (MRI), positron emission tomography (PET)/CT, single-photon emission CT (SPECT), and SPECT/CT have been used successfully over the years in the evaluation of patients with neuroendocrine tumors (NET). Detection of distant disease and the primary tumor is critical for optimal management of patients with this malignancy.[1] This article reviews the various imaging methods and their respective advantages and limitations for use in different types of NETs and in particular carcinoid tumors. The reader is also referred for additional information to several excellent recent reviews on this subject.[2–5]

CT/MRI

CT and MRI are typically the initial imaging techniques used in the evaluation of most patients with suspected NETs both for the detection of the primary tumor and for detection of possible local or distant metastases. CT and MRI are fairly sensitive for detection of many types of primary NETs.[6] Sensitivity, however, may be limited in some cases for recurrent or metastatic disease. MRI appears to be more sensitive than CT for liver and bone marrow metastases, but small nodal metastases may be

The authors have nothing to disclose.

[a] Division of Nuclear Medicine, Department of Radiology, University of Iowa Roy J. and Lucille A. Carver College of Medicine, 200 Hawkins Drive, Iowa City, IA 52242, USA

[b] Diagnostic Imaging and Radioisotope Therapy Service, Iowa City Veterans Administration Medical Center, Highway 6, Iowa City, IA 52244, USA

[c] Department of Nuclear Medicine/Center for Positron Emission Tomography, Pressekontakt: Katrin Gottwald, Zentralklinik Bad Berka GmbH, Robert-Koch-Allee 9, Bad Berka 99437, Germany

* Corresponding author. Division of Nuclear Medicine, Department of Radiology, University of Iowa Roy J. and Lucille A. Carver College of Medicine, 200 Hawkins Drive, Iowa City, IA 52242.

E-mail address: david-bushnell@uiowa.edu

Endocrinol Metab Clin N Am 40 (2011) 153–162
doi:10.1016/j.ecl.2010.12.002
0889-8529/11/$ – see front matter. Published by Elsevier Inc.

endo.theclinics.com

missed by either type of examination. Because these techniques primarily detect altered anatomy, they have only modest specificity.[6]

Most NETs are depicted on CT or MRI as enhancing lesions during the arterial phase of contrast delivery.[7] This is true for both the primary tumor and most metastases. Noncontrast images typically demonstrate low-density mass lesions on CT for either the primary or for metastases. Metastatic lesions often demonstrate low signal intensity on T1 weighted images versus high signal intensity on T2 weighted noncontrast images; however, there is significant patient-to-patient variability in this regard.[8] In general, multiphasic imaging, including the noncontrast phase, is required for optimal accuracy in this setting with either imaging method.[9]

SPECT/CT

The value of combining CT with SPECT in a single procedure cannot be overemphasized when imaging patients with the radiopharmaceuticals that will be discussed. When a SPECT/CT machine is not available, careful image correlation with standalone CT should be performed.[10]

Localization of a focus of uptake from either of these radiopharmaceuticals to a particular organ or structure in the body can mean the difference between a false-positive and a true-negative result. Moreover, at times subtle uptake that otherwise might be written off as insignificant may be deemed important by recognition of its location on CT. A good example of this is in abdominal or mesenteric lymph nodes, where metastatic disease can be recognized by seeing that there is even mild tracer uptake in a normal-appearing node on CT or MRI.

I-123 OR I-131 METAIODOBENZYLGUANIDINE

Metaiodobenzylguanidine (MIBG) is a norepinephrine analog that is actively concentrated in neuroendocrine tumor cells via the type 1 uptake mechanism. In most NET tumor cells, this molecule is then stored in neurosecretory granules. Originally, MIBG was labeled with I-131 for imaging, and subsequently therapy of pheochromocytoma. Over time its utility has been expanded to other NETs. The imaging properties of I-123 are notably superior to I-131, and clinical comparison studies make it clear that I-123 MIBG should be used in place of I-131 MIBG for imaging.[11] Perhaps most importantly, the use of I-123 makes it possible to obtain high-quality SPECT images, which significantly improves sensitivity. When combined with CT as SPECT/CT, specificity is improved as well.[12,13] In one study, for example, an additional 8% of lesions were conspicuous on I-123 MIBG images compared with I-131 MIBG in patients with pheochromocytoma.[11] Fig. 1 shows an example of a patient with pheochromocytoma imaged with SPECT/CT using I-123 MIBG.

The normal organ pattern of MIBG distribution includes salivary glands, liver, bladder, and faint uptake in kidneys. The heart also may show substantial uptake of MIBG. The thyroid gland is generally not seen if patients have been adequately prepared with SSKI or Lugols solution to block free I-123 or I-131 uptake in this organ. Brown fat accumulates MIBG as well and is particularly notable in the winter and more common in children. While the base of the neck and mediastinum are perhaps the most common sites for brown fat, other locations include perirenal and perispinal regions.[14] An often overlooked cause for false-positive findings with MIBG is physiologic contralateral adrenal hypertrophy following adrenalectomy.[15]

MIBG uptake in tumor cells may be inhibited by certain medications, including sympathomimetics such as pseudoephedrine, or other drugs including reserpine, calcium channel blockers, tricyclic antidepressants, and labetalol.[16] It is generally

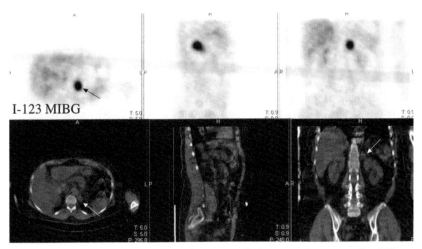

Fig. 1. Single-photon emission computed tomography/computed tomography (CT) examination with I-123 metaiodobenzylguanidine (MIBG) from a patient with a left adrenal pheochromocytoma. Tumor is depicted by white arrows on CT and black arrow on MIBG images.

advised that patients should discontinue these medications 3 to 4 days before administration of MIBG if clinically feasible.

Finally, NETs of the pancreas are not often MIBG positive; therefore there is probably no role for this agent in patients who have these tumor types.[17]

IN-111 PENTETREOTIDE (OCTRE OSCAN)

Somatostatin (SST) is a 28 amino acid peptide that has a variety of endocrine regulatory functions mediated through binding of this peptide to specific receptors on target cells throughout the body. There are five known SST receptor subtypes. Octreotide is an 8 amino acid cyclic peptide derivative of SST that binds primarily to SST receptor types 2 and 5. In-111 linked by a chelating agent to this peptide is marketed under the trade name Octreoscan (In-111 pentetreotide).

Most NETs express SST receptors, predominately type 2. Scintigraphic imaging with In-111 pentetreotide has become one of the standard methods for detection of NETs. Both sensitivity and specificity are improved with SPECT/CT when imaging with In-111 pentetreotide.[18] Imaging at 4 hours helps to avoid interfering with bowel uptake that is typically present at 24 hours. However, at 24 hours after injection the target (tumor)-to-background signal ratio is usually optimal. In patients on chronic therapy, it is advisable to withdraw cold octreotide immediate-release formulation 24 hours before scintigraphy. In patients treated with long-acting formulations, SRS imaging should be performed just before the next long-acting formulation administration.[19]

The normal pattern with In-111 pentetreotide includes intense activity in bladder, kidneys, and spleen, with lesser concentration in normal liver and bowel. Other less common sites of physiologic uptake include gallbladder, thyroid, and rarely pituitary. It is important for clinicians to keep in mind that certain inflammatory lesions will also concentrate this radiopharmaceutical. This is due to the fact that activated lymphocytes express SST receptors. Additionally, other types of malignancies may express these cell surface receptors, including some of the lymphomas.[20]

PET/CT

A number of PET radiopharmaceuticals have been studied as agents for detection of NETs. This section will focus on three in particular: fluorodeoxyglucose (F-18 FDG), which is widely available; Ga-68 octreotide, and F-18 fluorodehydroxyphenylalanine (DOPA). Nearly all modern health care facilities have access to PET or preferably PET/CT. PET has several advantages over imaging methods that use gamma-emitting radiopharmaceuticals such as In-111 pentetreotide or I-123 MIBG, including improved spatial and contrast resolution.

FDG

F-18FDG is an analog of glucose labeled with the positron emitting radioisotope fluorine-18, well known for its use with PET in many types of malignancy. Highly metabolic tumors, reflected by high FDG signal on PET images, tend to be more clinically aggressive. In general, this is true for NETs also. Very often when NETs exhibit strong affinity for FDG, the corresponding level of In-111 pentetreotide uptake or Ga-68 DOTATOC is low or absent, and conversely, when uptake is high with a radiolabeled SST analog, FDG activity in the tumor is low or absent.[21–24]

DOPA AND DOPAMINE

F-18DOPA, originally developed to image the dopaminergic system in the brain, has taken on a new role as a PET imaging agent for detection of neuroendocrine tumors. DOPA represents an intermediary molecule in the synthesis of norepinephrine and other chetacholamines. F-18DOPA is concentrated by neuroendocrine tumors through an amino acid transport system that is upregulated and highly active in the cells of these tumors. Metabolites of this tracer then are trapped in intracellular storage vesicles. Normal image patterns with this agent include high uptake in kidneys and urinary collecting systems. Preparation of patients with Carbidopa before imaging will increase tumor-to-background ratios.[25] Dopamine can similarly be labeled and imaged with F-18. PET/CT imaging using F-18DOPA or F-18 dopamine appears to have a very high sensitivity and specificity for carcinoid tumors and pheochromocytoma while being somewhat less sensitive for detection of pancreatic NETs.[26–31]

GA-68 DOTATOC/TATE/NOC

Ga-68 is a positron emitter that can be tightly labeled to the octreopeptide/chelator complex known as DOTATOC. Ga-68 DOTATOC has notably greater binding affinity for SST receptor 2 than does In-111 pentetreotide.[5] In addition, further small modifications to the octreopeptide molecule yield the other important SST receptor analogs DOTATATE and DOTANOC. DOTATATE has a modestly greater binding affinity for SST receptor 2 than does DOTATOC. The level of affinity for SST receptor 2 is summarized as: DOTATATE>DOTATOC>DOTANOC, and all demonstrate affinity greater than In-111 pentetreotide. DOTANOC has the advantage of better SST receptor 3 and 5 affinity than DOTATOC, DOTATATE, or In-111 pentetreotide.[5]

Several have confirmed the expected improved accuracy of Ga-68 DOTATOC PET/CT compared with SPECT or SPECT/CT imaging with In-111 pentetreotide in patients with NETs.[32–34]

IMAGING CARCINOID TUMORS

The most common among the neuroendocrine tumors, carcinoids have been detected with relatively high sensitivity and specificity for nearly 20 years using In-111 pentetreotide.[35] Modern SPECT imaging with this radiopharmaceutical yields sensitivities in excess of 80% for carcinoid tumor metastases.[36] For detection of radiologically occult primary tumors, the sensitivity is probably somewhat less. In-111 pentetreotide tumor uptake is useful to predict prognosis in patients with disseminated disease. In a large series of patients with metastatic well-differentiated endocrine carcinomas, lack of In-111 pentetreotide tumor uptake was associated with a significantly poorer overall survival.[37] In general, specificity is excellent, particularly when SPECT/CT is used. False-positive results are most commonly observed in inflammatory or infectious lesions and uncommonly in other tumor types.[20] **Fig. 2** shows an example of SPECT/CT with In-111 pentetreotide in a patient with lung carcinoid tumor.

Although sensitivity for detecting carcinoid tumors is notably less with MIBG (on the order of 50% to 60%) compared with In-111 pentetreotide, this radiopharmaceutical may still play a role in the care of some patients with carcinoid tumors.[38] It has become clear that there is a small fraction of patients with tumors that are MIBG-positive and In-111 pentetreotide-negative.[39] Importantly, in one series of 92 metastatic carcinoid patients, nearly 50% had at least one tumor site that was positive with MIBG and negative with In-111 pentetreotide and vice versa.[40] The highest sensitivity with I-123 MIBG generally is seen in the midgut carcinoid tumor subgroup.[41] In patients with advanced stage carcinoid tumors who have negative, or weakly positive, In-111 pentetreotide results, MIBG imaging may be used for selection of patients who might benefit from treatment with large doses of I-131 MIBG.[42]

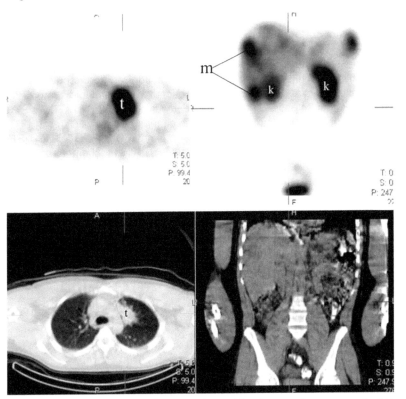

Fig. 2. SPECT/CT Octreoscan images from a patient with primary pulmonary carcinoid tumor metastatic to the liver. Note the liver metastases are not discernible on the noncontrast CT. k, kidneys; m, liver metastases; t, lung carcinoid tumor.

Poorly differentiated carcinoid tumors often do not concentrate either pentetreotide or MIBG in amounts adequate for detection. For these tumors, F-18FDG PET imaging is very likely to be positive.[22–24] **Fig. 3** demonstrates this imaging pattern. The likelihood of FDG tumor positivity on PET images is to some degree related to the ki-67 tumor proliferation index. In one study where octreopeptide imaging was accomplished with Ga-68 DOTATATE and compared with FDG PET findings, the authors found high FDG uptake and low Ga-68 DOTATATE uptake in NET tumors with high Ki-67, whereas they demonstrated low FDG uptake and high DOTATATE uptake in lesions with low ki67 results.[24]

FDG PET/CT in patients with NET, and specifically carcinoid tumors, has the ability to predict patient prognosis. In a study of 98 patients with NETs, 45 of which were intestinal carcinoid tumors, tumor affinity for FDG was strongly associated with poor outcome independent of the results of the Ki67 index.[43] In this study, progression-free survival was dramatically shorter for patients with FDG-positive versus FDG-negative tumors.

PET/CT imaging using F-18DOPA has a high sensitivity and specificity for detection of carcinoid tumors relative to other imaging techniques.[28,29] A large series of patients with carcinoid tumors found a sensitivity for PET DOPA of 96% on a per lesion basis.[26] Further work with this radiopharmaceutical has demonstrated substantial impact on patient management in carcinoid patients, particularly those with occult tumors.[27] In another study, 18F-DOPA PET alone detected more tumor sites than the combination of CT and SPECT octreotide imaging together.[30] In a smaller study, primary tumors were detected by F-18 DOPA in 13 patients (11 had carcinoid tumors), and these tumors were not conspicuous with In-111 pentetreotide or CT/MRI.[31]

Results from Ga-68 labeled octreopeptides imaged with PET also indicate a very high overall sensitivity and specificity for neuroendocrine tumors.[32,44] Ga-68 DOTA-TOC PET shows a significantly higher tumor detection rate than conventional SST receptor scintigraphy or diagnostic CT in patients with carcinoid tumors. In one comparison study of 84 patients, tumor sensitivity using Ga-68 DOTATOC was found to be 97%, which was significantly higher than either stand-alone CT or SPECT with In-111 pentetreotide.[32] In another comparison study, G-68 DOTATOC-PET was more sensitive in all locations of the body relative to In-111 pentetreotide SPECT except for the liver, where the two methods were found to be essentially equivalent.[33]

Overall, the management of carcinoid patients appears to be improved using PET with Ga-68 octreopeptides. In 64 patients with NET, predominately carcinoid, Ga-68 DTATOC PET/CT changed management in 38% of subjects. The authors noted that the CT component was important, as there were a significant number of lesions

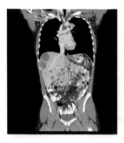
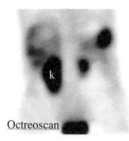
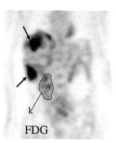

Fig. 3. Example of a patient with dedifferentiated carcinoid tumor liver metastases depicted on CT that do not concentrate, or minimally concentrate, in In -111 pentetreotide. In contrast, these tumors are strongly fluorodeoxyglucose avid on positron emission tomography (*arrows*). k, kidney.

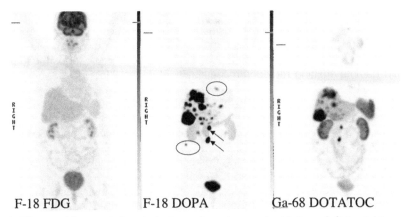

F-18 FDG   F-18 DOPA   Ga-68 DOTATOC

Fig. 4. 55 year-old man s/p hemicolectomy for colon carcinoid. From left to right, volume rendered PET images of F-18 FDG , F-18 fluorodehydroxyphenylalanine (DOPA), and Ga-68 DOTATOC. The FDG study does not demonstrate tumor activity. In contrast both DOPA and DOTATOC are for the most part strongly positive in liver metastases, peripancreatic nodal metastases (*arrows* on DOPA images) mediastinal lymph node (*upper oval*) and mesenteric node (*lower oval*). In this case, however, DOPA images clearly demonstrate stronger signal from almost all tumor sites compared with DOTATOC. Note mild normal pancreatic activity seen on DOPA image.

seen on CT that were not conspicuous on Ga-68 DOTATOC images.[34] Importantly, in this study CT was performed using triple-phase contrast-enhanced imaging. Similar findings relating to improved management of patients with carcinoid tumors also have been reported for other Ga-68 labeled octreotide agents imaged with PET.[45] PET images from three different radiopharmaceuticals are shown in a patient with metastatic carcinoid in **Fig. 4**.

CT and MRI play important roles in evaluating patients with carcinoid tumors. MRI in particular is highly sensitive for detecting carcinoid bone marrow metastases, with a sensitivity approaching 100% in one study.[46] Primary ileal tumors are often seen on CT as small stellate or spiculated masses. CT images may show mesenteric fibrosis near the tumor related to the release of serotonin or other bioactive amines.[47] In many cases, the tumor will be seen containing areas of calcification on CT.[48]

SUMMARY

In summary, functional imaging methods should be combined with CT or MRI to obtain maximal information in patients with NETs. PET/CT is the superior methodology for staging and detection of primary tumors of undetermined location. SPECT imaging (and preferably SPECT/CT) with In-111 pentetreotide or I-123 MIBG will likely be replaced in the coming years by PET/CT with Ga-68 labeled octreopeptides and either F-18 DOPA or F-18 dopamine. Likewise, MIBG imaging will at some point probably be performed with PET/CT using the positron emitter I-124 MIBG. Finally, octreopeptide and MIBG imaging will continue to also play important roles in establishing eligibility for therapy with either Y-90 or Lu-177 labeled DOTA octreopeptides or I-131 MIBG.

REFERENCES

1. Zuetenhorst JM, Taal BG. Metastatic carcinoid tumors: a clinical review. Oncologist 2005;10(2):123–31.

2. Koopmans KP, Neels ON, Kema IP, et al. Molecular imaging in neuroendocrine tumors: molecular uptake mechanisms and clinical results. Crit Rev Oncol Hematol 2009;71(3):199–213.

3. Bombardieri E, Coliva A, Maccauro M, et al. Imaging of neuroendocrine tumours with gamma-emitting radiopharmaceuticals. Q J Nucl Med Mol Imaging 2010; 54(1):3–15.

4. Scarsbrook AF, Ganeshan A, Statham J, et al. Anatomic and functional imaging of metastatic carcinoid tumors. Radiographics 2007;27(2):455–77.

5. Rufini V, Calcagni ML, Baum RP. Imaging of neuroendocrine tumors. Semin Nucl Med 2006;36(3):228–47.

6. Rockall AG, Reznek RH. Imaging of neuroendocrine tumours (CT/MR/US). Best Pract Res Clin Endocrinol Metab 2007;21(1):43–68.

7. Paulson EK, McDermott VG, Keogan MT, et al. Carcinoid metastases to the liver: role of triple-phase helical CT. Radiology 1998;206(1):143–50.

8. Bader TR, Semelka RC, Chiu VC, et al. MRI of carcinoid tumors: spectrum of appearances in the gastrointestinal tract and liver. J Magn Reson Imaging 2001;14:261–9.

9. Tamm EP, Kim EE, Ng CS. Imaging of neuroendocrine tumors. Hematol Oncol Clin North Am 2007;21(3):409–32.

10. Amthauer H, Denecke T, Rohlfing T, et al. Value of image fusion using single photon emission computed tomography with integrated low-dose computed tomography in comparison with retrospective voxel-based method in neuroendocrine tumors. Eur Radiol 2005;15(7):1456–62.

11. Furata N, Kiyota H, Yoshigoe F, et al. Diagnosis of pheochromocytoma using [123I]-compared with [131I]-metaiodobenzylguanidine scintigraphy. Int J Urol 1999;6(3):119–24.

12. Meyer-Rochow GY, Schembri GP, Benn DE, et al. The utility of metaiodobenzylguanidine single photon emission computed tomography/computed tomography (MIBG SPECT/CT) for the diagnosis of pheochromocytoma. Ann Surg Oncol 2010;17(2):392–400.

13. Rozovsky K, Koplewitz BZ, Krausz Y, et al. Added value of SPECT/CT for correlation of MIBG scintigraphy and diagnostic CT in neuroblastoma and pheochromocytoma. AJR Am J Roentgenol 2008;190(4):1085–90.

14. Okuyama C, Ushijima Y, Kubota T, et al. 123I-metaiodobenzylguanidine uptake in the nape of the neck of children: likely visualization of brown adipose tissue. J Nucl Med 2003;44(9):1421–5.

15. Boersma HH, Wensing JW, Kho TL, et al. Transient enhanced uptake of 123I-metaiodobenzylguanidine in the contralateral adrenal region after resection of an adrenal pheochromocytoma. N Engl J Med 2000;342(19):1450–1.

16. Khafagi FA, Shapiro B, Fig LM, et al. Labetalol reduces iodine-131 MIBG uptake by pheochromocytoma and normal tissues. J Nucl Med 1989;30(4):481–9.

17. Kaltsas G, Korbonits M, Heintz E, et al. Comparison of somatostatin analog and metaiodobenzylguanidine radionuclides in the diagnosis and localization of advanced neuroendocrine tumors. J Clin Endocrinol Metab 2001;86(2): 895–902.

18. Oberg K, Eriksson B. Nuclear medicine in the detection, staging, and treatment of gastrointestinal carcinoid tumors. Best Pract Res Clin Endocrinol Metab 2005; 19(2):265–76.

19. Oberg K, Kvols L, Caplin M, et al. Consensus report on the use of somatostatin analogs for the management of neuroendocrine tumors of the gastroenteropancreatic system. Ann Oncol 2004;15(6):966–73.

20. Bushnell DL, Menda Y, Madsen MT, et al. [99mTc] Depreotide tumour uptake in patients with non-Hodgkin's lymphoma. Nucl Med Commun 2004;25(8):839–43.
21. Kayani I, Conry BG, Groves AM, et al. A comparison of 68Ga-DOTATATE and 18F-FDG PET/CT in pulmonary neuroendocrine tumors. J Nucl Med 2009; 50(12):1927–32.
22. Intenzo CM, Jabbour S, Lin HC, et al. Scintigraphic imaging of body neuroendocrine tumors. Radiographics 2007;27(5):1355–69.
23. Menda Y, O'Dorisio T, Floresca J, et al. Detection of primary and recurrent carcinoid tumors with F-18-FDG PET: comparison with In-111-pentetreotide. J Nucl Med 2003;44:72P.
24. Kayani I, Bomanji JB, Groves A, et al. Functional imaging of neuroendocrine tumors with combined PET/CT using 68Ga-DOTATATE (DOTA-Dphe1, Tyr3-octreotate) and 18F-FDG. Cancer 2008;112(11):2447–55.
25. Imani F, Agopian VG, Auerbach MS, et al. 18F-FDOPA PET and PET/CT accurately localize pheochromocytomas. J Nucl Med 2009;50(4):513–9.
26. Koopmans KP, de Vries EG, Kema IP, et al. Staging of carcinoid tumors with 18F-DOPA PET: a prospective, diagnostic accuracy study. Lancet Oncol 2006; 7(9):728–34.
27. Montravers F, Kerrou K, Nataf V, et al. Impact of fluorohydroxy-phenylalanine-18F positron emission tomography on management of adult patients with documented or occult digestive endocrine tumors. J Clin Endocrinol Metab 2009; 94(4):1295–301.
28. Hoegerle S, Altehoefer C, Ghanem N, et al. Whole-body 18F DOPA PET for detection of gastrointestinal carcinoid tumors. Radiology 2001;220(2):373–80.
29. Becherer A, Szabó M, Karanikas G, et al. Imaging of advanced neuroendocrine tumors with (18)F-FDOPA PET. J Nucl Med 2004;45(7):1161–7.
30. Koopmans KP, Neels OC, Kema IP, et al. Improved staging of patients with carcinoid and islet cell tumors with 18F-dihydroxy-phenyl-alanine and 11C-5-hydroxy-tryptophan positron emission tomography. J Clin Oncol 2008;26(9): 1489–95.
31. Ambrosini V, Tomassetti P, Rubello D, et al. Role of 18F-dopa PET/CT imaging in the management of patients with 111In-pentetreotide negative GEP tumours. Nucl Med Commun 2007;28(6):473–7.
32. Gabriel M, Decristoforo C, Kendler D, et al. 68Ga-DOTA-Tyr3-octreotide PET in neuroendocrine tumors: comparison with somatostatin receptor scintigraphy and CT. J Nucl Med 2007;48(4):508–18.
33. Buchmann I, Henze M, Engelbrecht S, et al. Comparison of 68Ga- DOTATOC PET and 111In-DTPAOC (Octreoscan) SPECT in patients with neuroendocrine tumours. Eur J Nucl Med Mol Imaging 2007;34(10):1617–26.
34. Ruf J, Hueck F, Schiefer J, et al. Impact of multiphase 68Ga-DOTATOC- PET/CT on therapy management in patients with neuroendocrine tumors. Neuroendocrinology 2010;91(1):101–9.
35. Krenning EP, Kwekkeboom DJ, Bakker WH, et al. Somatostatin receptor scintigraphy with [111In-DTPA-D-Phe1]-and [123I-Tyr3]-octreotide: the Rotterdam experience with more than 1000 patients. Eur J Nucl Med 1993;20(8):716–31.
36. Kaltsas G, Rockall A, Papadogias D, et al. Recent advances in radiological and radionuclide imaging and therapy of neuroendocrine tumours. Eur J Endocrinol 2004;151(1):15–27.
37. Asnacios A, Courbon F, Rochaix P, et al. Indium-111-pentetreotide scintigraphy and somatostatin receptor subtype 2 expression: new prognostic factors for malignant well-differentiated endocrine tumors. J Clin Oncol 2008;26(6):963–70.

38. Binderup T, Knigge U, Loft A, et al. Functional imaging of neuroendocrine tumors: a head-to-head comparison of somatostatin receptor scintigraphy, 123I-MIBG scintigraphy, and 18F-FDG PET. J Nucl Med 2010;51(5):704–12.

39. Taal BG, Hoefnagel CA, Valdés Olmos RA, et al. Combined diagnostic imaging with 131I-metaiodobenzylguanidine and 111In-pentetreotide in carcinoid tumours. Eur J Cancer Am 1996;32(11):1924–32.

40. Quigley AM, Buscombe JR, Gopinath G, et al. In-vivo characterization of the functional aspects of carcinoid tumors by imaging somatostatin receptors and amine uptake. J Nucl Med 2003;44(Suppl 5):74p.

41. Ezziddin S, Logvinski T, Yong-Hing C, et al. Factors predicting tracer uptake in somatostatin receptor and MIBG scintigraphy of metastatic gastroenteropancreatic neuroendocrine tumors. J Nucl Med 2006;47(2):223–33.

42. Safford SD, Coleman RE, Gockerman JP, et al. Iodine-131 metaiodobenzylguanidine treatment for metastatic carcinoid. Results in 98 patients. Cancer 2004; 101(9):1987–93.

43. Binderup T, Knigge U, Loft A, et al. 18F-fluorodeoxyglucose positron emission tomography predicts survival of patients with neuroendocrine tumors. Clin Cancer Res 2010;16(3):978–85.

44. Ambrosini V, Tomassetti P, Castellucci P, et al. Comparison between 68Ga- DOTA-NOC and 18F-DOPA PET for the detection of gastro-entero-pancreatic and lung neuroendocrine tumors. Eur J Nucl Med Mol Imaging 2008;35(8):1431–8.

45. Ambrosini V, Campana D, Bodei L, et al. 68Ga-DOTANOC PET/CT clinical impact in patients with neuroendocrine tumors. J Nucl Med 2010;51(5):669–73.

46. Meijerj WG, van der Veer E, Jager PL, et al. Bone metastases in carcinoid tumors: clinical features, imaging characteristics, and markers of bone metabolism. J Nucl Med 2003;44(2):184–91.

47. Horton KM, Kamel I, Hofmann L, et al. Carcinoid tumors of the small bowel: a multitechnique imaging approach. AJR Am J Roentgenol 2004;182(3):559–67.

48. Pantongrag-Brown L, Buetow PC, Carr NJ, et al. Calcification and fibrosis in mesenteric carcinoid tumor: CT findings and pathologic correlation. AJR Am J Roentgenol 1995;164(2):387–91.

Surgery for Gastro-enteropancreatic Neuroendocrine Tumors (GEPNETS)

J. Philip Boudreaux, MD[a,b,c,*]

KEYWORDS

- Carcinoid • Cytoreduction • Mesenteric encasement
- Gastric carcinoid • Midgut carcinoid • MEN
- Asymptomatic primary

The only therapy with the potential for complete cure of patients with gastroentero-pancreatic neuroendocrine tumors (GEPNETS) is complete surgical excision.[1] Surgical treatment for all patients with abdominal neuroendocrine tumors falls into four major categories: (1) resection of the primary tumor and its regional (nodal) draining basin with curative or palliative intent; (2) resection of regional or distant metastatic disease with cytoreductive intent; (3) resection of disease for palliation without cytoreductive intent (bleeding, obstruction, or perforation); and (4) resection for treatment of lesions associated with multiple endocrine neoplasia (MEN) syndromes.[2] These categories often overlap in clinical practice. Because of the usually slow and indolent nature of this disease, patients with GEPNETS may require surgical therapy in more than one or all of these categories during their lifetime. Multimodality treatment options in addition to standard surgical excision now include such things as radiofrequency ablation, chemoembolization, yttrium 90 microsphere embolization, 131-iodine MIBG therapy, numerous clinical trials, and other forms of systemic therapy.[2] Because of the availability of multiple treatment options, the sequencing of these therapies and the relationship and timing of operations to these therapies becomes important. These types of management decisions are often best made in specialized centers that have experience with the use of these modalities, their risks and benefits, and the limitations they may impose on subsequent therapies. The maximum benefits of a well-planned longitudinal treatment plan can be exploited with input from multispecialty team

[a] Section of Endocrine Surgery, Department of Surgery, Louisiana State University Health Sciences Center, 200 West Esplanade Avenue, Suite 200, Kenner, LA 70065, USA
[b] Section of Surgical Oncology, Department of Surgery, Louisiana State University Health Sciences Center, 200 West Esplanade Avenue, Suite 200, Kenner, LA 70065, USA
[c] Section of Transplant Surgery, Department of Surgery, Louisiana State University Health Sciences Center, 200 West Esplanade Avenue, Suite 200, Kenner, LA 70065, USA
* Neuroendocrine Tumor Clinic, 200 West Esplanade, Suite 200, Kenner, LA 70065.
E-mail address: jboudr4@lsuhsc.edu

Endocrinol Metab Clin N Am 40 (2011) 163–171
doi:10.1016/j.ecl.2010.12.004
0889-8529/11/$ – see front matter © 2011 Elsevier Inc. All rights reserved.

members whose focus is primarily the diagnosis and management of patients with neuroendocrine tumors. Several such centers that can offer expert advice counseling and treatment options currently exist around the country.[2]

Surgical options per se are often dictated by the tumor's site of origin, degree of tumor burden, and overall health or debility of the individual patient. This article considers different options based on the type of tumor and site of origin.

GASTRIC CARCINOIDS

Gastric carcinoids are generally thought of as belonging to one of three types. Type I gastric carcinoids arise from the enterochromaffin-like cells of the stomach lining. They develop in response to elevated gastrin levels, such as encountered in patients with autoimmune gastritis and achlorhydria. These patients typically have an elevated gastric pH. Type II gastric carcinoids arise in 23% to 29% of patients with MEN-1 syndrome, hypergastrinemia secondary to the Zollinger-Ellison syndrome gastrinoma.[3,4] Sporadic gastrinomas give rise to Type II gastric carcinoid in only 1% to 3% of cases.[3,4] Gastric pH is usually low. Type III or sporadic gastric carcinoids arise spontaneously in the presence of normal gastric pH and normal gastrinemia.

In Type I, the performance of a gastric pH at the time of endoscopy assists the clinician in determining the type of carcinoid present. A high gastric pH with elevated gastrin levels indicates a Type I tumor. These are usually multiple and small. Endoscopic ultrasound (EUS) helps to determine the thickness and size of the lesions. Transendoscopic excision of a few (<6) small tumors with periodic surveillance is an acceptable form of therapy.[5] Pathologic examination for degree of differentiation, presence of lymphovascular invasion, and completeness of excision helps the surgeon decide if a more aggressive resection is required. Patients who have frequent recurrences or numerous tumors caused by the persistence of elevated gastrin levels should be considered for antrectomy, because this maneuver removes the source of gastrin and is curative in approximately 80% of cases.[2] Residual tumors in the body and cardia of the stomach often resolve after antrectomy. Tumors larger than 3 cm have a higher malignant potential and metastatic rate[3,6] and should be completely excised. These tumors, although often multiple and small, have a potential for hemorrhage and should be removed if feasible. The metastatic rate for gastric carcinoids Type I is approximately 10% to 30%, even though most of the tumors are small in the 1- to 2-cm range.[5] This indicates that close surveillance is required, because the potential for metastasis and lethality exits. Recalcitrant and recurrent lesions should lead one to consider a more aggressive therapy than endoscopic excision alone. Transmural invasion by the tumor seen on EUS is an indication for surgical resection and should not be attempted endoscopically. Frequent repeat endoscopy is usually indicated for both Types I and II in an ongoing surveillance program.[5]

Type III (spontaneous) gastric carcinoids are found in the presence of normal gastrin and normal pH. These tumors have a higher mitotic rate and a higher propensity to metastasize early. They behave more like adenocarcinoma of the stomach, tend to be greater than 2 cm in size at the time of diagnosis, and should not be observed. They should be excised along standard oncologic surgical principles for gastric cancer with total or subtotal gastrectomy and lymph node dissection.[5,6]

PANCREATIC NEUROENDOCRINE TUMORS

The most common pancreatic islet cell neuroendocrine tumor is the insulinoma,[7,8] which secretes insulin or, less commonly, proinsulin leading to hypoglycemia. Most insulinomas are benign (90%) and solitary (90%). They are more commonly small, less than 2 cm, and single. Approximately 10% of insulinomas are malignant.[7,8] Long-term survival is good (88% at 10 years)[7] with the exception of patients with MEN-1. Insulinomas in these patients have a tendency to recur or metastasize. The only known cure for insulinoma is complete surgical excision. Cure rates approach 100% for non-MEN patients, depending on the stage at presentation and adequacy of resection.[2] Improved outcomes and higher cure rates have been consistently reported at dedicated tertiary centers.[9] Once the diagnosis is confirmed, the difficulty arises, as with most small pancreatic islet cell tumors, in localizing the lesion preoperatively. For pancreatic head and body tumors, contrast-enhanced EUS with tattooing or marking of the lesion facilitates surgical excision and seems to be a more sensitive method than CT scanning, MRI, or transabdominal ultrasound.[7,10–12]

The weakness of endoscopic EUS lies in the inability to obtain good visualization of the distal body and tail of the pancreas. Detection rates in this region range from 37% to 60% versus 83% to 100% detection for proximal pancreatic tumors.[2,13] Transhepatic selective portal venous sampling and selective arterial calcium stimulation has been shown to be highly effective in localizing tumors to a given region of the pancreas when EUS is nondiagnostic and aids the surgeon in focusing exploration to a particular portion of the pancreas.[2] An additional useful tool is intraoperative ultrasound (IUS) coupled with careful bimanual palpation of the entire gland when preoperative attempts at localization are not precise. By combining IUS with preoperative portal venous sampling and selective arterial calcium injection, detection rates approach 95%.[14] Radical blind pancreatic resection has been replaced with pancreas-sparing enucleation, avoiding ductal and vascular structures with the use of IUS. In selective cases, insulinoma enucleation can be accomplished laparoscopically in experienced hands.[2,5]

RARE FUNCTIONING PANCREATIC NETS

Gastrinomas, non–MEN-1 (VIPomas), glucagonomas, carcinoid tumors, somatostatinomas, ACTHomas, calcitonin-secreting tumors, and other peptide-secreting tumors are much less common than insulinomas. Unlike insulinomas, however, these tumors are most often malignant, presenting with metastatic disease at the time of diagnosis. Lymph node and liver metastases are also common and attempts at R0 curative resections are recommended whenever possible.[2,5] Palliative cytoreduction for hormonal and symptom control is a secondary but worthwhile goal and plays a major role in patient management. Staged resections, radiofrequency ablation, and other cytoreductive therapies may all play a role in the surgical strategy and should be performed in specialized centers as part of an overall treatment regimen.[2,5] Surgical debulking can facilitate radionuclide therapy or chemotherapy for symptom control. Staged resections, bilateral adrenalectomies for Cushing syndrome, and liver transplantation in the absence of extrahepatic disease have all been used.[5]

MULTIPLE ENDOCRINE NEOPLASIA TYPE I

Duodenal and pancreatic NETs in MEN-1 syndrome can present as functioning or nonfunctioning. Fifty-five percent are nonfunctioning.[4,5] The two most common functional pancreatic NETs in MEN-1 are gastrinomas (Zollinger-Ellison syndrome) and insulinomas. Both gastrinomas and insulinomas are often multiple. Gastrinomas are often submucosal, occurring in the duodenum or situated in the head of the pancreas. EUS with tattooing is helpful in the preoperative localization for these tumors. The only cure for these tumors is surgical and approximately 50% of the lesions are benign. Duodenal tumors are found by duodenotomy and palpation and can be locally excised if small. Larger lesions of the duodenum and pancreas, especially those greater than 2 cm, require a more extensive resection and lymph node dissection because malignant potential is greater. An R0 resection is preferred, but recurrences are likely. Total pancreatectomy is controversial and is not routinely recommended.[5,15] Liver resection for metastatic disease after Whipple resection carries an increased risk of liver abscess and biliary sepsis, but may be required to control hormonal secretion. Debulking may aid in palliation and improve survival.[3–5] The nonfunctioning pancreatic neuroendocrine tumors are usually malignant. Well-differentiated nonfunctional tumors are more difficult to diagnose at an earlier stage, but palliative, non-R0 resections provide benefit by decreasing local regional complications (pain, bleeding, and obstruction). Only R0 resections have demonstrated survival benefit in non–MEN-1 patients. For MEN-1 patients, lesions larger than 2 cm again have a higher malignancy rate and nonfunctional pancreatic NETs cause up to 20% of MEN-1–related deaths.[16] The surgical strategy ranges from enucleation to aggressive resection (subtotal pancreatectomy) as prophylaxis against tumor recurrence. Recurrent lesions can be reresected in otherwise healthy patients.[16] Hepatic debulking for metastatic disease should include cholecystectomy to avoid the potential complication of cholecystitis from long-term octreotide therapy and the complication of biliary necrosis from chemoembolization or yttrium 90 microsphere embolization. A 90% hepatic debulking can lead to 47% to 65% 5-year survival[16,17] versus a 30% to 40% 5-year survival for unresected patients.

POORLY DIFFERENTIATED NONFUNCTIONING NETS OF THE FOREGUT (STOMACH, DUODENUM, PANCREAS)

Patients with these rare tumors are candidates for surgery only if R0 resection can be achieved or if their tumor demonstrates responsiveness to systemic therapies. These tumors tend to be fast-growing with high mitotic index and therapy for nonresectable tumors is primarily medical. Partial debulking in surgery for metastatic disease is associated with poorer outcomes[15,18] and generally not recommended.

MIDGUT CARCINOIDS OF THE JEJUNOILEUM

The only known cure for midgut carcinoids is surgical. Many patients are diagnosed at the time of an operation for some other reason or as a result of an evaluation for chronic gastrointestinal blood loss, obstruction, or as a result of evaluation for metastatic disease.[6] The findings of a gut-based neuroendocrine tumor should be followed by an in-depth search for additional primary tumors, because these tumors are often small and multiple. They can only be detected by close inspection and palpation in many cases. Laparoscopic resections have the potential for being inadequate because the ability to evaluate the entire small bowel in a tactile manner is negated and carries the risk of incomplete resection. I have encountered several patients in this category and have found as many as 70 tumors along a length of bowel after prior laparoscopic resection for carcinoma.[2,19] The extent of surgical resection should proceed along sound oncologic principles with excision of the draining nodal basin. Resection of the mesenteric lymph nodes encasing the mesenteric vessels should be undertaken by experienced surgeons familiar with the technique of debulking these metastases to prevent the disastrous complication of intestinal ischemia or infarction, either as a result of tumor progression or as a result of surgical misadventure.[2,9,20] Approximately 50% of the patients referred to our center with bulky mesenteric vascular encasement were declared unresectable or were operated elsewhere and could be successfully decompressed.

LYMPHATIC MAPPING

The ileocecal valve can be spared in up to 40% of patients with terminal ileal tumors by using a technique of intraoperative lymphatic mapping.[20] The technique used is similar to that for sentinel node mapping with lymphazurin blue or methylene blue dye. If the lymphatic drainage of the subserosal lymphatics from the tumor closest to the ileocecal valve crosses the ileocecal valve onto the cecum, it is advised to resect the colon and associated draining lymphatic nodal basin along with the distal small bowel. Every effort should be made to save the ileocecal valve in syndromic patients, because they are already challenged with diarrhea as a result of their tumor secretions and may already be at risk for having shortened gut.[20] If the subserosal lymphatics do not cross the ileocecal valve, one can often spare the ileocecal valve and still do an adequate lymph node resection.

Lymphatic mapping may also explain the relationship between the primary tumor and multiple small bowel primary tumors. I have found longitudinal lymphatic spread to extend beyond 20 cm from an individual tumor along the intestinal wall,[20] often in the presence of bulky mesenteric nodal metastases and proximal lymphatic obstruction. This may explain why multiple primary carcinoid tumors in the small bowel have been shown to be of monoclonal origin,[21,22] perhaps caused by the longitudinal lymphatic intramural spread of drop metastases when central lymphatic drainage roots are occluded by tumor and the desmoplastic reaction.[20] These drop metastases may also explain the phenomenon of local recurrence at or near the previous resection margin. Subserosal lymphatics that are mapped by the blue dye may represent the true resection margin rather than an arbitrary 5-cm margin from the tumor border.

ASYMPTOMATIC PRIMARY TUMOR

An asymptomatic primary tumor is usually not asymptomatic forever and is not a contraindication for operation, even in the presence of distant metastases. On the contrary, by the time the primary tumor in the gut becomes symptomatic, the patient may become a higher risk for surgery as when emergency operations for bleeding, obstruction, or intestinal ischemia are performed in an overall debilitated patient secondary to a chronic carcinoid syndrome and malnutrition.[2,9] I have found as many as 33% of patients who were referred for progressive carcinoid syndrome with worsening abdominal pain, distention, and episodic diarrhea were actually suffering from occult intestinal obstruction caused by their "unknown primary" in the small bowel. An additional subgroup of patients were suffering from intestinal ischemia caused by progressive desmoplastic reaction, fibrosis, and vascular encasement from bulky mesenteric nodal disease.[20] It was often difficult to sort out their symptomatology from obstruction ischemia versus poorly controlled syndrome.

A delay in resection of an intestinal primary may make later attempts at resection more difficult, if not impossible.[23] Patients with an "unknown primary" and liver and mesenteric metastases had a small bowel tumor found at operation in 50% to 70% of cases.[24] At the time of operation, cholecystectomy is recommended, because many of these patients are on long-term octreotide therapy.[2,9,15,20] Both functioning and nonfunctioning tumors and their metastases can sometimes be found at operation by gamma probe radioguided surgery after injection of ^{111}In-labeled octreotide or ^{123}I-MIBG.[25,26] I have found this technique of radioguided surgery useful in evaluating the liver, ovaries, pelvis, retroperitoneum, and nodal basins of the head and neck, upper mediastinum, and pelvis. I have also found that waiting 7 days after injection of ^{111}In octreotide facilitated results by allowing the background radiation levels to decay low enough so as not to overwhelm the handheld gamma probe.

APPENDICEAL AND COLONIC CARCINOIDS

Most appendiceal carcinoids are cured by appendectomy if (1) the tumor is less than 1 cm and located at the tip, (2) the base of resection is not involved by tumor, (3) there is no invasion of the mesoappendix, (3) there is no lymphovascular invasion, and (4) the mitotic index is low.[6] Careful pathologic examination of the specimen is required. If tumor is present at the base, lymphovascular or mesoappendiceal invasion is present, or the mitotic index is high, right hemicolectomy and formal node resection should be undertaken.[2,23] Cecal and colonic carcinoids behave more like adenocarcinomas and aggressive surgical resection is required with en bloc removal of associated lymph node draining basin. These tumors are often metastatic at the time of diagnosis.[6] A rare variant adenocarcinoid, also called "goblet cell" carcinoma, behaves very aggressively with mucin production and a propensity to metastasize, similar to that for adenocarcinoma. Lymphatic mapping may assist in completeness of regional lymphadenectomy. The mortality for colonic carcinoids and appendiceal carcinoids is directly related to tumor size and the presence or absence of metastases. Tumors larger than 2.5 cm should be considered malignant.[2,15]

RECTAL CARCINOIDS

Resection of the primary tumor and associated regional lymph nodes is the only curative therapy for rectal and hindgut carcinoids typically associated with the descending colon.[10] Local excision or endoscopic excision of small rectal carcinoids is justified if transrectal ultrasound shows no invasion of the muscularis propria and no pathologic lymph nodes. Pathologic examination should show no lymphovascular invasion and a well-differentiated tumor. Patients treated with local excision require periodic surveillance and repeat EUS. Patients with lymphovascular invasion, invasion through the muscularis propria, or lymph node metastases require low anterior resection and total mesorectal excision. Malignancy is greater when lesions are greater than 2.5 cm or when unfavorable pathology, such as a poorly differentiated lesion, is encountered.[27,28]

HEPATIC METASTASES

Liver resection for metastatic GEPNETS can be for curative or palliative intent. The most common cause of death in carcinoid patients is liver failure, followed by bowel obstruction or ischemia. Tumor burden, hormonal control, and overall physiologic state of the patient and the presence or absence of options for adjunctive therapies and the ability to control the primary tumor, along with anatomic considerations, all play a role in the surgical strategy for liver resection.[2,15–17,20,23,29] Cytoreductive ablative therapies, in addition to surgical resection, can offer improved survival and quality of life exceeding that of nonoperated patients (70%–90% vs 50% at 5 years) in selected series.[2,15–17,20,23,29] Patients should not be deemed inoperable until they have been evaluated by an experienced center with a multispecialty team. Sometimes nonsurgical candidates can be rendered operable by adjunctive therapies, such as preoperative yttrium 90 microspheres, chemoembolization, ^{123}I-MIBG therapy, chemotherapy, or other modalities. Conversely, surgical resection may sometimes render these modalities more effective. Proper sequencing of these therapies and operative management is best performed in dedicated tertiary centers.[2,9,14,19,20,23]

LIVER TRANSPLANTATION

Liver transplantation for unresectable metastatic GEPNETS is the only acceptable indication for liver replacement for metastatic disease. The current recommendations regarding liver transplantation for patients with metastatic neuroendocrine tumors include the following inclusion criteria: (1) low mitotic index tumors (Ki67≤10%), (2) absence of extrahepatic disease, (3) the primary tumor should be drained by the portal venous system, (4) the patient should be stable for at least 6 months during the pretransplant waiting period, (5) generally less than 55 years old, (6) metastatic tumor burden to liver ratio is less than 50%; and (6) no unresectable extrahepatic disease. When these criteria (Milan criteria) are met, the 5-year survival rates exceed 75% and the recurrence rates are as low as 30%.[28] Nonselective series of orthotopic liver transplantation have reported poorer outcomes with 45% survival at 5 years and recurrence rates approaching 75%.[30] Clearly, recipient selection and tumor biology play a role in overall success rates and disease-free survival. In this era of organ shortage, proper recipient selection plays an increasing role in the appropriate use of a scarce resource. Some centers are pursuing the option of living donor liver transplantation to circumvent the scarce donor organ problem. There are additional unanswered questions regarding liver transplantation for metastatic GEPNETS: (1) which tumor type carries the best prognosis for disease-free survival and long-term survival, (2) what is the best immunosuppressive regimen to follow that would minimize the risk of tumor recurrence, and (3) how can the complication rate be reduced with simultaneous en bloc primary tumor resection with multivisceral liver transplantation. Morbidity and mortality are increased when liver transplantation is combined with more aggressive and extensive resections. It is now known that quality of life is definitely increased for syndromic patients who have hypersecretion syndromes after orthotopic liver transplantation.[28]

CARCINOID CRISIS

The prevention of carcinoid crisis and other hypersecretion syndromes can be mitigated by use of continuous-infusion octreotide. It is best used in the preoperative, intraoperative, and postoperative setting and is recommended for any syndromic patient, such as the carcinoid syndrome, undergoing a major surgical procedure. Carcinoid crises can be precipitated by any surgical procedure, but especially during manipulation of the liver when bulky tumor burden is present. Carcinoid crisis can also be caused by physiologic or emotional stress, or even relatively minor procedures, such as biopsy, endoscopy, or bronchoscopy.[5] I currently use a 250- to 500-μg bolus of octreotide followed by a 250- to 500-μg per hour continuous infusion, which is tapered over 4 to 48 hours, depending on the magnitude of the procedure. Epinephrine and other vasopressors worsen rather than correct the hypotension of carcinoid crisis, unless the patient is covered with high-dose octreotide before administration of vasopressor substances. Vasopressors, such as epinephrine, can cause degranulation of the amines containing the tumor cells and can lead to vasomotor collapse.[2] Vasopressors have been used successfully during cardiac valvular procedures in carcinoid syndrome patients under octreotide infusion coverage.[26] Other hypersecretion syndromes may also be ameliorated by continuous octreotide infusion during surgical extirpations. Acute exacerbations of carcinoid crises can be treated with additional 500- to 1000-μg boluses until stabilization occurs. Careful preoperative planning with the anesthesiologist and surgical team is required for successful operations in patients with carcinoid syndrome. Often the operation must be halted until the patient stabilizes, additional octreotide is administered, and blood pressure improves. The operation can then resume under increased octreotide coverage.

SUMMARY

Overall, with the advent of newer and more complex treatment options for patients with GEPNETS, a well thought out treatment plan, sequencing, and explanation of options is best performed in an experienced tertiary center with dedicated multispecialty teams for the care of patients with these rare tumors. The treatment plan can often be performed at home in conjunction with the patient's local physician, except when specialized skills or equipment are required.

REFERENCES

1. Plockinger U, Rindi G, Arnold R, et al. Guidelines for the diagnosis and treatment of neuroendocrine gastrointestinal tumors. Neuroendocrinology 2005;80(6): 394–424.
2. Woltering E, Cundiff J, Lyons J. Neuroendocrine tumors of the gastroenteropancreatic axis. In: Silberman H, Silberman A, editors. Principles and practice of surgical oncology. Philadelphia (PA): Lippincott Williams & Wilkins; 2010. p. 769–800.
3. Gibril F, Schumann M, Pace A, et al. Multiple endocrine neoplasia type I and the Zollinger-Ellison syndrome. A prospective study of 107 cases and comparison with 1009 cases from the literature. Medicine 2004;83:43–83.
4. Norton JA, Melcher ML, Gibril F, et al. Gastric carcinoid tumors in multiple endocrine neoplasia type I patients with Zollinger-Ellison syndrome can be symptomatic, demonstrate aggressive growth and require surgical treatment. Surgery 2004;136:1267–74.
5. Rusznewski P, Fave GD, Cadiot G, et al. European Neuroendocrine Society Guidelines (ENETS). Well differentiated gastric tumors/carcinomas. Neuroendocrinology 2006;84:158–64.
6. Modlin LM, Lye KD, Kidd A. A five decade analysis of 13,715 carcinoid tumors. Cancer 2003;97:934–59.
7. Tucker ON, Crotty PL, Conlon KC. The management of insulinoma. Br J Surg 2006;93:264–75.
8. Geoghegan JG, Jackson JE, Leno MP, et al. Localization and surgical management of insulinoma. Br J Surg 1994;81:1025–8.
9. Ramage JK, Davies AH, Ardill J, et al. Guidelines for the management of gastroenteropancreatic (including carcinoid) neuroendocrine tumors. Gut 2005;54: 1–16.
10. Kasono K, Hyodo T, Suminaga Y, et al. Contrast-enhanced endoscopic ultrasonography improves the preoperative localization of insulinomas. Endocr J 2002;49:517–22.
11. Gress FG, Barawi M, Kim D, et al. Preoperative localization of neuroendocrine tumor of the pancreas with endoscopic ultrasound-guided fine needle tattooing. Gastrointest Endosc 2002;55:594–7.
12. Gouya H, Vignaux O, Augie J, et al. CT endoscopic sonography and a combined protocol for preoperative evaluation of pancreatic insulinomas. AJR Am J Roentgenol 2003;181:987–92.
13. Gorma B, Charboneau JW, James EM, et al. Benign pancreatic insulinoma, preoperative and intraoperative sonographic localization. AJR Am J Roentgenol 1986;147:929–34.
14. Hirimoto J, Feldstein VA, LaBerge JM, et al. Intraoperative ultrasound and preoperative localization detects all occult insulinomas. Arch Surg 2001;136:1020–6.

15. National Comprehensive Cancer Network, (NCCN): Practice guidelines in oncology. Web 2010. Available at: www.NCCN.org, V.1.2010. Accessed December 17, 2010.

16. Falconi M, Plockinger U, Kwekkeboom DJ, et al. ENETS Guidelines. Well differentiated nonfunctioning pancreatic tumor/carcinoma. Neuroendocrinology 2006;84: 196–211.

17. Sarmiento JM, Heywood G, Rubin J, et al. Surgical treatment of neuroendocrine metastases to the liver: a plea for resection to increase survival. J Am Coll Surg 2003;197(1):29–37.

18. Nilsson O, Cutsem EV, Fave GD, et al. Poorly differentiated tumors of the foregut (gastric, duodenal, pancreatic). ENETS Guidelines. Neuroendocrinology 2006; 84:212–5.

19. Makridis C, Oberg K, Juhlin C, et al. Surgical treatment of midgut carcinoid tumors. World J Surg 1990;14:377–82.

20. Wang YZ, Boudreaux JP, Joseph S, et al. Lymphatic mapping helps to define resection margins for midgut carcinoids. Surgery 2009;146:993–7.

21. Guo Z, Li Q, Wilander E, et al. Clonality analysis of multifocal carcinoid tumors of the small intestine by X chromosome inactivation analysis. J Pathol 2000;190: 76–9.

22. Kobayashi K, Katsuma T, Yoshizawa S, et al. Indications for endoscopic polypectomy for rectal carcinoid tumors and clinical usefulness of endoscopic ultrasound. Dis Colon Rectum 2005;48(2):285–91.

23. Marouin J, Cocha H, Kvols L, et al. Guidelines for the diagnosis and management of carcinoid tumors from the Canadian National Carcinoid Expert Group. Acta Oncol 2004;43:626–36.

24. Boudreaux JP, Putty B, Frey DJ, et al. Surgical treatment of advanced stage carcinoid tumors, lessons learned. Ann Surg 2005;241:839–46.

25. Yuksel M, Eziddin S, Ladwein E. ^{111}In-Pentatreotide and ^{123}I-MIBG for detection and resection of lymph node metastases of a carcinoid not visualized by CT, MRI, or FDG-PET. Ann Nucl Med 2005;19:611–5.

26. Benevento A, Dominioni L, Carcano G, et al. Intraoperative localization of gut endocrine tumors with radiolabeled somatostatin analogues and a gamma-detecting probe. Semin Surg Oncol 1998;15(4):239–44.

27. Fahy BN, Tang LH, Klimstra D, et al. Carcinoid of the rectum and risk stratification (CaRRS): a strategy for preoperative outcome assessment. Ann Surg Oncol 2007;14(2):396–404.

28. Mazzaferro V, Pulvirenti A, Coppa J. Neuroendocrine tumors metastatic to the liver: how to select patients for liver transplant. J Hepatol 2007;47:454–75.

29. Makidis C, Rostad J, Oberg K, et al. Progression of metastasis and symptom improvement from laparotomy in midgut carcinoid tumors. World J Surg 1996; 20:900–90.

30. Que FG, Sarmiento JM, Nagorney D. Hepatic surgery for metastatic gastrointestinal neuroendocrine tumors. Cancer Control 2002;9(1):67–79.

Somatostatin Receptor-Targeted Radionuclide Therapy in Patients with Gastroenteropancreatic Neuroendocrine Tumors

Dik J. Kwekkeboom, MD, PhD[a,*], Wouter W. de Herder, MD, PhD[b], Eric P. Krenning, MD, PhD[a]

KEYWORDS

- Peptide receptor radionuclide therapy • Somatostatin receptor
- Targeted radionuclide therapy
- Gastroenteropancreatic neuroendocrine tumor

Peptide receptor scintigraphy in humans started with the in vivo demonstration of somatostatin receptor-positive tumors in patients using a radioiodinated somatostatin analog.[1] Later, other radiolabeled somatostatin analogs were developed, and two of these subsequently became commercially available. Also, over the past decade positron emission tomography (PET) tracers for somatostatin receptor imaging were developed, and the superiority of the image quality as well as the increased sensitivity in tumor site detection using these newer tracers and PET cameras, has been reported by various research groups.

Starting in the 1990s, attempts at treatment with radiolabeled somatostatin analogs were undertaken in patients with inoperable or metastasized neuroendocrine tumors. Improvements, particularly in the peptides used (with higher receptor affinity) and the radionuclides that were applied (with beta instead of gamma emission), together with precautions to limit the radiation dose to the kidneys and the bone marrow, led to better results with a low percentage of serious adverse events.

The unique features of peptide receptor radionuclide therapy (PRRT) are the high specific binding of the radiolabeled hormone analog to its target, the somatostatin receptor on the tumor cells; the relatively fast clearance of residual radioactivity; and the long retention of the radioactivity in the tumor cells. With all this, PRRT has

[a] Department of Nuclear Medicine, Erasmus Medical Center, 's Gravendijkwal 230, 3015 CE Rotterdam, The Netherlands
[b] Department of Internal Medicine, Erasmus Medical Center, 's Gravendijkwal 230, 3015 CE Rotterdam, The Netherlands
* Corresponding author.
E-mail address: d.j.kwekkeboom@erasmusmc.nl

Endocrinol Metab Clin N Am 40 (2011) 173–185
doi:10.1016/j.ecl.2010.12.003
0889-8529/11/$ – see front matter © 2011 Elsevier Inc. All rights reserved.

great advantages over external beam irradiation or systemic chemotherapy, being more effective on the tumor cell level, and having less systemic side-effects.

This article deals with somatostatin receptor-based radionuclide therapy. The authors attempt to summarize the results obtained with the currently accepted standards or "state of the art" methods.

PRRT WITH [^{111}INDIUM-DIETHYLENETRIAMINE PENTAACETIC ACID^0]OCTREOTIDE

Because at that time no other chelated somatostatin analogs labeled with beta-emitting radionuclides were available, early studies in the mid- to late 1990s used [^{111}Indium (In)-diethylenetriamine pentaacetic acid (DTPA)^0]octreotide for PRRT. Initial studies with high dosages of [^{111}In-DTPA^0]octreotide in patients with metastasized neuroendocrine tumors were encouraging with regard to symptom relief, but partial remissions (PRs) were the exception. Two out of 26 patients with gastroenteropancreatic neuroendocrine tumors (GEPNETs) who were treated with high dosages of [^{111}In-DTPA^0]octreotide, and received a total cumulative dose of more than 550 milliCurie (mCi) (20 GigaBequerel [GBq]), had a decrease in tumor size of in between 25% and 50%, as measured on CT scans.[2] None, however, had PR (**Table 1**). In another study in 27 patients with GEPNETs, PR was reported in 2 out of 26 patients with measurable disease (see **Table 1**).[3] Both series had relatively high numbers of patients who were in a poor clinical condition upon study entry. Also, many had progressive disease when entering the study. The most common toxicity in both series was due to bone marrow suppression. Serious side-effects consisted of leukemia and myelodysplastic syndrome (MDS) in three patients who had been treated with total cumulative doses of less than 3.7 Ci (100 GBq) (and estimated bone marrow radiation doses of more than 3 Gy).[2] One of these patients had also been treated with chemotherapy, which may have contributed to or caused this complication. Anthony and colleagues[3] reported renal insufficiency in one patient that was probably not treatment-related, but due to preexistent retroperitoneal fibrosis. Transient liver toxicity was observed in three patients with widespread liver metastases. Although in both series favorable effects on symptomatology were reported, CT scan-assessed tumor regression was observed only in rare cases. This is not surprising, since ^{111}In-coupled peptides are not ideal for PRRT because of the small particle range and therefore short tissue penetration.

PRRT WITH [^{90}YTTRIUM-DOTA^0, TYROSINE^3]OCTREOTIDE

The next generation of somatostatin receptor-mediated radionuclide therapy used a modified somatostatin analog, tyrosine^3 [Tyr^3]octreotide, with a higher affinity for the somatostatin receptor subtype-2, and a different chelator, 1,4,7,10-Tetraazacyclododecane-1,4,7,10-tetra-acetic acid (DOTA) instead of DTPA, to ensure a more stable binding of the intended beta-emitting radionuclide ^{90}Yttrium (^{90}Y). Using the [^{90}Y-DOTA^0, Tyr^3]octreotide compound (OctreoTher, Novartis, Basel, Switzerland; Onalta, Molecular Insight Pharmaceuticals, Cambridge, MA, USA), different phase-1 and phase-2 PRRT trials have been performed.

Otte and colleagues[4] and Waldherr and colleagues[5,6] (Basel, Switzerland) reported different phase-1 and phase-2 studies in patients with GEPNETs. In their first reports, using a dose escalating scheme of four treatment sessions up to a cumulative dose of 160 mCi (6 GBq)/m^2, at which time renal protection with amino acid infusion was not performed in half of the patients, renal insufficiency developed in 4 out of 29 patients. The overall response rate in patients with GEPNETs who were either treated with 160 mCi (6 GBq)/m^2,[5] or, in a later study, with 200 mCi (7.4GBq)/m^2 in 4 doses,[6] was 24% (see **Table 1**). In a subsequent study, with the same dose of 200 mCi (7.4 GBq)/m^2

Table 1
Tumor responses in patients with GEPNETs, treated with different radiolabeled somatostatin analogs

Center (References)	Tumor Response Ligand	Patient Number	CR	PR	MR	SD	PD	CR + PR
Rotterdam[2]	[^{111}In-DTPA^0]octreotide	26	0	0	5 (19%)	11 (42%)	10 (38%)	0%
New Orleans[3]	[^{111}In-DTPA^0]octreotide	26	0	2 (8%)	NA	21 (81%)	3 (12%)	8%
Basel[5,6]	[^{90}Y-DOTA^0,Tyr^3]octreotide	74	3 (4%)	15 (20%)	NA	48 (65%)	8 (11%)	24%
Basel[7]	[^{90}Y-DOTA^0,Tyr^3]octreotide	33	2 (6%)	9 (27%)	NA	19 (57%)	3 (9%)	33%
Milan[10]	[^{90}Y-DOTA^0,Tyr^3]octreotide	21	0	6 (29%)	NA	11 (52%)	4 (19%)	29%
Multicenter[11]	[^{90}Y-DOTA^0,Tyr^3]octreotide	58	0	5 (9%)	7 (12%)	33 (61%)	10 (19%)	9%
Multicenter[14]	[^{90}Y-DOTA^0,Tyr^3]octreotide	90	0	4 (4%)	NA	63 (70%)	11 (12%)	4%
Rotterdam[22]	[^{177}Lu-DOTA^0,Tyr^3]octreotate	310	5 (2%)	86 (28%)	51 (16%)	107 (35%)	61 (20%)	29%

Response percentages that do not add up to 100% are due to patients with unevaluable disease.

administered in two sessions, complete and partial remissions were found in one third of 36 patients[7] (see **Table 1**). It should be emphasized, however, that this was not a randomized trial comparing two dosing schemes.

Chinol and colleagues[8] (Milan, Italy), described dosimetric and dose-finding studies with [^{90}Y-DOTA^0,Tyr^3]octreotide with and without the administration of kidney protecting agents. No major acute reactions were observed up to an administered dose of 150 mCi (5.6 GBq) per cycle. Reversible grade 3 hematological toxicity was found in 43% of patients injected with 140 mCi (5.2 GBq), which was defined as the maximum tolerated dose per cycle. None of the patients developed acute or delayed kidney failure, although follow-up was short. Partial and complete remissions were reported by the same group in 28% of 87 patients with neuroendocrine tumors.[9]

In a more detailed publication from the same group, Bodei and colleagues[10] report the results of a phase-1 study in 40 patients with somatostatin receptor-positive tumors, of whom 21 had GEPNETs. Cumulative total treatment doses ranged from 160 to 300 mCi (5.9–11.1 GBq), given in two treatment cycles. Six of 21 (29%) patients had tumor regression (see **Table 1**). Median duration of the response was 9 months.

Another study with [^{90}Y-DOTA^0,Tyr^3]octreotide is a multicenter phase-1 study that was performed in Rotterdam, The Netherlands; Brussels, Belgium; and Tampa, FL, USA, in which 58 patients received escalating doses up to 400 mCi (14.8 GBq)/m^2 in four cycles or up to 250 mCi (9.3 GBq)/m^2 single dose, without reaching the maximum tolerated single dose.[11] The cumulative radiation dose to the kidneys was limited to 27 Gy. All received amino acids concomitant with [^{90}Y-DOTA^0,Tyr^3]octreotide for kidney protection. Three patients had dose-limiting toxicity: one liver toxicity, one thrombocytopenia grade 4 (<25*10^9/L), and one MDS. Five out of 58 (9%) patients had PR, and 7 (12%) had a minor response (MR) (25%–50% tumor volume reduction) (see **Table 1**). The median time to progression in the 44 patients who had either stable disease (SD), MR, or PR was 30 months.[12]

Bushnell and colleagues[13] (Iowa City, IA, USA) reported a favorable clinical response as determined by a scoring system that included weight, patient-assessed health score, Karnofsky score, and tumor-related symptoms, in 14 out of 21 patients who were treated with a total cumulative dose of 360 mCi [^{90}Y-DOTA^0,Tyr^3]octreotide in three treatment cycles.

Finally, there is a recent report on a multicenter study in 90 patients with documented disease progression, using a fixed dose of 3*4.4 GBq (3*120 mCi) [^{90}Y-DOTA^0,Tyr^3]octreotide.[14] Four patients had PR (4%), and 63 had SD (70%) (see **Table 1**). Median overall survival in this study was 27 months.

Despite differences in protocols used, complete plus partial remissions in most of the different studies with [^{90}Y-DOTA^0,Tyr^3]octreotide are in the same range, between 10% and 30%, and, therefore, better than those obtained with [^{111}In-DTPA^0]octreotide.

PRRT WITH [^{177}LUTETIUM-DOTA^0,TYR^3]OCTREOTATE

The somatostatin analog [DTPA^0,Tyr^3]octreotate, differs from [DTPA^0,Tyr^3]octreotide only in that the C-terminal threoninol is replaced with threonine. Compared with [DTPA^0,Tyr^3]octreotide, it shows an improved binding to somatostatin receptor positive tissues in animal experiments.[15] Also, its DOTA-coupled counterpart, [DOTA^0,Tyr^3]octreotate, labeled with the beta- and gamma-emitting radionuclide ^{177}Lutetium (^{177}Lu), was reported very successful in terms of tumor regression and animal survival in a rat model.[16] Reubi and colleagues[17] reported a ninefold increase in affinity for the somatostatin receptor subtype 2 for [DOTA^0,Tyr^3]

Table 2
Affinity profiles (IC50) for human sst_1–sst_5 receptors of a series of somatostatin analogs

Peptide	sst_1	sst_2	sst_3	sst_4	sst_5
Somatostatin-28	5.2(0.3)	2.7(0.3)	7.7(0.9)	5.6(0.4)	4.0(0.3)
Octreotide	>10,000	2.0(0.7)	187(55)	>1000	22(6)
DTPA-octreotide	>10,000	12(2)	376(84)	>1000	299(50)
In-DTPA-octreotide	>10,000	22(3.6)	182(13)	>1000	237(52)
DOTA-[Tyr^3]octreotide	>10,000	14(2.6)	880(324)	>1000	393(84)
DOTA-[Tyr^3]octreotate	>10,000	1.5(0.4)	>1000	453(176)	547(160)
DOTA-lanreotide	>10,000	26(3.4)	771(229)	>10,000	73(12)
Y-DOTA-[Tyr^3]octreotide	>10,000	11(1.7)	389(135)	>10,000	114(29)
Y-DOTA-[Tyr^3]octreotate	>10,000	1.6(0.4)	>1000	523(239)	187(50)
Y-DOTA-lanreotide	>10,000	23(5)	290(105)	>10,000	16(3.4)

All values are half maximal inhibitory concentration (IC50) (SEM) in nM.
Data from Reubi JC, Schaer JC, Waser B, et al. Affinity profiles for human somatostatin receptor sst_1-sst_5 of somatostatin radiotracers selected for scintigraphic and radiotherapeutic use. Eur J Nucl Med 2000;27:273–82.

octreotate if compared with [DOTA^0,Tyr^3]octreotide, and a six- to sevenfold increase in affinity for their Yttrium-loaded counterparts (**Table 2**).

In a comparison in patients, it was found that the uptake of radioactivity, expressed as percentage of the injected dose of [^{177}Lu-DOTA^0,Tyr^3]octreotate, was comparable to that after [^{111}In-DTPA^0]octreotide for kidneys, spleen, and liver, but was three- to fourfold higher for four of five tumors.[18] Therefore, [^{177}Lu-DOTA^0,Tyr^3]octreotate potentially represents an important improvement because of the higher absorbed doses that can be achieved to most tumors with about equal doses to potentially dose-limiting organs and because of the lower tissue penetration range of ^{177}Lu if compared with ^{90}Y, which may be especially important for small tumors. Also, when the authors compared the residence time in tumors for [^{177}Lu-DOTA^0,Tyr^3]octreotide and [^{177}Lu-DOTA^0,Tyr^3] octreotate in the same patients in a therapeutic setting, a factor 2.1 in favor of [^{177}Lu-DOTA^0,Tyr^3]octreotate was found.[19] Therefore, the authors think that ^{177}Lu-octreotate is the radiolabeled somatostatin analog of choice when performing PRRT.

Consistent with two earlier reports,[20,21] an analysis of the side-effects and treatment outcome of [^{177}Lu-DOTA^0,Tyr^3]octreotate therapy was described in 504 and 310 patients with neuroendocrine gastroenteropancreatic (GEP) tumors, respectively.[22] In the 504 patients, acute side-effects occurring within 24 hours after the administration of the radiopharmaceutical were: nausea after 25% of administrations, vomiting after 10%, and abdominal discomfort or pain after 10% of administrations. Six patients were hospitalized within 2 days of the administration of the radiopharmaceutical because of hormone-related crises.[23] All patients recovered after adequate care.

Subacute, hematological toxicity, World Health Organization (WHO) toxicity grade 3 or 4, occurred 4 to 8 weeks after 3.6% of administrations, or, expressed patient-based, after at least one of several treatments in 9.5% of patients. Factors that were associated with a higher frequency of hematological toxicity grade 3 or 4 were: age over 70 years at treatment start, a history with previous chemotherapy treatment, creatinine clearance (estimated with Cockroft's formula) less than or equal to 60 mL/min, and the presence of bone metastases. When these factors were tested together in multivariate logistic regression, low creatinine clearance was a significant factor for grades 3 or 4 thrombocytopenia ($P<.001$), as for any hematological grade 3 or 4 toxicity ($P<.001$), whereas a history with previous chemotherapy was less significant in predicting thrombocytopenia ($P<.05$). Creatinine clearance less than or equal to 60 mL/min was significantly more frequent in patients aged 70 or more ($P<.001$, Chi-square test). Temporary hair loss (WHO grade 1; no baldness) occurred in 62% of patients.

Serious delayed toxicities were observed in 9 out of 504 patients. There were two cases of renal insufficiency, both of which were probably unrelated to ^{177}Lu-octreotate treatment. There were three patients with serious liver toxicity, two of which were probably treatment-related. Lastly, MDS occurred in four patients, and was potentially treatment-related in three patients.

Treatment responses according to tumor type at 3 months after the last therapy cycle were analyzed in 310 patients. Overall objective tumor response rate, comprising complete remission (CR), PR, and MR, was 46%. An example is given in **Fig. 1**. Prognostic factors for predicting tumor remission (CR, PR, or MR) as treatment outcome were high uptake on the OctreoScan ($P<.01$), and Karnofsky Performance Score (KPS) less than 70 ($P<.05$).

A small percentage of patients who had either SD or MR at their first two evaluations after therapy, had a further improvement in categorized tumor response at 6 months and 12 months follow-up, occurring in 4% of patients and 5% of patients, respectively.

Median time to progression was 40 months from start of treatment. Median overall survival was 46 months (median follow-up 19 months; 101 deaths). Median disease related survival was greater than 48 months (median follow-up 18 months; 81 deaths). Median progression-free survival was 33 months. The most important factor predicting survival was treatment outcome. Low KPS and liver involvement were very significant negative predicting factors.

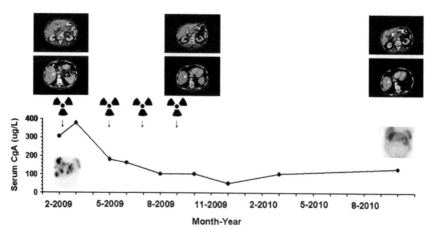

Fig. 1. Serial CT scans (*upper two rows*), and serum chromogranin-A levels (graph) in a 78 years old male patient with well-differentiated metastatic pancreatic neuroendocrine tumor. Arrows point at the pancreatic tumor (*upper row*) and liver metastases (*second row*) that show shrinkage (PR) after PRRT. Four cycles of treatment with 200 mCi [^{177}Lu-DOTA[0],Tyr[3]]octreotate are indicated with symbols and arrows. OctreoScan images of the abdomen (anterior views) at start of therapy and 1 year after completion of therapy, showing dramatic improvement, are projected in the graph.

QUALITY OF LIFE

Another study evaluated the quality of life (QoL) in the authors first 50 Dutch patients with metastatic somatostatin receptor-positive GEP tumors treated with [^{177}Lu-DOTA^0,Tyr^3]octreotate.[24] The patients completed the European Organization for the Research and Treatment of Cancer Quality of Life Questionnaire C30 before therapy and at follow-up visit 6 weeks after the last cycle. A significant improvement in the global health status-QoL scale was observed after therapy with [^{177}Lu-DOTA^0,Tyr^3] octreotate. Furthermore, significant improvement was observed in the role, emotional, and social function scales. The symptom scores for fatigue, insomnia, and pain decreased significantly. Patients with proven tumor regression most frequently had an improvement of QoL domains.

COMPARISON OF TREATMENT WITH [^{177}LU-DOTA^0,TYR^3]OCTREOTATE WITH OTHER PRRT

Treatment with radiolabeled somatostatin analogs is a promising new tool in the management of patients with inoperable or metastasized neuroendocrine tumors. The results that were obtained with [^{90}Y-DOTA^0,Tyr^3]octreotide and [^{177}Lu-DOTA^0,Tyr^3] octreotate are very encouraging, although a direct, randomized comparison between the various treatments is lacking. Also, the reported percentages of tumor remission after [^{90}Y-DOTA^0,Tyr^3]octreotide treatment vary. This may have several causes. The administered doses and dosing schemes differ: some studies use dose-escalating schemes, whereas others use fixed doses. Also, there are several patient and tumor characteristics that determine treatment outcome, such as amount of uptake on the OctreoScan, the estimated total tumor burden, and the extent of liver involvement. Therefore, differences in patient selection may play an important role in determining treatment outcome. Other factors that can have contributed to the different results that were found in the different centers performing trials with the same compounds, may be differences in tumor response criteria, and centralized versus decentralized follow-up CT scoring.

From our analysis in patients treated with [^{177}Lu-DOTA^0,Tyr^3]octreotate, the authors learned that the two significant factors predicting favorable treatment outcome were high patient performance score and high uptake on the pretreatment OctreoScan. It is obvious that different studies can only be reliably compared if stratification for these factors is applied. From the published data, such stratified comparison cannot be performed. Also, to establish which treatment scheme and which radiolabeled somatostatin analogs or combination of analogs is optimal, randomized trials are needed.

Chelated Lanreotide, another somatostatin analog, labeled with ^{111}In for diagnostic purposes and with ^{90}Y for therapeutic use, has been advocated because of its better binding than [^{111}In-DTPA^0]octreotide to the somatostatin receptor subtypes 3 and 4.[25] This claim can be questioned.[17] Although this compound has been used to treat patients with GEP tumors, it shows poorer affinity than radiolabeled [DOTA^0, Tyr^3] octreotide or octreotate for the somatostatin receptor subtype-2, which is predominantly overexpressed in GEP tumors (see **Table 2**).[17]

Wehrmann and colleagues[26] compared the biodistribution of [^{177}Lu-DOTA^0]octreotate and [^{177}Lu-DOTA^0]-1-Nal^3-octreotide in patients, and concluded that tumor uptake and absorbed dose were comparable for both radioligands, whereas wholebody retention was lower for [^{177}Lu-DOTA^0]octreotate, and therefore the authors advocate the use of [^{177}Lu-DOTA^0]octreotate.

Preliminary data have been presented from a study using ^{90}Y-labelled [DOTA^0,Tyr^3] octreotate.[27,28] However, the treatment protocols vary and the way of response evaluation was not clearly defined. The reported results were an objective response rate

(PR) of 37% (28/75) and a stabilization of the disease in 39 out of 75 patients (52%). In the same study the intra-arterial use of [^{90}Y-DOTA^0,Tyr^3]octreotate in five patients was described. However, no detailed results for this application were provided. An important issue is that, to date, reliable dosimetry for [^{90}Y-DOTA^0,Tyr^3]octreotate is lacking.

COMPARISON OF SURVIVAL DATA

Because the treatment with [^{177}Lu-DOTA^0,Tyr^3]octreotate is still open for new patients, and median follow-up in relation to survival is relatively short, the authors also analyzed the local, Dutch patients separately with subgroups that had longer follow-up. The results from these analyses point out that both overall and disease-specific survival time are consistently at or above 48 months. These numbers compare favorably to those reported in the literature. Clancy and colleagues[29] reported a significantly shorter survival in patients with elevated serum alkaline phosphatase concentrations at referral compared with those who had normal values. The authors found the same, but in patients treated with ^{177}Lu-octreotate, survival from referral was longer. Even more striking was the difference in median overall survival from diagnosis: 128 months versus 72 months, despite the fact that in this group mean serum alkaline phosphatase concentration was higher, indicating more advanced liver involvement and worse prognosis. Comparing survival data in this group, either from time of diagnosis or from time of referral, with data from different epidemiologic studies or studies pertaining to a specific intervention, and limiting the data to similar subgroups of patients, the authors found a benefit in overall survival for patients treated with ^{177}Lu-octreotate, which ranged from 40 to 72 months from diagnosis.[29–32] The authors are aware that comparisons with historical controls should be interpreted with caution, but we also think that such a consistent difference with many other reports in similar patient groups cannot be ignored, and is most probably caused by a real difference in survival.

TIMING OF TREATMENT

In patients treated with [^{177}Lu-DOTA^0,Tyr^3]octreotate, median overall survival (OS) was shorter in patients having a poor performance score and those having extensive liver involvement. This implies that treatment with [^{177}Lu-DOTA^0,Tyr^3]octreotate should preferably be started early in the disease evolution. Because GEPNETs can be clinically stable for years, however, it is, in the authors' opinion, good clinical practice to wait for signs of disease progression if the tumor load is moderate. Such signs should not be restricted to CT-assessed tumor growth, but also include rises in serum tumor markers, increase in symptoms, or involuntary weight loss. In patients with very limited tumor load and in whom cure is potentially possible, treatment should be initiated without further delay, and the same holds true for patients with extensive tumor load, hepatomegaly, or those with significant weight loss, when waiting for formally assessed tumor progression would place these patients in an unfavourable starting position for treatment or would even qualify them as ineligible.

RETREATMENT

Recently, data on retreatment with two cycles of 7.4 GBq (200 mCi) of [^{177}Lu-DOTA^0, Tyr^3]octreotate in 33 patients was reported.[33] Twenty-eight of these had had a radiological response (at least MR) after the regular treatment with usually four cycles of [^{177}Lu-DOTA^0,Tyr^3]octreotate, and five had experienced a significant clinical improvement. All had CT-assessed tumor progression before the start of retreatment. In seven patients (24%) renewed tumor size reduction was observed, and seven (24%) had SD at follow-up. No major side-effects were observed during a median follow-up of 16 months. It was concluded that in the absence of treatment alternatives this salvage therapy is safe and can be effective in selected patients.

OPTIONS TO IMPROVE PRRT

From animal experiments, it can be inferred that ^{90}Y-labeled somatostatin analogs may be more effective for larger tumors, whereas ^{177}Lu-labeled somatostatin analogs may be more effective for smaller tumors, but their combination may be the most effective.[34] Therefore, apart from comparisons between radiolabeled octreotate and octreotide, and between somatostatin analogs labeled with ^{90}Y or ^{177}Lu, PRRT with combinations of [90]Y- and ^{177}Lu-labeled analogs should also be evaluated.

Future directions to improve this therapy may also include the use of radiosensitizing chemotherapeutical agents. Chemosensitization with 5-fluorouracil (5-FU) in combination with ^{90}Y-labeled antibody radioimmunotherapy is feasible and safe.[35] Also, chemosensitization with 5-FU, combined with [^{111}In-DTPA]octreotide treatment resulted in symptomatic response in 71% of patients with neuroendocrine tumors,[36] whereas other studies using only [^{111}In-DTPA]octreotide treatment reported such responses in lower percentages.[2,3] Numerous trials to the effects of combined chemotherapy and (fractionated) external beam radiotherapy have been performed. In many of these, 5-FU was used. More recent trials used the prodrug of 5-FU, capecitabine, which has the advantage of oral administration. Also with the combination of radiotherapy and capecitabine, an increased efficacy in terms of tumor growth control was reported if compared with radiotherapy as single treatment modality.[37] If capecitabine is used in relatively low doses (1600–2000 mg/m^2/day), grade 3 hematologic or other toxicity is rare.[37,38] For these reasons, after proving the safety of the combined therapy,[39] the authors started a randomized multicenter trial comparing treatment with ^{177}Lu-octreotate with and without capecitabine in patients with GEPNETs.

Also, attempts to improve the results of this type of therapy may focus on further reducing the radiation absorbed dose to normal tissues and organs, like kidneys and bone marrow, or at increasing the receptor density on the tumors, for instance via receptor upregulation. Both strategies may increase the therapeutic window.

Intra-arterial treatment in selected patients with a predominant tumor load in the liver has been reported to be safe and effective. McStay and colleagues,[40] using [^{90}Y-DOTA[0],Tyr[3]]lanreotide for hepatic artery administration (mostly 2 times 1 GBq) in 23 patients, reported PR in 3 and SD in 12. However, two of the three patients with PR had also had concomitant embolization. Clinical improvement and a decrease of serum tumor markers was observed in 60% of patients. Limouris and colleagues,[41] using [^{111}In-DTPA[0]]octreotide, 6.3 GBq per injection and with a maximum of 12 injections per patient, reported CR and PR in 9 of 17 patients. Lastly, Kratochwil and colleagues,[42] found a fourfold higher uptake after intra-arterial administration of [^{68}Ga-DOTA[0],Tyr[3]] octreotide if compared with intravenous administration in the same patients. Therefore, in selected cases this type of administration seems advantageous.

Lastly, individualized dosimetry for each patient is desirable. Kidney-absorbed radiation dose varies widely between patients treated with [^{177}Lu-DOTA[0],Tyr[3]] octreotate.[18] Based on calculations performed in six patients with a limited tumor load, the authors initially found that the radiation dose to the bone marrow does not vary much between patients and can be estimated at a mean of 260 mGy/100 mCi (range 200–290 mGy/100 mCi). Therefore, allowing a maximum of 2 Gy for the absorbed dose to the bone marrow, the resulting cumulative dose that can be given was fixed at 800 mCi.[18] A later study in 15 patients, however, demonstrated that the dose to the bone marrow also shows variability between patients, and that in most patients this dose is lower than 260 mGy/100 mCi.[43] Also, in 53% of 334 patients in whom kidney dosimetry was performed, the upper limit of 23 Gy for the kidney-absorbed dose would be reached with a total cumulative administered dose of 900 mCi or more (Dik J. Kwekkeboom, MD, PhD, unpublished data, 2008). This means that with fixed dose regimens that show relatively few side-effects, a proportion of patients is undertreated. This is also clear from a study by Valkema and colleagues,[44] who reported a relatively mild loss in creatinine clearance in patients treated with [^{177}Lu-DOTA^0,Tyr^3]octreotate (median 3.8% per year), and a higher loss in patients treated with [^{90}Y-DOTA^0,Tyr^3]octreotide (median 7.3% per year). More important, however, is the observation from this study that a creatinine clearance loss of more than 25% per year is required to develop end-stage renal disease within 5 years. This was found in only 1 of 37 patients treated with [^{177}Lu-DOTA^0,Tyr^3]octreotate. Also, hypertension and diabetes were found to be risk factors for developing kidney function loss after PRRT.[44,45] If these comorbidities are present, one could consider to lower the upper limit for the absorbed dose to the kidneys, as suggested by Bodei and colleagues.[45] Lastly, both the upper limits for the absorbed dose to the kidneys that are accepted in PRRT and the calculation methods that are used for dosimetry may be questioned. The accepted upper limit for the kidney dose of 23 Gy is derived from experience in external beam irradiation, which uses much higher dose rates than PRRT. Also, the heterogeneous distribution of radioactivity in the kidneys after PRRT invalidates the Medical Internal Radiation DOSE-based dosimetry models for low-energy emitting radionuclides like ^{177}Lu.[46] With the limitations of the currently available methods for dosimetry after PRRT, however, individual dosimetry for the absorbed doses to both bone marrow and kidneys seems desirable, because of the huge variation between patients. Tailored dosimetry, currently based on urine collection, repeated imaging and blood sampling after therapy, is time-consuming. However, such an individualized calculation of the maximum cumulative doses that can be given to a certain patient may, in a considerable number of the patients, result in higher cumulative doses that can safely be administered.

SUMMARY

Treatment with radiolabeled somatostatin analogs is a promising new tool in the management of patients with inoperable or metastasized neuroendocrine tumors. Symptomatic improvement may occur with all ^{111}In, ^{90}Y, or ^{177}Lu-labeled somatostatin analogs that have been used for PRRT. The results that were obtained with [^{90}Y-DOTA^0, Tyr^3]octreotide and [^{177}Lu-DOTA^0,Tyr^3]octreotate are very encouraging in terms of tumor regression. Also, if kidney protective agents are used, the side-effects of this therapy are few and mild, and the duration of the therapy response for both radiopharmaceuticals is more than 30 months. The patients' self-assessed quality of life increases significantly after treatment with [^{177}Lu-DOTA^0,Tyr^3]octreotate. Lastly, compared with historical controls, there is a benefit in overall survival of several years from time of diagnosis in patients treated with [^{177}Lu-DOTA^0,Tyr^3]octreotate. These data compare favorably with the limited number of alternative treatment approaches. If more widespread use of PRRT can be guaranteed, such therapy may well become the therapy of first choice in patients with metastasized or inoperable GEPNETs.

REFERENCES

1. Krenning EP, Bakker WH, Breeman WA, et al. Localization of endocrine related tumors with radioiodinated analogue of somatostatin. Lancet 1989;1:242–5.

2. Valkema R, de Jong M, Bakker WH, et al. Phase I study of peptide receptor radio-nuclide therap1y with [^{111}In-DTPA^0]Octreotide: the Rotterdam experience. Semin Nucl Med 2002;32:110–22.

3. Anthony LB, Woltering EA, Espanan GD, et al. Indium-111-pentetreotide prolongs survival in gastroenteropancreatic malignancies. Semin Nucl Med 2002;32: 123–32.

4. Otte A, Herrmann R, Heppeler A, et al. Yttrium-90 DOTATOC: first clinical results. Eur J Nucl Med 1999;26:1439–47.

5. Waldherr C, Pless M, Maecke HR, et al. The clinical value of [^{90}Y-DOTA]-D-Phe^1-Tyr^3-octreotide (^{90}Y-DOTATOC) in the treatment of neuroendocrine tumours: a clinical phase II study. Ann Oncol 2001;12:941–5.

6. Waldherr C, Pless M, Maecke HR, et al. Tumor response and clinical benefit in neuroendocrine tumors after 7.4 GBq (90)Y-DOTATOC. J Nucl Med 2002;43: 610–6.

7. Waldherr C, Schumacher T, Maecke HR, et al. Does tumor response depend on the number of treatment sessions at constant injected dose using 90Yttrium-DOTATOC in neuroendocrine tumors? [abstract]. Eur J Nucl Med 2002; 29(Suppl 1):S100.

8. Chinol M, Bodei L, Cremonesi M, et al. Receptor-mediated radiotherapy with Y-DOTA-DPhe-Tyr-octreotide: the experience of the European Institute of Oncology group. Semin Nucl Med 2002;32:141–7.

9. Paganelli G, Bodei L, Handkiewicz Junak D, et al. 90Y-DOTA-D-Phe1-Tyr3-octreo-tide in therapy of neuroendocrine malignancies. Biopolymers 2002;66:393–8.

10. Bodei L, Cremonesi M, Zoboli S, et al. Receptor-mediated radionuclide therapy with ^{90}Y-DOTATOC in association with amino acid infusion: a phase I study. Eur J Nucl Med Mol Imaging 2003;30:207–16.

11. Valkema R, Pauwels S, Kvols LK, et al. Survival and response after peptide receptor radionuclide therapy with [90Y-DOTA0, Tyr3]octreotide in patients with advanced gastroenteropancreatic neuroendocrine tumors. Semin Nucl Med 2006;36:147–56.

12. Valkema R, Pauwels S, Kvols L, et al. Long-term follow-up of a phase 1 study of peptide receptor radionuclide therapy (PRRT) with [90Y-DOTA0, Tyr3]octreotide in patients with somatostatin receptor positive tumours [abstract]. Eur J Nucl Med Mol Imaging 2003;30(Suppl 2):S232.

13. Bushnell D, O'Dorisio T, Menda Y, et al. Evaluating the clinical effectiveness of ^{90}Y-SMT 487 in patients with neuroendocrine tumors. J Nucl Med 2003;44: 1556–60.

14. Bushnell DL Jr, O'Dorisio TM, O'Dorisio MS, et al. 90Y-Edotreotide for metastatic carcinoid refractory to octreotide. J Clin Oncol 2010;28:1652–9.

15. De Jong M, Breeman WA, Bakker WH, et al. Comparison of (111)In-labeled somatostatin analogues for tumor scintigraphy and radionuclide therapy. Cancer Res 1998;58:437–41.

16. Erion JL, Bugaj JE, Schmidt MA, et al. High radiotherapeutic efficacy of [Lu-177]-DOTA-Y(3)-octreotate in a rat tumor model [abstract]. J Nucl Med 1999; 40(Suppl):223P.

17. Reubi JC, Schaer JC, Waser B, et al. Affinity profiles for human somatostatin receptor sst1-sst5 of somatostatin radiotracers selected for scintigraphic and radiotherapeutic use. Eur J Nucl Med 2000;27:273–82.

18. Kwekkeboom DJ, Bakker WH, Kooij PP, et al. [177Lu-DOTA0Tyr3]octreotate: comparison with [111In-DTPA0]octreotide in patients. Eur J Nucl Med 2001;28: 1319–25.

19. Esser JP, Krenning EP, Teunissen JJ, et al. Comparison of [(177)Lu-DOTA(0), Tyr(3)]octreotate and [(177)Lu-DOTA(0), Tyr(3)]octreotide: which peptide is preferable for PRRT? Eur J Nucl Med Mol Imaging 2006;33:1346–51.

20. Kwekkeboom DJ, Bakker WH, Kam BL, et al. Treatment of patients with gastro-entero-pancreatic (GEP) tumours with the novel radiolabeled somatostatin analogue [177Lu-DOTA^0, Tyr^3]octreotate. Eur J Nucl Med Mol Imaging 2003;30:417–22.

21. Kwekkeboom DJ, Teunissen JJ, Bakker WH, et al. Treatment with the radiolabeled somatostatin analogue [^{177}Lu-DOTA^0, Tyr^3]octreotate in patients with gastro-entero-pancreatic (GEP) tumors. J Clin Oncol 2005;23:2754–62.

22. Kwekkeboom DJ, de Herder WW, Kam BL, et al. Treatment with the radiolabeled somatostatin analog [177Lu-DOTA0, Tyr3]octreotate: toxicity, efficacy, and survival. J Clin Oncol 2008;26:2124–30.

23. De Keizer B, van Aken MO, Feelders RA, et al. Hormonal crises following receptor radionuclide therapy with the radiolabeled somatostatin analogue [177Lu-DOTA0, Tyr3]octreotate. Eur J Nucl Med Mol Imaging 2008;35:749–55.

24. Teunissen JJ, Kwekkeboom DJ, Krenning EP. Quality of life in patients with gastroenteropancreatic tumors treated with [177Lu-DOTA0, Tyr3]octreotate. J Clin Oncol 2004;22:2724–9.

25. Virgolini I, Britton K, Buscombe J, et al. ^{111}In- and ^{90}Y-DOTA-Lanreotide: results and implications of the MAURITIUS trial. Semin Nucl Med 2002;32:148–55.

26. Wehrmann C, Senftleben S, Zachert C, et al. Results of individual patient dosimetry in peptide receptor radionuclide therapy with 177Lu DOTA-TATE and 177Lu DOTA-NOC. Cancer Biother Radiopharm 2007;22:406–16.

27. Baum RP, Soldner J, Schmucking M, et al. Peptidrezeptorvermittelte Radiotherapie (PRRT) neuroendokriner Tumoren Klinischen Indikationen und Erfahrung mit 90Yttrium-markierten Somatostatinanaloga. Der Onkologe 2004;10:1098–110 [in German].

28. Baum RP, Soldner J, Schmucking M, et al. Intravenous and intra-arterial peptide receptor radionuclide therapy (PRRT) using Y-90-DOTA-Tyr3-octreotate (Y-90-DOTA-TATE) in patients with metastatic neuroendocrine tumors [abstract]. Eur J Nucl Med 2004;31(Suppl 2):S238.

29. Clancy TE, Sengupta TP, Paulus J, et al. Alkaline phosphatase predicts survival in patients with metastatic neuroendocrine tumors. Dig Dis Sci 2006;51:877–84.

30. Janson ET, Holmberg L, Stridsberg M, et al. Carcinoid tumors: analysis of prognostic factors and survival in 301 patients from a referral center. Ann Oncol 1997; 8:685–90.

31. Quaedvlieg PF, Visser O, Lamers CB, et al. Epidemiology and survival in patients with carcinoid disease in The Netherlands. An epidemiological study with 2391 patients. Ann Oncol 2001;12:1295–300.

32. Mazzaglia PJ, Berber E, Milas M, et al. Laparoscopic radiofrequency ablation of neuroendocrine liver metastases: a 10-year experience evaluating predictors of survival. Surgery 2007;142:10–9.

33. Van Essen M, Krenning EP, Kam BL, et al. Salvage therapy with (177)Lu-octreotate in patients with bronchial and gastroenteropancreatic neuroendocrine tumors. J Nucl Med 2010;51:383–90.

34. De Jong M, Valkema R, Jamar F, et al. Somatostatin receptor-targeted radionuclide therapy of tumors: preclinical and clinical findings. Semin Nucl Med 2002; 32:133–40.

35. Wong JY, Shibata S, Williams LE, et al. A Phase I trial of 90Y-anti-carcinoembryonic antigen chimeric T84.66 radioimmunotherapy with 5-fluorouracil in patients with metastatic colorectal cancer. Clin Cancer Res 2003;9:5842–52.

36. Kong G, Lau E, Ramdave S, et al. High-dose In-111 octreotide therapy in combination with radiosensitizing 5-FU chemotherapy for treatment of SSR-expressing neuroendocrine tumors [abstract]. J Nucl Med 2005;46(Suppl 2):151P.
37. Rich TA, Shepard RC, Mosley ST. Four decades of continuing innovation with fluorouracil: current and future approaches to fluorouracil chemoradiation therapy. J Clin Oncol 2004;22:2214–32.
38. Dunst J, Reese T, Sutter T, et al. Phase I trial evaluating the concurrent combination of radiotherapy and capecitabine in rectal cancer. J Clin Oncol 2002;20: 3983–91.
39. Van Essen M, Krenning EP, Kam BL, et al. Report on short-term side effects of treatments with (177)Lu-octreotate in combination with capecitabine in seven patients with gastroenteropancreatic neuroendocrine tumours. Eur J Nucl Med Mol Imaging 2008;35:743–8.
40. McStay MK, Maudgil D, Williams M, et al. Large-volume liver metastases from neuroendocrine tumors: hepatic intraarterial 90Y-DOTA-lanreotide as effective palliative therapy. Radiology 2005;237:718–26.
41. Limouris GS, Chatziioannou A, Kontogeorgakos D, et al. Selective hepatic arterial infusion of In-111-DTPA-Phe1-octreotide in neuroendocrine liver metastases. Eur J Nucl Med Mol Imaging 2008;35:1827–37.
42. Kratochwil C, Giesel FL, López-Benítez R, et al. Intraindividual comparison of selective arterial versus venous 68Ga-DOTATOC PET/CT in patients with gastro-enteropancreatic neuroendocrine tumors. Clin Cancer Res 2010;16:2899–905.
43. Förrer F, Krenning EP, Kooij PP, et al. Bone marrow dosimetry in peptide receptor radionuclide therapy with [(177)Lu-DOTA(0), Tyr(3)]octreotate. Eur J Nucl Med Mol Imaging 2009;36:1138–46.
44. Valkema R, Pauwels SA, Kvols LK, et al. Long-term follow-up of renal function after peptide receptor radiation therapy with (90)Y-DOTA(0), Tyr(3)-octreotide and (177)Lu-DOTA(0), Tyr(3)-octreotate. J Nucl Med 2005;46(Suppl 1):83S–91S.
45. Bodei L, Cremonesi M, Ferrari M, et al. Long-term evaluation of renal toxicity after peptide receptor radionuclide therapy with 90Y-DOTATOC and 177Lu-DOTA-TATE: the role of associated risk factors. Eur J Nucl Med Mol Imaging 2008;35: 1847–56.
46. Konijnenberg M, Melis M, Valkema R, et al. Radiation dose distribution in human kidneys by octreotides in peptide receptor radionuclide therapy. J Nucl Med 2007;48:134–42.

Targeted Radiotherapy with Radiolabeled Somatostatin Analogs

Guillaume Nicolas, MD, Giampiero Giovacchini, MD, PhD, Jan Müller-Brand, MD, Flavio Forrer, MD, PhD*

KEYWORDS

- Neuroendocrine tumor • Carcinoid tumor
- Somatostatin receptor • Targeted radiopeptide therapy
- Internal radiotherapy • Peptide receptor radionuclide therapy

Five somatostatin receptor subtypes (sst) are known to date (sst_{1-5}). Most neuroendocrine tumors (NETs) feature a strong overexpression of these receptors, mainly of subtype 2 (sst_2). The density of these receptors is vastly higher than on nontumor tissues.[1,2] Therefore, sst are attractive targets for delivery of radioactivity via radiolabeled somatostatin analogs. Although long-lasting somatostatin analogs prolong time to progression and induce tumor stabilization in up to 50% of the patients with functionally active and inactive well-differentiated metastatic midgut NETs,[3–10] little is currently known about the functional role of sst.[11] The sst_2 has been shown to internalize into the cell in a fast, efficient, and reversible manner after specific binding of a receptor agonist.[12,13] This molecular process is likely to be responsible for the high and long-lasting uptake of radioactivity in the target cell after binding of the radiolabeled somatostatin analog.[14]

Introduced in the late 1980s, [^{111}In-DTPA^0]-octreotide (Octreoscan), the first available radiolabeled somatostatin analog, rapidly became the gold standard for diagnosis and staging of sst-positive NETs.[15,16] Although numerous peptide-based tracers targeting sst have been developed over the past decade,[17] Octreoscan along with Neotect are still the only 2 radiopeptide tracers on the market approved by the Food and Drug Administration, since 1994 and 1999, respectively. The chelator of Octreoscan (DTPA: diethylenetriaminepentaacetic acid) is not suitable for the β^--emitting radionuclides used for therapy, such as ^{90}Y and ^{177}Lu or for the β^+-emitting

Department of Radiology and Nuclear Medicine, University Hospital Basel, 4031 Basel, Switzerland
* Corresponding author.
E-mail address: forrerf@uhbs.ch

Endocrinol Metab Clin N Am 40 (2011) 187–204
doi:10.1016/j.ecl.2010.12.006
0889-8529/11/$ – see front matter © 2011 Elsevier Inc. All rights reserved.

endo.theclinics.com

radionuclides, (eg, ^{68}Ga and ^{64}Cu) for positron emission tomography (PET). Nowadays, different somatostatin analogs[17,18] are available not only for therapeutic purposes but also when labeled with β[+]-emitters for tumor imaging with integrated PET/CT scanners. The PET/CT technology provides a highly valuable combination of physiologic and anatomic information[19–23] and has been shown to impact significantly on the patient's management.[24] Consequently, diagnostic scans with radiolabeled somatostatin analogs are not only used for staging of patients, but also to identify suitable candidates for targeted radiopeptide therapy (TRT) and for the monitoring of the therapy.[25,26]

[111]In-octreotide, in addition to diagnostic purposes, has also been used for systemic therapy in high dosages in pilot trials.[27–29] Although promising results on tumor-related symptoms were obtained, objective tumor response was rarely achieved. It appears that ^{111}In is not a suitable radionuclide for receptor-mediated radionuclide therapy. The Auger electrons, which are emitted and expected to have a therapeutic effect, probably fail to reach and intercalate within the DNA helix.[30] Moreover, owing to their limited energy and range in tissues they do not cause cross-fire effect.[31] Later on, analogs with higher receptor affinity than octreotide, such as Tyr[3]-octreotide (TOC), Tyr[3]-octreotate (TATE), and lanreotide were developed and conjugated with the chelator 1,4,7,10-tetraazacyclododecane-1,4,7,10-tetraacetic acid (DOTA). These conjugates (DOTATOC, DOTATATE, and DOTA-lanreotide) allowed thermodynamically and kinetically stable chelation of the pure, high-energy β[−]-emitter ^{90}Y and of the intermediate energy β[−]-emitter [177]Lu. Currently, various somatostatin analogs labeled with these two radionuclides and different treatment protocols are used in numerous centers, mainly across Europe. In this article, a summary of the results yielded in clinical studies, as well as new approaches combining different radionuclides and analogs, are discussed.

RADIONUCLIDES USED IN TRT

Clinical trials evidenced large patient variability regarding target and nontarget uptake, individual differences in tumor mass, and inhomogeneity of uptake within tumor sites. These observations give rational explanations to the use of radionuclides with different physical properties. Over the past decade, the most frequently used radionuclides in TRT with somatostatin analogs were ^{111}In, ^{90}Y, and [177]Lu (Table 1). Their different physical characteristics influence the effects of the therapy (ie, different particles are emitted at different energies resulting in various tissue penetration ranges). [90]Y, a pure β[−]-emitter, emits electrons with a relatively high energy (E_{max} = 2.28 MeV), resulting in a tissue penetration range of up to 12 mm. Therefore, a pronounced "cross-fire effect" is found, which is beneficial in target organs because it allows irradiating tumor cells that are not directly targeted by

Table 1
Nuclear properties of the most commonly radionuclides used in targeted radiopeptide therapy

Isotope	Half-Life (days)	Decay Mode	E [keV]	Range (max)
[111]In	2.81	Auger	0.5–25	10 μm
		γ	171 (90%), 247 (94%)	
[90]Y	2.67	β[−]	2270 (max)/930 (mean) (100%)	12 mm
[177]Lu	6.71	β[−]	497 (max)/150 (mean) (79%)	1.5 mm
		γ	208 (11%), 113 (6%)	

the radiopharmaceutical. On the other hand, the long range of the ^{90}Y β^- particles appears to be less favorable concerning kidney toxicity.[32] ^{177}Lu emits intermediate-energy beta-particles (E_{max} = 0.5 MeV), resulting in tissue penetration range of up to 2 mm. In addition, ^{177}Lu has 2 gamma peaks, at 113 and 208 keV, which makes it suitable for imaging with a gamma camera and can be used for posttherapeutic dosimetry.[33–35]

Another difference between these radionuclides is their physical half-life. The half-lives of ^{111}In and ^{90}Y are almost identical with 67.4 and 64.1 hours respectively, whereas for ^{177}Lu it is more than double (6.7 days). Although the influence of the physical half-life is not fully understood yet, it is very likely that it influences the therapeutic results as well as the secondary effects.

When planning therapy with radiopeptides, dosimetry should be considered for the specific radiolabeled somatostatin analog used, as the peptide significantly influences the biokinetics. For a given peptide, to assess whether ^{177}Lu or ^{90}Y will offer better results, several radiobiological considerations should be taken into account.

DOSIMETRIC CONSIDERATIONS

The clinical impact of dosimetric calculations is debated. Clinical experience has shown that acute or delayed toxicity are rare but potentially serious. Laboratory parameters and/or clinical factors may be useful to identify patients at risk for toxicity[36]; however, the variability of adsorbed dose among patients is high and intersubject variability is much higher than intrasubject variability. Thus, if one could identify through pretherapeutic dosimetric measurements the intensity of tracer uptake in the different organs, it could be possible to personalize therapy. This would allow maximizing the therapeutic dose in patients with low risk for toxicity and reducing the dose in patients with high risk for toxicity. For these reasons, dosimetry has been considered useful for a successful therapy in all patients.

However, there is a poor relationship between the amount of adsorbed dose and clinical response with the current dosimetric means. In a preliminary report it was found that the median adsorbed dose was higher in responsive tumors than in nonresponsive tumors (230 Gy vs 40 Gy, respectively),[37] whereas a linear relationship between adsorbed dose and development of toxicity has not been observed. Many factors are important in determining organ toxicity, such as organ volume,[37] uniformity of uptake in the organ,[38] specific tissue radiosensitivity, dose rate, and fractionation, as well as associated risk factors[36] along with the physical characteristics of the tracer. These factors are well exemplified by kidney dosimetry. Applying the linear quadratic model to TRT with ^{90}Y, a correlation between the kidneys' biologic effective dose (BED) and renal toxicity has been found.[39,40]

The most commonly used ^{90}Y- and ^{177}Lu-labeled somatostatin analogs concord on some essential aspects[30]: (1) the pharmacokinetics data show very fast blood clearance and urinary elimination; (2) nontarget organs such as the spleen, kidneys, and liver receive the highest absorbed dose; (3) kidneys and bone marrow are the major dose-limiting organs for this treatment; and (4) there is wide intrapatient variability of the absorbed dose. However, because of the physical characteristics of the radionuclides, the absorbed doses with ^{90}Y-radiolabeled analogs are higher than those obtained with ^{177}Lu-radiolabeled peptides, for the same injected activity.

Although a promising example of Bremstrahlung images have recently been published with single-photon emission computed tomography (SPECT)/CT[41] and PET/CT,[42,43] quantification with ^{90}Y is considered to be difficult. To assess the biodistribution and quantify uptake for each ^{90}Y-labeled analog, alternative options have been considered using the similar half-life and pharmacologic behavior of the corresponding ^{111}In-radiolabeled somatostatin analogs (eg, ^{111}In-DOTATOC, ^{111}In-DOTATATE). Reliable dosimetry for ^{90}Y-DOTATATE is lacking and is currently extrapolated from ^{90}Y-DOTATOC. A study performed by Cremonesi and colleagues[44] showed that ratios of absorbed dose between the one delivered by the ^{90}Y-labeled analog and the one delivered by the ^{177}Lu counterpart was somehow constantly close to a factor of 4 for the nontarget organs, while highly variable in tumors (typically ranging from 2.0 to 4.5). Forrer and colleagues[45] showed that use of ^{111}In-DOTATOC and ^{111}In-DOTATATE as surrogate for the [90]Y- and ^{177}Lu-radiolabeled somatostatin analogs tumor-to-kidney dose ratios were advantageous with DOTATOC (5.91 ± 5.48) versus DOTATATE (4.32 ± 4.36). On the contrary, the residence time of radioactivity in the tumors evaluated by Esser and colleagues[46] was about twice as long with ^{177}Lu-DOTATATE than with ^{177}Lu-DOTATOC.

CLINICAL STUDIES

A number of Phase I and II therapy studies using different somatostatin analogs and different radionuclides have been published to date. The numerous variables, including different injected activity and dosing schemes, as well as the differences in the recruited population to be treated make it nearly impossible to properly compare the results of these studies. For example, the administered activity and the number of treatment cycles differ considerably; some studies use dose-escalating schemes, whereas others use fixed doses. Besides, there are several patient and tumor characteristics that determine treatment outcome, such as intensity of uptake on the ^{111}In-octreotide scintigraphy, the total tumor burden, and the extent of liver involvement.[47]

A number of studies using ^{90}Y-DOTATOC, ^{90}Y-DOTA-lanreotide, and ^{90}Y-DOTATATE,[48–55] as well as ^{177}Lu-DOTATATE and ^{177}Lu-DOTATOC, alone or in combination, have been published.[33,35,56] A short summary of clinical data on TRT, with these radiolabeled somatostatin analogs, is given in **Table 2**.

STUDIES USING [111]IN-OCTREOTIDE

[111]In-octreotide, developed initially for diagnosis,[15] was the first radiolabeled somatostatin analog used for TRT in cumulated injected activities ranging from 3.1 to 160 GBq.[29,57–59] Although treatment with high doses often led to symptomatic relief, tumor shrinkage was rarely achieved and the number of objective responses was low (see **Table 2**). Nevertheless, these results were encouraging, especially in the context of the results that can be achieved with other therapy modalities like chemotherapy.[60] Nonetheless, it appeared that the antitumor effect of ^{111}In-octreotide is not ideal for macroscopic tumors.

STUDIES USING ^{90}Y-DOTATOC, ^{90}Y-DOTA-LANREOTIDE, AND ^{90}Y-DOTATATE

The first radiolabeled somatostatin analog used for TRT that was labeled with ^{90}Y was ^{90}Y-DOTATOC. The first clinical results were reported at the end of the 1990s from the group at Basel University.[48,61] On a limited number of patients they showed an objective response rate (OR) of 6%, defined as complete remission (CR) and partial remission (PR). In the following studies, patients were treated with cumulated injected activities of 6.0 or 7.4 GBq/m^2 ^{90}Y-DOTATOC in 4 cycles. The ORs were 27% and 22%, respectively.[49,50] Similar results were found in a more extensive study that included 116 patients who were treated with the same activities (an OR of 27% was found).[51]

The research group from the European Cancer Institute in Milan used a higher range of cumulated injected activity (5.9 to 11.0 GBq in 2 cycles) in 21 patients with gastroenteropancreatic neuroendocrine tumors (GEP-NETs), achieving an OR of 29%

Table 2
Targeted radiotherapy with ^{90}Y- and ^{177}Lu-labeled somatostatin analogs in patients with gastroenteropancreatic neuroendocrine tumors

Authors	n	PD at Time of Inclusion	Response[a]					
			CR	PR	MR[b]	SD	PD	CR+PR
[^{111}In-DTPA] octreotide (^{111}In-DTPAOC)								
Valkema et al,[57] 2002	26	26/26	0	0	2/26 (8%)	15/26 (58%)	—	0/26 (0%)
Anthony et al,[58] 2002	26	—	0	2/26 (8%)	N/I	21/26 (81%)	—	2/26 (8%)
Buscombe et al,[114] 2003	12	—	0	2/12 (17%)	N/I	7/12 (58%)	3/12 (25%)	2/12 (17%)
Delpassand et al,[29] 2008	18	—	0	11%	N/I	—	—	0/26 (11%)
[^{90}Y-DOTA^0,Tyr^3] octreotide (^{90}Y-DOTATOC)								
Otte et al,[48] 1999	16	N/I	0	1 (6%)	N/I	14 (88%)	1 (6%)	1/16 (6%)
Waldherr et al,[49] 2001	37	34/37 (84%)	1 (3%)	9 (24%)	N/I	23 (62%)	4 (11%)	10/37 (27%)
Waldherr et al,[50] 2002	37	37/37 (100%)	1 (3%)	7 (19%)	N/I	6 (70%)	3 (8%)	8/37 (22%)
Bodei et al,[62] 2003	21	N/I	0	6 (29%)	N/I	11 (52%)	4 (19%)	6/21 (29%)
Valkema et al,[64] 2006	58	—	0	5 (9%)	7 (12%)	33 (61%)	10 (19%)	(9%)
[^{90}Y-DOTA]-lanreotide								
Virgolini et al,[52] 2002	39	39/39 (100%)	0	0	8 (20%)	17 (44%)	14 (36%)	0/39 (0%)
[^{90}Y-DOTA^0,Tyr^3] octreatate (^{90}Y-DOTATATE)								
Baum et al,[26] 2008c	75	67/75 (89%)	0	28c (37%)	N/I	39 (52%)	8c (11%)	28/75c (37%)
Cwikla et al,[53] 2010d	60	—	0	13 out 57 (23%)	N/I	44 out of 57 (77%)	3 out of 60 (5%)	13/57 (23%)c
[^{177}Lu-DOTA^0,Tyr^3] octreotate (^{177}Lu-DOTATATE)								
Kwekkeboom et al,[56] 2008	310	—	5 (2%)	86 (28%)	51 (16%)	107 (35%)	61 (20%)	(29%)

Abbreviation: N/I, not indicated.
a Criteria of tumor response (Southwest Oncology Group/World Health Organization [SWOG/WHO]): CR (complete remission), no evidence of disease; PR (partial remission), >50% reduction in tumor size; SD (stable disease), ±25% reduction or increase in tumor size; PD (progressive disease), >25% increase in tumor size.
b Modification of SWOG criteria including MR (minor remission), between 25% and 50% reduction in tumor size.
c Criteria for tumor response are not published in this study.
d Radiological response classified according to Response Evaluation Criteria in Solid Tumors (RECIST) criteria 6 months after completing therapy.

(see **Table 2**).[62] In a more recent study[63] including 141 patients with various sst-positive tumors, an OR of 23% to 32% was reported depending on the stage of the disease before therapy; however, these results were not subdivided for different tumor types.

Long-term follow-up and survival data for ^{90}Y-DOTATOC were published by Valkema and colleagues[64] (see **Table 2**). In this study, 58 patients were treated in a dose-escalating study with 1.7 to 32.8 GBq of ^{90}Y-DOTATOC. The response rates were comparable with other studies using ^{90}Y-labeled somatostatin analogs, but in addition to the encouraging response rates a significant longer overall survival (36.7 months) was shown compared with a group treated with ^{111}In-octreotide (median survival 12.0 months).[57]

The goal of a multicenter phase I study was to determine the maximum tolerated injected activity in a single cycle or in 4 cycles.[65,66] Escalating doses of ^{90}Y-DOTATOC up to 9.3 GBq/m^2 as a single injection and up to 14.8 GBq/m^2 in 4 cycles were administered in 60 patients, from which 54 could be treated with their maximum allowed activity. Objective response was achieved in 7%. The median time to progression was not reached at 26 months after the last treatment cycle. However, the maximum tolerated injected activity could not be determined because, based on [86]Y-DOTATOC dosimetry, the dose to the red marrow would have been too high.

The analog ^{90}Y-DOTA-lanreotide was investigated in a European multicenter trial (MAURITIUS), in 39 patients administered with a cumulative injected activity ranging from 1.9 to 8.6 GBq.[52] No objective response was noticed in this trial.

Clinical data on ^{90}Y-DOTATATE have been published by Baum and colleagues[26,67]; however, the treatment schemes were very inconsistent and the method to evaluate benefit was not defined. The reported results show an objective response rate (OR) of 37%. Recently, Seregni and colleagues[68] published their preliminary results on ^{90}Y-DOTATOC, whereas Cwikla and colleagues,[53] in a more detailed study, reported clinical results of 60 patients who received a mean cumulated administered activity of 11.2 GBq (range 4.1 to 16.2 GBq) in 2 to 4 cycles with an OR of 23% after 6 months.

In most of the studies using ^{90}Y-DOTATOC, the OR rates were 9% to 29% in patients with GEP-NET, despite the differences in the protocols used. These results along with the prolonged overall survival represent an improvement in therapeutic effectiveness compared with the studies using ^{111}In-octreotide.

STUDIES USING [177]LU-DOTATATE AND [177]LU-DOTATOC

In 2003, the first study using ^{177}Lu-DOTATATE was published.[33] In this trial, 35 patients with GEP-NET were treated with escalating activities up to a final cumulative injected activity of 22.2 to 29.6 GBq. An OR of 38% was found. In a more recent evaluation of 310 patients, an OR of 30% was reported (**Table 2**), whereas a significantly higher median overall survival of 48 months was reported.[56]

So far only 1 study has been published using ^{177}Lu-DOTATOC.[35] One of the inclusion criteria was relapse after ^{90}Y-DOTATOC treatment and only 1 therapy cycle was administrated because of the pretreatment. Even though the effectiveness of the treatment could be demonstrated, the results of the outcome cannot be compared owing to the different settings.

SIDE EFFECTS AND TOXICITY

Generally, TRT can be regarded as a safe treatment and severe side effects are rare, especially when compared with side effects of chemotherapy.[69,70] The side effects in TRT can be divided into acute side effects and more delayed effects caused by radiation toxicity. The acute effects occurring at the time of injection up to a few days after therapy include nausea, vomiting, and increased pain at tumor sites.[50,56,58] These side effects are generally mild, are minimized by a slow infusion, and can be prevented or reduced by symptomatic treatment.

Severe toxicity may occur as a result of the radiation absorbed dose in healthy organs. The organs at risk are mainly the kidneys, the bone marrow, and to a lower extent the liver.

Hematological Toxicity

Essentially, all studies investigating TRT report hematological toxicity. It appears that the absorbed radiation dose to the bone marrow is mainly caused by the circulation of the radioactivity in the blood,[71] which limits the options to reduce the absorbed dose. Severe but reversible hematological toxicity (>grade 2 for hemoglobin, white blood cells, and platelets) has been reported in up to 15% of the patients who received TRT.[48,49,58,72] According to our experience, only limited cases of patients have developed a myelodysplastic syndrome (MDS). This observation has also been reported by other groups.[56,57,64] The cause for MDS cases is difficult to be defined, as most of the patients had received chemotherapy and/or external beam radiation before TRT. Currently, a maximum absorbed radiation dose to the bone marrow of 2 Gy is assumed to be safe.[73] Hematological toxicity following TRT is frequent but generally mild and transient. MDS may occur, but the limited data on long-term follow-up does not allow a reliable, precise estimation of the risk to date.

Renal Toxicity

The radiation absorbed dose to the kidney is dose-limiting in TRT. The radiopeptides are filtered by the glomeruli and although they are mainly excreted into the urine, they are partially taken up in proximal tubule cells, leading to a considerable radiation dose to the kidneys.[32,45,64] The localization in the kidney is not homogeneous, but predominantly in the cortex, with most of the radioactivity centered in the inner cortical zone.[74] The megalin/cubulin system seems to be essential for a major part of the uptake in the proximal tubules.[75] For ligands binding to megalin via their cationic sites, coadministration of basic compounds can inhibit their renal reabsorption.[76] The administration of cationic amino acids, especially arginine and lysine, significantly reduces the renal uptake of radiolabeled somatostatin analogs by about 40% to 60%.[73,77,78] Amino acids are infused slowly over 4- to 10-hours in TRT. However, amino acids may have some side effects especially at high doses.[73,79] An alternative strategy is the use of polypeptide-based succinylated gelatin (GELO) plasma expander Gelofusine or Haemaccel, which induces low-molecular-weight proteinuria and therefore reduces tubular reabsorption. It was shown to reduce renal uptake in animals and patients.[80–82] However, the benefit in patients during TRT remains to be proven. Amifostine is the first drug investigated for TRT not to reduce renal uptake but to reduce systemically the toxic effects of the radiation, as it acts as a radical scavenger.[83] Animal studies have shown that a combination of amifostine with drugs that reduce the renal uptake is most promising.[83]

In a phase I study to define the maximal tolerated dose of ^{90}Y-DOTATOC that was performed without amino acid coadministration, 2 of 16 patients developed renal toxicity grade IV.[48] Renal biopsies of patients who developed renal toxicity revealed histologic changes comparable to the changes that occur after external beam radiation.[84] Despite the coadministration of amino acids, a number of later studies also reported renal toxicity.[36,85,86] Individual dosimetry might be helpful to avoid kidney failure.[36] An absorbed dose of 23 Gy to the whole kidney is generally accepted to be safe. This dose threshold is based on observations during external beam radiotherapy[87] and is therefore not indisputable. No renal toxicity was reported after therapeutic application of ^{111}In-octreotide,[57] whereas for ^{177}Lu-DOTATATE only 1 patient of 201 patients was reported with renal insufficiency[88] This is an indication that the physical characteristics of the radionuclide may have a significant impact on renal toxicity.

Several more detailed studies investigated kidney toxicity after TRT.[36,37,89] It was shown that along with the total absorbed dose to the kidney, the dose volume, fractionation rate, and clinical parameters like hypertension, diabetes, and age play an important role for the development of kidney failure. Especially, the fractionation influenced significantly the biologic effect of internally deposited radiation on the kidneys.[37] Theoretic considerations, applying the linear-quadratic model to dosimetry supported a higher tolerability when multiplying the number of therapy cycles. A renal cortex–sparing dose of 18 to 22 Gy with ^{90}Y-DOTATOC (2–6 cycles), and 7 to 12 Gy with ^{177}Lu-DOTATATE (4–8 cycles) may be achieved.[30]

If renal toxicity occurs, it cannot be regarded as fixed kidney damage. It appears rather that the loss of function is a continuous process with a defined pace of progression that can be expressed as loss of clearance per year.[37] However, this observation needs to be confirmed by other groups.

Liver Toxicity

Because most patients who are treated with TRT suffer from liver metastases, physiologic uptake in normal liver tissue also occurs. The physiologic and the specific tumor uptake can result in a considerable radiation absorbed dose to the liver.[44] However, because the tumor load in the liver shows high interpatient variability, it is difficult to generalize radiation absorbed doses to the liver.

A significant increase in liver enzymes after administration of ^{90}Y-DOTATOC has been reported in 2 studies.[59,64] It was concluded that patients with diffuse sst-positive hepatic metastases could be treated with a cumulative administered activity of 13.2 GBq of ^{90}Y-DOTATOC with only a small chance of developing mild acute or subacute liver failure. In the case of ^{177}Lu-DOTATATE, significantly increased liver function parameters (grade 4 liver toxicity) was evident in 2 patients after the first cycle of treatment.[88]

Liver toxicity is very rare and if it occurs, it is mostly mild and reversible. However, extensive liver metastases seem to be a risk factor for liver impairment after TRT. Most of the time, in these patients, it is difficult to distinguish between real toxicity caused by radiation and effects by the metastases themselves.

PATIENT SELECTION

In patients with metastatic neuroendocrine tumors in whom loco-regional approaches are no longer an option, TRT appears to be the most effective therapeutic option with limited side effects. TRT with radiolabeled somatostatin analogs allows treating all sst-positive tumors. However, because of the potential morbidity of TRT, patients should be carefully selected. The selection is mainly based on the sst_2 overexpression in targeted tumor tissue displayed in somatostatin receptor imaging. Kidney failure and severe thrombocytopenia represent the 2 major exclusion criteria. Inclusion criteria for most studies were tumor uptake equal or higher than liver uptake on the ^{111}In-octreotide scintigraphy.[28] Although positivity on sst imaging is a necessary condition, it is not sufficient as the only inclusion criteria.

An important issue is to determine the negative and positive prognostic factors relevant for therapy response and survival. This allows identifying patients susceptible to benefit from more intensive treatment schemes. A clinical staging and grading system is therefore required. Risk factors have been identified as affecting survival and therapy response. Poorer prognosis is reported for patients having decreased performance status, extensive liver involvement, and elevated alkaline phosphatase concentrations in serum[56,90]; however, these parameters are subject to interpretation and lack of sensitivity. A Tumor-Node-Metastasis classification including grading features of tumors has been proposed by Rindi and colleagues[91] for GEP-NET and was recently validated,[92,93] confirming the independent predicting value for outcome of the staging (localized vs metastasized) and the grading (well vs poorly differentiated or Ki-67 index $\leq$2% or >20%) of the disease. The variation in tumor differentiation results in highly variable rates of progression.

The stage of disease at the time of diagnosis is highly variable. It ranges from a small localized primary tumor to advanced or even end-stage disease. The intensity of uptake on the ^{111}In-octreotide scintigraphy is a prognostic factor for predicting tumor remission (complete [CR], partial [PR], or minor [MR]).[56] On the other hand, it has been demonstrated in patients with well-differentiated NETs that a negative ^{111}In-octreotide scintigraphy is correlated with a poor prognosis.[94] Recently PET imaging with radio-labeled somatostatin analogs (eg, ^{68}Ga-DOTATOC, -DOTATATE, or -DOTANOC) became available and might be used alternatively to ^{111}In-octreotide scintigraphy for staging. In a recent study, Ambrosini and colleagues[24] showed that ^{68}Ga-DOTA-NOC PET/CT compared with conventional imaging modalities (CT, MRI, ultrasound [US], and endoscopy) affected either staging of the disease or modified the therapy approach in 50 (55.5%) of 90 patients. It was also found that the major impact of PET findings was on the therapeutic management rather than stage modifications.

Garin and colleagues[95] showed, in a prospective study including 38 patients with well-differentiated NET, that fluorine-18 fluorodeoxyglucose (^{18}F-FDG) PET can be used to recognize patients who have a rapidly progressive tumor and that ^{18}F-FDG PET results were independently predictive of progression-free survival. Another prospective study[96] confirmed this finding, showing a strong prognostic value of ^{18}F-FDG PET for prediction of the overall survival of patients with NETs in which a hazard ratio of 10 for risk-of-death was found for patients with ^{18}F-FDG PET-positive foci compared with ^{18}F-FDG PET-negative patients, exceeding the prognostic value of traditionally used parameters such as Ki-67, Chromogranin A level, and the presence of liver metastases.

The best time point for initiating TRT remains uncertain up to now. The "wait-and-see" approach often still remains the mainstay of initial management in patients with unresectable well-differentiated and slow-growing disease. The natural course of GEP tumors can be indolent for many years and the well-being of patients, even with metastasized tumors, can be unchanged for a long period. However, the reported studies on TRT clearly indicate that patients with documented progressive disease or a substantial increase in symptoms benefit in a high percentage from radiopeptide therapy. In a study in which the relationship between delay of diagnosis, extent of disease, and survival in 115 patients with carcinoid was studied, a mean delay in the diagnosis of 66 months was found.[97] It was concluded that the diagnosis of carcinoid is difficult, and therefore a delay of diagnosis by physicians is common. Strikingly, the delay of the diagnosis did not correlate with the extent of the disease. However, the extent of the disease did correlate with survival. It underscores the need for earlier diagnosis and for improved systemic therapies for advanced disease. Although there are no guidelines yet for the initiation of TRT, there are certain hints that the treatment is more effective when given in an earlier stage. The degree of liver involvement is inversely related to the chance of remission.[34] In a trial with ^{111}In-octreotide it was reported that a beneficial effect of TRT is less likely in end-stage patients than in patients with less tumor burden and in better general condition.[57,98] Furthermore, it was clearly shown that patients benefit in quality of life after TRT.[50,99] This justifies treating all symptomatic patients who fulfill the inclusion criteria and are no longer responsive to treatment with non-radiolabeled somatostatin analogs.

Another argument for an earlier treatment is that NETs can dedifferentiate over time. Dedifferentiation is commonly associated with a decrease in sst expression. In turn, TRT using radiolabeled somatostatin analogs will be less effective or even impossible. The administration of TRT in an early stage does not exclude patients from a later repetition of the treatment. It was shown that patients can be retreated. A good response after the first treatment cycles was found to be a positive predictor for the effectiveness of the retreatment.[35]

A randomized study comparing the long-term survival of patients with malignant, unresectable neuroendocrine tumors that undergo TRT compared with a "wait and see" strategy is lacking. Keeping in mind the latest follow-up data of patients treated with ^{177}Lu-DOTATATE (median time to progression >36 months)[33,56] makes, however, such a study disputable from an ethical point of view.

FUTURE DEVELOPMENTS

Although the results of TRT in the treatment of a heterogeneous group of patients compare favorably with other systemic approaches,[100] there is place for improvement of the therapy protocols. Based on the histologic grading and the characterization of the tumors by imaging, several centers are currently attempting to optimize and individualize their therapy protocol.

Future research to improve TRT with radiolabeled somatostatin analogs consists of 5 main directions.

- Improving the vehicle, ie, the peptide, is a highly interesting approach. Many new somatostatin analogs with a higher affinity for sst_2 or with a wider affinity profile for several sst subtypes have already been introduced into the preclinic.[101] Recently, somatostatin receptor antagonists have also been characterized preclinically. Although they do not internalize into sst_2-expressing cells after binding to the receptor, they find significantly more binding sites on the receptor than agonists.[102] In clinics, the somatostatin-based antagonist called ^{111}In-DOTA-BASS was compared with ^{111}In-octreotide. The receptor antagonist detected 42 lesions, whereas ^{111}In-octreotide scintigraphy detected only 24 lesions.[103] Moreover, ^{111}In-DOTABASS showed an approximately 3 times higher tumor-to-kidney uptake ratio than ^{111}In-octreotide.
- Simultaneously, investigations have been made to increase the delivery of the radiopharmaceutical to the target. This includes the way of application, eg, intra-arterially, at a slower rate, with different peptide concentrations, or fractionated. Moreover, the improvement of the availability of the target by modulation of the receptor with drugs could be a way to further improve TRT.[104,105]
- Furthermore, the most suitable radionuclide will have to be defined. In preclinical studies comparing ^{90}Y and ^{177}Lu, it appeared that ^{90}Y was more effective for larger tumors, whereas with ^{177}Lu fewer relapses occurred when treating smaller lesions.[65,75] Besides the effects on the tumor, the different physical properties cause differences in microdosimetry, which in turn will influence the toxicity profile of a compound.[30,32] Besides the commonly used ^{90}Y and ^{177}Lu, a number of other radionuclides with different physical characteristics including alpha-emitters are under investigation.[106,107]

- In external beam radiation, the application of radio-sensitizers to improve the antitumor effect of the radiation is established.[108] In TRT, the introduction of combination therapies will open a whole new field of research to improve the treatment. Conventional chemotherapy and external radiotherapy either alone or in a variety of permutations are of minimal efficacy and should be balanced against the decrease in quality of life often caused by such agents.[109] A preliminary study of a therapy protocol combining ^{177}Lu-DOTA-TATE with capecitabine has been published recently on a small group of patients with GEP-NET showing the feasibility and moderate additional short-term toxicity of this scheme.[110] However, a randomized controlled study is lacking to date.
- Finally, the improvement of the toxicity profile of the current radiopeptides is an important issue. Especially with respect to the reduction of the kidney absorbed dose, several studies were recently published, and also other strategies to reduce radiation toxicity in general are under investigation.[80,81,83,111] An important step toward a better understanding of the deterministic effect provided by the variable dose rate delivered in TRT has been recently evidenced.[40] Applying the linear quadratic radiobiological formalism, as well as improved dosimetry methods (voxelwise dosimetry, multiregion model for a suborgan dosimetry, and individual organ masses determination)[32,36,112] to explain the renal toxicity after fractionated ^{90}Y-DOTATOC therapy, a trend toward correlation has been found between the biologically effective dose (BED) delivered to the kidneys and the expected effect derived from the external beam radiation therapy BED-effect curve.[113]

SUMMARY

TRT has been proven to be an effective and safe treatment alternative for sst-positive, unresectable NETs. Currently, the maximum tolerated injected activity is defined by the absorbed radiation dose to the critical organs, kidney, and bone marrow. It is likely that the dose can be increased in the future by the introduction of new protective agents, different treatment schemes, and radionuclides.

The present data in the literature do not allow defining the most suitable peptide and radionuclide for the treatment of NETs. Especially concerning the radionuclide, there is emerging evidence that a combination of nuclides with different physical characteristics might be more effective.

The principle of targeted treatment has a number of obvious advantages over unspecific systemic treatments. Therefore, TRT, along with the discovery of new molecular targets, holds great promise for the future.

REFERENCES

1. Reubi JC. Peptide receptors as molecular targets for cancer diagnosis and therapy. Endocr Rev 2003;24:389–427.
2. Reubi JC, Waser B, Schaer JC, et al. Somatostatin receptor sst1-sst5 expression in normal and neoplastic human tissues using receptor autoradiography with subtype-selective ligands. Eur J Nucl Med 2001;28:836–46.
3. Rinke A, Muller HH, Schade-Brittinger C, et al. Placebo-controlled, double-blind, prospective, randomized study on the effect of octreotide LAR in the control of tumor growth in patients with metastatic neuroendocrine midgut tumors: a report from the PROMID Study Group. J Clin Oncol 2009;27:4656–63.

4. Aparicio T, Ducreux M, Baudin E, et al. Antitumour activity of somatostatin analogues in progressive metastatic neuroendocrine tumours. Eur J Cancer 2001;37:1014–9.

5. Arnold R, Trautmann ME, Creutzfeldt W, et al. Somatostatin analogue octreotide and inhibition of tumour growth in metastatic endocrine gastroenteropancreatic tumours. Gut 1996;38:430–8.

6. Bajetta E, Di Leo A, Biganzoli L, et al. Phase II study of vinorelbine in patients with pretreated advanced ovarian cancer: activity in platinum-resistant disease. J Clin Oncol 1996;14:2546–51.

7. Ducreux M, Ruszniewski P, Chayvialle JA, et al. The antitumoral effect of the long-acting somatostatin analog lanreotide in neuroendocrine tumors. Am J Gastroenterol 2000;95:3276–81.

8. Faiss S, Pape UF, Bohmig M, et al. Prospective, randomized, multicenter trial on the antiproliferative effect of lanreotide, interferon alfa, and their combination for therapy of metastatic neuroendocrine gastroenteropancreatic tumors—the International Lanreotide and Interferon Alfa Study Group. J Clin Oncol 2003;21:2689–96.

9. Saltz L, Trochanowski B, Buckley M, et al. Octreotide as an antineoplastic agent in the treatment of functional and nonfunctional neuroendocrine tumors. Cancer 1993;72:244–8.

10. Shojamanesh H, Gibril F, Louie A, et al. Prospective study of the antitumor efficacy of long-term octreotide treatment in patients with progressive metastatic gastrinoma. Cancer 2002;94:331–43.

11. Strowski MZ, Blake AD. Function and expression of somatostatin receptors of the endocrine pancreas. Mol Cell Endocrinol 2008;286:169–79.

12. Bodei L, Paganelli G, Mariani G. Receptor radionuclide therapy of tumors: a road from basic research to clinical applications. J Nucl Med 2006;47:375–7.

13. Waser B, Tamma ML, Cescato R, et al. Highly efficient in vivo agonist-induced internalization of sst2 receptors in somatostatin target tissues. J Nucl Med 2009;50:936–41.

14. Reubi JC, Waser B, Liu Q, et al. Subcellular distribution of somatostatin sst2A receptors in human tumors of the nervous and neuroendocrine systems: membranous versus intracellular location. J Clin Endocrinol Metab 2000;85: 3882–91.

15. Krenning EP, Kwekkeboom DJ, Bakker WH, et al. Somatostatin receptor scintigraphy with [111In-DTPA-D-Phe1]- and [123I-Tyr3]-octreotide: the Rotterdam experience with more than 1000 patients. Eur J Nucl Med 1993;20:716–31.

16. Kwekkeboom D, Krenning EP, de Jong M. Peptide receptor imaging and therapy. J Nucl Med 2000;41:1704–13.

17. Schottelius M, Wester HJ. Molecular imaging targeting peptide receptors. Methods 2009;48:161–77.

18. Rufini V, Calcagni ML, Baum RP. Imaging of neuroendocrine tumors. Semin Nucl Med 2006;36:228–47.

19. Hofmann M, Maecke H, Borner R, et al. Biokinetics and imaging with the somatostatin receptor PET radioligand (68)Ga-DOTATOC: preliminary data. Eur J Nucl Med 2001;28:1751–7.

20. Maecke HR, Hofmann M, Haberkorn U. (68)Ga-labeled peptides in tumor imaging. J Nucl Med 2005;46(Suppl 1):172S–8S.

21. Wester HJ, Schottelius M, Scheidhauer K, et al. PET imaging of somatostatin receptors: design, synthesis and preclinical evaluation of a novel 18F-labelled, carbohydrated analogue of octreotide. Eur J Nucl Med Mol Imaging 2003;30: 117–22.

22. Gabriel M, Decristoforo C, Kendler D, et al. 68Ga-DOTA-Tyr3-octreotide PET in neuroendocrine tumors: comparison with somatostatin receptor scintigraphy and CT. J Nucl Med 2007;48:508–18.
23. Buchmann I, Henze M, Engelbrecht S, et al. Comparison of 68Ga-DOTATOC PET and 111In-DTPAOC (Octreoscan) SPECT in patients with neuroendocrine tumours. Eur J Nucl Med Mol Imaging 2007;34:1617–26.
24. Ambrosini V, Campana D, Bodei L, et al. 68Ga-DOTANOC PET/CT clinical impact in patients with neuroendocrine tumors. J Nucl Med 2010;51:669–73.
25. Gabriel M, Oberauer A, Dobrozemsky G, et al. 68Ga-DOTA-Tyr3-octreotide PET for assessing response to somatostatin-receptor-mediated radionuclide therapy. J Nucl Med 2009;50:1427–34.
26. Baum RP, Prasad V, Hommann M, et al. Receptor PET/CT imaging of neuroendocrine tumors. Recent Results Cancer Res 2008;170:225–42.
27. Mariani G, Bodei L, Adelstein SJ, et al. Emerging roles for radiometabolic therapy of tumors based on auger electron emission. J Nucl Med 2000;41:1519–21.
28. Krenning EP, de Jong M, Kooij PP, et al. Radiolabelled somatostatin analogue(s) for peptide receptor scintigraphy and radionuclide therapy. Ann Oncol 1999;10(Suppl 2):S23–9.
29. Delpassand ES, Sims-Mourtada J, Saso H, et al. Safety and efficacy of radionuclide therapy with high-activity In-111 pentetreotide in patients with progressive neuroendocrine tumors. Cancer Biother Radiopharm 2008;23:292–300.
30. Cremonesi M, Botta F, Di Dia A, et al. Dosimetry for treatment with radiolabelled somatostatin analogues. A review. Q J Nucl Med Mol Imaging 2010;54:37–51.
31. Capello A, Krenning E, Bernard B, et al. 111In-labelled somatostatin analogues in a rat tumour model: somatostatin receptor status and effects of peptide receptor radionuclide therapy. Eur J Nucl Med Mol Imaging 2005;32:1288–95.
32. Konijnenberg MW, Bijster M, Krenning EP, et al. A stylized computational model of the rat for organ dosimetry in support of preclinical evaluations of peptide receptor radionuclide therapy with (90)Y, (111)In, or (177)Lu. J Nucl Med 2004;45:1260–9.
33. Kwekkeboom DJ, Bakker WH, Kam BL, et al. Treatment of patients with gastro-entero-pancreatic (GEP) tumours with the novel radiolabelled somatostatin analogue [177Lu-DOTA(0), Tyr3]octreotate. Eur J Nucl Med Mol Imaging 2003;30:417–22.
34. Kwekkeboom DJ, Teunissen JJ, Bakker WH, et al. Radiolabeled somatostatin analog [177Lu-DOTA0, Tyr3] octreotate in patients with endocrine gastroentero-pancreatic tumors. J Clin Oncol 2005;23:2754–62.
35. Forrer F, Uusijarvi H, Storch D, et al. Treatment with 177Lu-DOTATOC of patients with relapse of neuroendocrine tumors after treatment with 90Y-DOTATOC. J Nucl Med 2005;46:1310–6.
36. Barone R, Borson-Chazot F, Valkema R, et al. Patient-specific dosimetry in predicting renal toxicity with (90)Y-DOTATOC: relevance of kidney volume and dose rate in finding a dose-effect relationship. J Nucl Med 2005;46(Suppl 1):99S–106S.
37. Pauwels S, Barone R, Walrand S, et al. Practical dosimetry of peptide receptor radionuclide therapy with (90)Y-labeled somatostatin analogs. J Nucl Med 2005;46(Suppl 1):92S–8S.
38. Konijnenberg M, Melis M, Valkema R, et al. Radiation dose distribution in human kidneys by octreotides in peptide receptor radionuclide therapy. J Nucl Med 2007;48:134–42.

39. Dale R. Use of the linear-quadratic radiobiological model for quantifying kidney response in targeted radiotherapy. Cancer Biother Radiopharm 2004;19:363–70.

40. Wessels BW, Konijnenberg MW, Dale RG, et al. MIRD pamphlet No. 20: the effect of model assumptions on kidney dosimetry and response—implications for radionuclide therapy. J Nucl Med 2008;49:1884–99.

41. Fabbri C, Sarti G, Cremonesi M, et al. Quantitative analysis of 90Y Bremsstrahlung SPECT-CT images for application to 3D patient-specific dosimetry. Cancer Biother Radiopharm 2009;24:145–54.

42. Lhommel R, Goffette P, Van den Eynde M, et al. Yttrium-90 TOF PET scan demonstrates high-resolution biodistribution after liver SIRT. Eur J Nucl Med Mol Imaging 2009;36:1696.

43. Werner MK, Brechtel K, Beyer T, et al. PET/CT for the assessment and quantification of (90)Y biodistribution after selective internal radiotherapy (SIRT) of liver metastases. Eur J Nucl Med Mol Imaging 2010;37:407–8.

44. Cremonesi M, Ferrari M, Bodei L, et al. Dosimetry in peptide radionuclide receptor therapy: a review. J Nucl Med 2006;47:1467–75.

45. Forrer F, Uusijarvi H, Waldherr C, et al. A comparison of (111)In-DOTATOC and (111)In-DOTATATE: biodistribution and dosimetry in the same patients with metastatic neuroendocrine tumours. Eur J Nucl Med Mol Imaging 2004;31:1257–62.

46. Esser JP, Krenning EP, Teunissen JJ, et al. Comparison of [(177)Lu-DOTA(0), Tyr(3)]octreotate and [(177)Lu-DOTA(0), Tyr(3)]octreotide: which peptide is preferable for PRRT? Eur J Nucl Med Mol Imaging 2006;33:1346–51.

47. Kwekkeboom DJ, Krenning EP, Scheidhauer K, et al. ENETS consensus guidelines for the standards of care in neuroendocrine tumors: somatostatin receptor imaging with (111)In-pentetreotide. Neuroendocrinology 2009;90:184–9.

48. Otte A, Herrmann R, Heppeler A, et al. Yttrium-90 DOTATOC: first clinical results. Eur J Nucl Med 1999;26:1439–47.

49. Waldherr C, Pless M, Maecke HR, et al. The clinical value of [90Y-DOTA]-D-Phe1-Tyr3-octreotide (90Y-DOTATOC) in the treatment of neuroendocrine tumours: a clinical phase II study. Ann Oncol 2001;12:941–5.

50. Waldherr C, Pless M, Maecke HR, et al. Tumor response and clinical benefit in neuroendocrine tumors after 7.4 GBq (90)Y-DOTATOC. J Nucl Med 2002;43: 610–6.

51. Forrer F, Waldherr C, Maecke HR, et al. Targeted radionuclide therapy with 90Y-DOTATOC in patients with neuroendocrine tumors. Anticancer Res 2006;26: 703–7.

52. Virgolini I, Britton K, Buscombe J, et al. In- and Y-DOTA-lanreotide: results and implications of the MAURITIUS trial. Semin Nucl Med 2002;32:148–55.

53. Cwikla JB, Sankowski A, Seklecka N, et al. Efficacy of radionuclide treatment DOTATATE Y-90 in patients with progressive metastatic gastroenteropancreatic neuroendocrine carcinomas (GEP-NETs): a phase II study. Ann Oncol 2010;21: 787–94.

54. Aloj L, D'Ambrosio L, Aurilio M, et al. First line Y-90 DOTATATE treatment in patients with well differentiated, inoperable neuroendocrine tumors. Eur J Nucl Med Mol Imaging 2009;36(Suppl 2):S218.

55. Kunikowska J, Krolicki L, Hubalewska-Dydejczyk A, et al. Comparison between clinical results of PRRT with 90Y-DOTATATE and 90Y/177Lu-DOTATATE. Eur J Nucl Med Mol Imaging 2009;36(Suppl 2):S219.

56. Kwekkeboom DJ, de Herder WW, Kam BL, et al. Treatment with the radiolabeled somatostatin analog [177 Lu-DOTA 0, Tyr3]octreotate: toxicity, efficacy, and survival. J Clin Oncol 2008;26:2124–30.

57. Valkema R, De Jong M, Bakker WH, et al. Phase I study of peptide receptor radionuclide therapy with [In-DTPA] octreotide: the Rotterdam experience. Semin Nucl Med 2002;32:110–22.
58. Anthony LB, Woltering EA, Espenan GD, et al. Indium-111-pentetreotide prolongs survival in gastroenteropancreatic malignancies. Semin Nucl Med 2002;32:123–32.
59. Bushnell D, Menda Y, Madsen M, et al. Assessment of hepatic toxicity from treatment with 90Y-SMT 487 (OctreoTher(TM)) in patients with diffuse somatostatin receptor positive liver metastases. Cancer Biother Radiopharm 2003;18: 581–8.
60. Oberg K, Eriksson B. Endocrine tumours of the pancreas. Best Pract Res Clin Gastroenterol 2005;19:753–81.
61. Otte A, Jermann E, Behe M, et al. DOTATOC: a powerful new tool for receptor-mediated radionuclide therapy. Eur J Nucl Med 1997;24:792–5.
62. Bodei L, Cremonesi M, Zoboli S, et al. Receptor-mediated radionuclide therapy with 90Y-DOTATOC in association with amino acid infusion: a phase I study. Eur J Nucl Med Mol Imaging 2003;30:207–16.
63. Bodei L, Handkiewicz-Junak D, Grana C, et al. Receptor radionuclide therapy with 90Y-DOTATOC in patients with medullary thyroid carcinomas. Cancer Biother Radiopharm 2004;19:65–71.
64. Valkema R, Pauwels S, Kvols LK, et al. Survival and response after peptide receptor radionuclide therapy with [90Y-DOTA0, Tyr3] octreotide in patients with advanced gastroenteropancreatic neuroendocrine tumors. Semin Nucl Med 2006;36:147–56.
65. De Jong M, Valkema R, Jamar F, et al. Somatostatin receptor-targeted radionuclide therapy of tumors: preclinical and clinical findings. Semin Nucl Med 2002; 32:133–40.
66. Smith MC, Liu J, Chen T, et al. OctreoTher: ongoing early clinical development of a somatostatin-receptor-targeted radionuclide antineoplastic therapy. Digestion 2000;62(Suppl 1):69–72.
67. Baum RP, Söldner J, Schmüching M, et al. [Peptidrezeptorvermittelte radiotherapie (prrt) neuroendokriner tumoren klinischen indikationen und erfahrung mit 90yttrium-markierten somatostatinanaloga.] Der Onkologe 2004;10:1098–110 [in German].
68. Seregni E, Maccauro M, Coliva A, et al. Treatment with tandem [90Y]DOTA-TATE and [177Lu] DOTA-TATE of neuroendocrine tumors refractory to conventional therapy: preliminary results. Q J Nucl Med Mol Imaging 2010;54:84–91.
69. Moertel CG, Hanley JA. Combination chemotherapy trials in metastatic carcinoid tumor and the malignant carcinoid syndrome. Cancer Clin Trials 1979;2: 327–34.
70. Engstrom PF, Lavin PT, Moertel CG, et al. Streptozocin plus fluorouracil versus doxorubicin therapy for metastatic carcinoid tumor. J Clin Oncol 1984;2:1255–9.
71. Cremonesi M, Ferrari M, Zoboli S, et al. Biokinetics and dosimetry in patients administered with (111)In-DOTA-Tyr(3)-octreotide: implications for internal radiotherapy with (90)Y-DOTATOC. Eur J Nucl Med 1999;26:877–86.
72. Virgolini I, Kurtaran A, Angelberger P, et al. "MAURITIUS": tumour dose in patients with advanced carcinoma. Ital J Gastroenterol Hepatol 1999;31(Suppl 2): S227–30.
73. Rolleman EJ, Valkema R, de Jong M, et al. Safe and effective inhibition of renal uptake of radiolabelled octreotide by a combination of lysine and arginine. Eur J Nucl Med Mol Imaging 2003;30:9–15.

74. De Jong M, Valkema R, Van Gameren A, et al. Inhomogeneous localization of radioactivity in the human kidney after injection of [(111)In-DTPA] octreotide. J Nucl Med 2004;45:1168–71.
75. de Jong M, Breeman WA, Valkema R, et al. Combination radionuclide therapy using 177Lu- and 90Y-labeled somatostatin analogs. J Nucl Med 2005;46(Suppl 1):13S–7S.
76. Mogensen CE, Solling. Studies on renal tubular protein reabsorption: partial and near complete inhibition by certain amino acids. Scand J Clin Lab Invest 1977; 37:477–86.
77. Behr TM, Goldenberg DM, Becker W. Reducing the renal uptake of radiolabeled antibody fragments and peptides for diagnosis and therapy: present status, future prospects and limitations. Eur J Nucl Med 1998;25:201–12.
78. Barone R, Pauwels S, De Camps J, et al. Metabolic effects of amino acid solutions infused for renal protection during therapy with radiolabelled somatostatin analogues. Nephrol Dial Transplant 2004;19:2275–81.
79. Bernard BF, Krenning EP, Breeman WA, et al. D-lysine reduction of indium-111 octreotide and yttrium-90 octreotide renal uptake. J Nucl Med 1997;38:1929–33.
80. Vegt E, Wetzels JF, Russel FG, et al. Renal uptake of radiolabeled octreotide in human subjects is efficiently inhibited by succinylated gelatin. J Nucl Med 2006; 47:432–6.
81. van Eerd JE, Vegt E, Wetzels JF, et al. Gelatin-based plasma expander effectively reduces renal uptake of 111In-octreotide in mice and rats. J Nucl Med 2006;47:528–33.
82. Vegt E, van Eerd JE, Eek A, et al. Reducing renal uptake of radiolabeled peptides using albumin fragments. J Nucl Med 2008;49:1506–11.
83. Rolleman EJ, Forrer F, Bernard B, et al. Amifostine protects rat kidneys during peptide receptor radionuclide therapy with [177Lu-DOTA0, Tyr3] octreotate. Eur J Nucl Med Mol Imaging 2007;34:763–71.
84. Moll S, Nickeleit V, Mueller-Brand J, et al. A new cause of renal thrombotic microangiopathy: yttrium 90-DOTATOC internal radiotherapy. Am J Kidney Dis 2001; 37:847–51.
85. Cybulla M, Weiner SM, Otte A. End-stage renal disease after treatment with 90Y-DOTATOC. Eur J Nucl Med 2001;28:1552–4.
86. Otte A, Mueller-Brand J, Dellas S, et al. Yttrium-90-labelled somatostatin-analogue for cancer treatment. Lancet 1998;351:417–8.
87. Emami B, Lyman J, Brown A, et al. Tolerance of normal tissue to therapeutic irradiation. Int J Radiat Oncol Biol Phys 1991;21:109–22.
88. Kwekkeboom DJ, Mueller-Brand J, Paganelli G, et al. Overview of results of peptide receptor radionuclide therapy with 3 radiolabeled somatostatin analogs. J Nucl Med 2005;46(Suppl 1):62S–6S.
89. Valkema R, Pauwels SA, Kvols LK, et al. Long-term follow-up of renal function after peptide receptor radiation therapy with (90)Y-DOTA(0), Tyr(3)-octreotide and (177)Lu-DOTA(0), Tyr(3)-octreotate. J Nucl Med 2005;46(Suppl 1):83S–91S.
90. Clancy TE, Sengupta TP, Paulus J, et al. Alkaline phosphatase predicts survival in patients with metastatic neuroendocrine tumors. Dig Dis Sci 2006;51:877–84.
91. Rindi G, Kloppel G, Alhman H, et al. TNM staging of foregut (neuro)endocrine tumors: a consensus proposal including a grading system. Virchows Arch 2006;449:395–401.
92. Pape UF, Jann H, Muller-Nordhorn J, et al. Prognostic relevance of a novel TNM classification system for upper gastroenteropancreatic neuroendocrine tumors. Cancer 2008;113:256–65.

93. Garcia-Carbonero R, Capdevila J, Crespo-Herrero G, et al. Incidence, patterns of care and prognostic factors for outcome of gastroenteropancreatic neuroendocrine tumors (GEP-NETs): results from the National Cancer Registry of Spain (RGETNE). Ann Oncol 2010;21:1794–803.
94. Asnacios A, Courbon F, Rochaix P, et al. Indium-111-pentetreotide scintigraphy and somatostatin receptor subtype 2 expression: new prognostic factors for malignant well-differentiated endocrine tumors. J Clin Oncol 2008;26:963–70.
95. Garin E, Le Jeune F, Devillers A, et al. Predictive value of 18F-FDG PET and somatostatin receptor scintigraphy in patients with metastatic endocrine tumors. J Nucl Med 2009;50:858–64.
96. Binderup T, Knigge U, Loft A, et al. 18F-fluorodeoxyglucose positron emission tomography predicts survival of patients with neuroendocrine tumors. Clin Cancer Res 2010;16:978–85.
97. Toth-Fejel S, Pommier RF. Relationships among delay of diagnosis, extent of disease, and survival in patients with abdominal carcinoid tumors. Am J Surg 2004;187:575–9.
98. Oberg K, Norheim I, Lundqvist G, et al. Cytotoxic treatment in patients with malignant carcinoid tumors. Response to streptozocin—alone or in combination with 5-FU. Acta Oncol 1987;26:429–32.
99. Teunissen JJ, Kwekkeboom DJ, Krenning EP. Quality of life in patients with gastroenteropancreatic tumors treated with [177Lu-DOTA0, Tyr3] octreotate. J Clin Oncol 2004;22:2724–9.
100. Kwekkeboom DJ, Kam BL, van Essen M, et al. Somatostatin receptor-based imaging and therapy of gastroenteropancreatic neuroendocrine tumors. Endocr Relat Cancer 2010;17:R53–73.
101. Ginj M, Chen J, Walter MA, et al. Preclinical evaluation of new and highly potent analogues of octreotide for predictive imaging and targeted radiotherapy. Clin Cancer Res 2005;11:1136–45.
102. Ginj M, Zhang H, Waser B, et al. Radiolabeled somatostatin receptor antagonists are preferable to agonists for in vivo peptide receptor targeting of tumors. Proc Natl Acad Sci U S A 2006;103:16436–41.
103. Wild D, Fani M, Behe M, et al. First clinical evaluation of a somatostatin receptor antagonist for imaging of neuroendocrine tumors (NETs). Nuklearmedizin 2010; 49:A16.
104. Breeman WA, van der Wansem K, Bernard BF, et al. The addition of DTPA to [177Lu-DOTA0, Tyr3] octreotate prior to administration reduces rat skeleton uptake of radioactivity. Eur J Nucl Med Mol Imaging 2003;30:312–5.
105. Froidevaux S, Hintermann E, Torok M, et al. Differential regulation of somatostatin receptor type 2 (sst 2) expression in AR4-2J tumor cells implanted into mice during octreotide treatment. Cancer Res 1999;59:3652–7.
106. Uusijarvi H, Bernhardt P, Rosch F, et al. Electron- and positron-emitting radiolanthanides for therapy: aspects of dosimetry and production. J Nucl Med 2006;47:807–14.
107. Norenberg JP, Krenning BJ, Konings IR, et al. 213Bi-[DOTA0, Tyr3] octreotide peptide receptor radionuclide therapy of pancreatic tumors in a preclinical animal model. Clin Cancer Res 2006;12:897–903.
108. van Putten JW, Price A, van der Leest AH, et al. A Phase I study of gemcitabine with concurrent radiotherapy in stage III, locally advanced non-small cell lung cancer. Clin Cancer Res 2003;9:2472–7.
109. Modlin IM, Latich I, Kidd M, et al. Therapeutic options for gastrointestinal carcinoids. Clin Gastroenterol Hepatol 2006;4:526–47.

110. van Essen M, Krenning EP, Kam BL, et al. Report on short-term side effects of treatments with 177Lu-octreotate in combination with capecitabine in seven patients with gastroenteropancreatic neuroendocrine tumours. Eur J Nucl Med Mol Imaging 2008;35:743–8.

111. Forrer F, Rolleman E, Bijster M, et al. From outside to inside? Dose-dependent renal tubular damage after high-dose peptide receptor radionuclide therapy in rats measured with in vivo (99m)Tc-DMSA-SPECT and molecular imaging. Cancer Biother Radiopharm 2007;22:40–9.

112. Bouchet LG, Bolch WE, Blanco HP, et al. MIRD Pamphlet No 19: absorbed fractions and radionuclide S values for six age-dependent multiregion models of the kidney. J Nucl Med 2003;44:1113–47.

113. Emami B, Myerson RJ, Scott C, et al. Phase I/II study, combination of radiotherapy and hyperthermia in patients with deep-seated malignant tumors: report of a pilot study by the Radiation Therapy Oncology Group. Int J Radiat Oncol Biol Phys 1991;20:73–9.

114. Buscombe JR, Caplin ME, Hilson AJ. Long-term efficacy of high-activity 111in-pentetreotide therapy in patients with disseminated neuroendocrine tumors. J Nucl Med 2003;44:1–6.

Neuroendocrine Tumors: Current Recommendations for Diagnosis and Surgical Management

Saju Joseph, MD[a,b], Yi-Zarn Wang, MD[a,c],
J. Philip Boudreaux, MD[a,c,d], Lowell B. Anthony, MD[e,f],
Richard Campeau, MD[g,h], Daniel Raines, MD[i],
Thomas O'Dorisio, MD[j], Vay Liang Go, MD[k],
Aaron I. Vinik, MD, PhD, FCP, MACP[l], Jason Cundiff, MD[a],
Eugene A. Woltering, MD[a,c],*

KEYWORDS

- Neuroendocrine tumors • Imaging • Surgery • Chemotherapy
- Radiation therapy • Foregut • Hindgut • Midgut
- Biochemical markers • Tumor markers

[a] Section of Endocrine Surgery, Department of Surgery, Louisiana State University Health Sciences Center, 200 West Esplanade Avenue, Suite 200, Kenner, LA 70065, USA
[b] Section of Hepatobiliary Surgery, Department of Surgery, Louisiana State University Health Sciences Center, 200 West Esplanade Avenue, Suite 200, Kenner, LA 70065, USA
[c] Section of Surgical Oncology, Department of Surgery, Louisiana State University Health Sciences Center, 200 West Esplanade Avenue, Suite 200, Kenner, LA 70065, USA
[d] Section of Transplant Surgery, Department of Surgery, Louisiana State University Health Sciences Center, 200 West Esplanade Avenue, Suite 200, Kenner, LA 70065, USA
[e] Section of Hematology and Oncology, Department of Medicine, Louisiana State University Health Sciences Center, 200 West Esplanade Avenue, Suite 200, Kenner, LA 70065, USA
[f] Section of Medical Oncology, Department of Medicine, Louisiana State University Health Sciences Center, 200 West Esplanade Avenue, Suite 200, Kenner, LA 70065, USA
[g] Section of Radiation Oncology, Department of Radiology, Louisiana State University Health Sciences Center, 200 West Esplanade Avenue, Suite 200, Kenner, LA 70065, USA
[h] Section of Radiation Oncology, Department of Medicine, Louisiana State University Health Sciences Center, 200 West Esplanade Avenue, Suite 200, Kenner, LA 70065, USA
[i] Section of Gastroenterology, Department of Medicine, Louisiana State University Health Sciences Center, 200 West Esplanade Avenue, Suite 200, Kenner, LA 70065, USA
[j] Carver College of Medicine at the University of Iowa, University of Iowa Hospitals and Clinics, 200 Hawkins Drive E419GH, Iowa City, IA 52242, USA
[k] UCLA Center for Excellence in Pancreatic Diseases, David Geffen School of Medicine at UCLA, 900 Veteran Avenue, 13-146 Warren Hall, Los Angeles, CA 90095–1742, USA
[l] Eastern Virginia Medical School, Strelitz Diabetes Center, 855 West Brambleton Avenue, Norfolk, VA 23510, USA
* Corresponding author. 200 West Esplanade Avenue, Suite 200, Kenner, LA 70065.
E-mail address: ewolte@lsuhsc.edu

Endocrinol Metab Clin N Am 40 (2011) 205–231
doi:10.1016/j.ecl.2010.08.004
0889-8529/11/$ – see front matter © 2011 Elsevier Inc. All rights reserved.

endo.theclinics.com

The diverse clinical and histologic nature of neuroendocrine tumors (NETs) and the relative paucity of adequately powered studies make it difficult to formulate a consistent diagnosis and treatment strategy. In addition, the rapid emergence and incorporation of new technologies into the clinical arena makes defining a "static" gold standard for diagnosis or treatment difficult.

Based on the expertise of the Inter-Science Institute's GI council and the expertise of the Louisiana State University Neuroendocrine tumor group's extensive experience, the authors compiled recommendations for the diagnostic work-up of patients with suspected NETs. These recommendations are presented in tabular form to make it easier for clinical reference. The guidelines help serve as an aggregate of the available consensus reports and reflect a practical, but academically oriented, approach to these tumors. These recommendations are from diverse areas of clinical practice including surgery, endocrinology, oncology, and gastroenterology.

TUMOR CLASSIFICATION

The most recent World Health Organization classification described three general categories of NETs: (1) well-differentiated NETs, which exhibit uncertain malignant potential; (2) well-differentiated NE carcinomas, which are low-grade malignancies; and (3) poorly differentiated NE carcinomas, which are high-grade malignancies.[1] Currently, the term "carcinoid" is commonly used to refer to well-differentiated tumors of the bronchus, thymus, ovary, or gut. The term "islet cell tumor" commonly refers to well-differentiated adenoma-like lesions that behave in a benign fashion. Likewise, the term "islet cell carcinoma" commonly refers to a well-differentiated neuroendocrine carcinoma that arises from the pancreas or periampullary region.[2] In all of these tumors, therapeutic decisions are influenced by the degree of cellular differentiation. The standard criteria for classifying these tumors are based on the histologic characteristics of the tumor. The microscopic assessment of tumor differentiation is commonly supplemented by immunohistochemical stains, such as Ki-67, chromogranin A (CgA), and synaptophysin. Other stains, such as neuron-specific enolase and specific stains for multiple peptides in pancreatic or duodenal tumors, are commonly used in the classification of NETs. Ultimately, the rationale for classification of these tumors is to provide the clinician with a framework for the prediction of a tumor's behavior. These "islet" cell tumors commonly stain positively for gastrin, glucagon, somatostatin, vasoactive intestinal peptide, pancreatic polypeptide, insulin, and C-peptide. It is critical to note that the presence of a positive peptide or amine stain in these pancreatic-duodenal tumors often leads to the mistaken diagnosis of a specific functional tumor type. The ultimate diagnosis of the functionality of these tumors is solely dependent on hypersecretion of peptide being documented in the serum, plasma, or urine. All NETs should undergo histologic evaluation by an experienced pathologist with extensive experience in NETs. These pathologists should determine the tumor's degree of differentiation. This should be determined by visual examination of the tumor and the selective use of stains, such as Ki-67, CgA, synaptophysin, and others as needed to assist the pathologist in determination of the proper classification.[1]

More recently, within the appendiceal carcinoid specimens, the terms "adenocarcinoid" or "mucinous carcinoid" have been used. It is the authors' opinion that these tumors represent a subset of carcinoid tumors that exhibit macroscopic similarities to carcinoids but morphologically also possess glandular structures that produce mucin. Their behavior mimics that of a classic adenocarcinoma rather than an NET.

BIOCHEMICAL MARKERS

Clinically suspicious symptoms or radiographic findings suggestive of an NET necessitate biochemical testing for hypersecreted peptides or amines or their metabolic by-products. Determination of peptide-amine levels requires attention to pre–blood draw (fasting) requirements and the cessation of specific foods or medications to yield optimal sensitivity and accuracy. Specific blood drawing techniques, such as the use of a tourniquet, tubes with special preservatives, specific specimen handling, and strict adherence to proper transportation requirements, are critical to ensure that the reported values are as accurate as possible.[3]

It is important to use laboratories that have specific expertise in the determination of peptide levels. Not all laboratories "normal" value ranges for a peptide or amine are the same and results from various laboratories' are not directly comparable. Split sample testing is the only way to ensure that two laboratory's normal values are identical or at least comparable (parallel values but consistently higher or lower by a given fraction).

Serotonin (5-HT) is commonly secreted by mid-gut NETs. This amine is costored with CgA in secretory granules in NET cells. Both are released on stimulation.[4] Common stimuli for the release of serotonin is the 5 "E's": (1) epinephrine, (2) exercise, (3) emotions, (4) ethanol, and (5) eating. Determination of plasma levels of 5-HT has not been generally useful in clinical practice, unlike its by-product, 5-hydroxy indole acetic acid (5-HIAA).[4]

The rate-limiting step for the synthesis of serotonin is the conversion of tryptophan into 5-HTP, catalyzed by the enzyme tryptophan hydroxylase. In midgut NETs, 5-HTP is rapidly converted to 5-HT by the enzyme dopa-decarboxylase. 5-HT is either stored in the neurosecretory granules or may be secreted directly into the vascular compartment. Most of the secreted 5-HT is taken up by platelets and stored in secretory granules. The rest remains free in the plasma, and circulating 5-HT is then largely converted into the urinary metabolite 5-HIAA by the enzyme monoamine oxidase and by aldehyde dehydrogenase. These enzymes are abundant in the kidney, and the urine of a patient with a symptomatic midgut carcinoid typically contains large amounts of 5-HIAA. In contrast, in patients with foregut tumors, the urine contains relatively little 5-HIAA but can contain large amounts of 5-HTP. It is presumed that these tumors are deficient in dopa-decarboxylase, which impairs the conversion of 5-HTP into 5-HT, leading to 5-HTP secretion into the vascular compartment. Some 5-HTP, however, is converted to 5-HT and 5-HIAA, resulting in the modest increase in these metabolites.

The normal range for 5-HIAA secretion is 2 to 8 mg per 24 hours, and the quantitation of serotonin and all of its metabolites usually permit the detection of 84% of patients with carcinoid tumors. No single marker measurement detects all cases of carcinoid syndrome, although the urine 5-HIAA seems to be the best screening procedure for patients suspected of having a mid-gut carcinoid.

In addition to specific peptides, secretory granules of neuroendocrine cells typically contain CgA-secretogranin (Sg) proteins.[5,6] These acidic peptides belong to a unique family of secretory proteins that share biochemical properties and are exclusively localized in neuronal and neuroendocrine secretory granules.[7] The name is derived from its original identification in the catecholamine-containing chromaffin granules of the adrenal medulla.[8]

The three major Cg-Sg proteins are currently designated as CgA and CgB and Sg11. CgA is the predominant protein in this family used as a biochemical marker. The levels of CgA are significantly elevated in most types of NETs, but particularly high levels are encountered in classical midgut NETs where levels of CgA may increase 100- to 1000-fold.[7] Because it does not rely on serotonin secretion, serum CgA is a more sensitive and broadly applicable marker than urinary 5-HIAA and may be used not only in patients with foregut and midgut NETs, but also in patients with bronchial and rectal carcinoid tumors in whom urinary 5-HIAA levels are less likely to be elevated.

The widespread use of proton pump inhibitors limits the usefulness of CgA as a screening tool for NETs. Chronic proton pump inhibitors use elevates CgA levels to similar levels as seen with patients with NETs, thus making it hard to interpret results.

Pancreastatin, a fragment of CgA, useful in several studies, is believed by some authors to be a more sensitive marker of tumor volume than the intact CgA molecule.[9,10] This is caused by intracellular and extracellular processing of CgA by prohormone convertase 1.[10] The authors recommend that any patient with a suspected NET have CgA and pancreastatin blood levels checked after cessation of proton pump inhibitors. They also suggest that all patients have a 24-hour urine collection for 5-HIAA. Furthermore, depending on history the location and symptomatology of most patients NETs can be identified. This can assist in the decision of what other tumor markers should be checked at the time of blood testing (**Tables 1** and **2**).

IMAGING

The preliminary work-up of an NET often includes plain abdominal radiographs and CT. These tests are often used nonspecifically because of the presence of vague symptom complexes. Once the NETs diagnosis is suspected, more specific means of imaging are typically used. For detecting the primary NET tumor, a multimodality approach is best and may include CT, MRI, somatostatin receptor scintigraphy (SRS), endoscopic ultrasound (EUS), endoscopy, digital selective angiography, and venous sampling. There is little difference in sensitivity between CT and MRI, although CT is probably superior for localizing the primary tumor, mesenteric invasion, and thoracic lesions, whereas MRI may be superior in characterizing liver lesions.[11] EUS combined with biopsy is the most sensitive method to detect pancreatic NETs.[12]

The most sensitive imaging modality for detecting metastatic disease in NETs is SRS (OctreoScan). This technique is based on the tumor's expression of somatostatin receptor type 2 (sst2). Five somatostatin receptor subtypes exist; however, tumors may not express all types of this receptor. Thus, some NETs are not visualized because of the lack of sst2 receptor.

The use of positron emission tomography scanning in undifferentiated tumors or small cell-like lesions of the bronchus or thymus is highly effective. The role of positron emission tomography scanning for well-differentiated NETs is less well delineated. Results suggest that these well-differentiated tumors are seen by ^{18}F positron emission tomography scans in about 10% to 20% of patients.[13]

After a gut-based NETs is suspected, barium studies or endoscopy may be helpful to localize the primary tumor. Capsule endoscopy and double-balloon push-pull enteroscopy have been useful in some cases of midgut-based NETs. The authors currently use a multimodality approach to the imaging of NET patients. Visualization of the primary tumor can be done with endoscopy, EUS, or barium studies; however, these do not provide information about the nodal or organ metastasis status. They routinely use CT scanning for the evaluation of mesenteric and mediastinal nodal basins and to search for metastatic disease. All patients should undergo SRS imaging to document if the tumor has the sst2 receptors and to help identify occult disease that can be missed by other imaging techniques. The authors reserve

MRI with gadolinium contrast administration for patients found to have liver metastasis that may be amenable to surgical excision. Newer contrast agents for liver imaging may be helpful for identification of occult metastasis; however, this is still experimental (**Tables 3** and **4**).

SYMPTOMATIC TREATMENT

Long-acting somatostatin analogs have been proved to provide reliable control of peptide and amine-mediated symptoms. The current generation of approved somatostatin analogs predominantly recognizes sst2 and sst5. These somatostatin analogs bind to membrane-bound somatostatin receptors, turn on the inhibitory subunit of the G-protein, and subsequently trigger the activation a number of postreceptor signal transduction pathways, such as IP-3, c-AMP, and adenylate cyclase. The result of somatostatin analog therapy is the inhibition of amine and peptide hypersecretion.[2]

The two commercially available somatostatin analogs are octreotide and lanreotide. Aqueous octreotide has a 90- to 120-minute half-life and requires subcutaneous injection three times per day. Currently, it is limited to use as "rescue medication" for breakthrough symptoms of carcinoid syndrome, as intravenous infusion to prevent carcinoid crisis in patients undergoing operative or stressful medical examinations, or as a continuous subcutaneous infusion in patients who wish to avoid monthly injection of octreotide LAR. Typical starting doses for the aqueous form of octreotide are 150 to 500 μg three times a day. When used as a continuous infusion, common doses of aqueous octreotide range from 1000 to 2000 μg per day (30–60 mg/month).[14] Finally, to prevent carcinoid crisis during operation, the authors recommend a 500-μg intravenous bolus 2 hours before the surgical procedure followed by a 500-μg per hour intravenous infusion. This infusion is tapered off in the immediate postoperative period. In cases where carcinoid crisis still occurs, 1- to 5-mg boluses of octreotide may be useful.

Several experts have advocated use of higher monthly doses of octreotide LAR in patients with breakthrough symptoms. Most clinicians prefer to use 30-mg doses at shorter dosing intervals rather than using multiple injections once a month. Trough plasma octreotide levels can be used to evaluate the circulating octreotide levels in patients with poorly controlled symptoms, rising biomarker values, or progressive tumor growth.[15,16] The authors believe that the optimum saturation of the sst2 receptor should occur at plasma levels of approximately 10,000 pg/mL (1×10^{-8} M). These plasma levels are approximately 10 times the K_d for octreotide and the sst2 receptor. These measurements may become increasingly important because it has been shown that the optimum antiproliferative effects of somatostatin analogs occur in similar concentration ranges.[17,18]

Traditionally, somatostatin analog therapy has been considered to be useful only for the control of symptoms and was thought not to have a proved benefit on survival. Recently, a randomized prospective multiinstitutional trial has shown a survival benefit for the use of octreotide LAR. In this study the authors showed a significant increase in progression-free survival in those patients who used LAR.[19]

Lanreotide (Somatuline Depot Ipsen, Brisbane, CA) is a long-acting somatostatin analog that is available in 60-, 90-, and 120-mg doses. These doses can be administered by deep subcutaneous injection. Currently, Somatuline Depot is available in the United States for the treatment of acromegly; however, it can be used as an "out of indication" medication by physicians wishing to offer their patients an alternative to octreotide LAR.

The use of long-acting somatostatin analog therapy varies by the disease process. Doses of octreotide LAR (30 mg/every 2–4 weeks) are commonly associated with

Table 1
Recommendations of the Inter Science Institute Gastrointestinal Council on the use of biomarkers for diagnosis and treatment of neuroendocrine tumors (carcinoid and islet cell)

| Marker | Consensus Recommendation | | Individual Recommendations: Physician/Specialty | | | | | | | |
| | Tumor Type | Rec | EAW Surgery | | TMO Endocrinology | | AIV Endocrinology | | WG Gastroenterology | |
			Type	Rec	Type	Rec	Type	Rec	Type	Rec
5-HIAA	C	M	C	M	C	M	C	M	B	M
CGA	B	M	B	M	B	M	B	M	B	M
Substance P	C	P	C	P	C	M	C	P	N	P
Neurokinin A	C	P	C	P	C	P	C	P	N	P
Secretin	N	NR	N	NR	N	NR	N	NR	N	NR
Gastrin	B	P	B	P	B	P	IC	M	IC	P
Parietal cell Ab	C	P	C	P	C	P	C	P	IC	P
PP	IC	P	IC	P	IC	P	IC	P	IC	P
Blood glucose	B	M	B	M	B	M	B	M	B	M
Fasting insulin	IC	M	IC	M	IC	M	IC	M	IC	M
Proinsulin	IC	M	IC	M	IC	M	IC	M	IC	M
C-peptide	IC	M	IC	M	IC	M	IC	M	IC	M
VIP	IC	R	IC	M	IC	P	B	M	IC	P
Glucagon	IC	R	IC	M	IC	R	IC	M	IC	P

Somatostatin	IC	P	IC	M	IC	P	B	P	M	N	NR
PTH	IC	R	B	R	IC	R	IC	R	M	IC	P
Ca++	B	M	B	R	B	R	B	R	M	B	M
Calcitonin	B	P	B	P	B	P	B	P	M	B	P
Prolactin	IC	P	IC	P	IC	R	IC	P	P	IC	P
ACTH	B	P	B	P	B	R	B	P	P	B	P
PSA	N	NR	N	NR	N	NR	N	NR	NR	N	NR
AFP	N	NR	N	NR	N	NR	N	NR	NR	N	NR
CEA	N	NR	N	NR	N	NR	N	NR	NR	N	NR
Chemistry	B	M	B	M	B	R	B	M	M	B	M
CBC	B	M	B	M	B	R	B	M	M	B	M

Tumor type: B, both; C, carcinoid; IC, islet cell; N, neither.

Recommendation: M, mandatory; NR, not recommended; P, potentially useful; R, recommended.

Physicians making recommendations: AIV, Aaron Vinik; EAW, Eugene Woltering; TMO, Thomas O'Dorisio; WG, Vay Liang (Bill) Go.

Abbreviations: Ab, antibody (parietal cell antibody); ACTH, adrenocorticotropic hormone; AFP, alpha-fetoprotein; Ca++, calcium ion; CBC, complete blood count; CEA, carcinoembryonic antigen; CGA, chromogranin A; 5-HIAA, 5-hydroxyindoleacetic acid; PP, pancreatic polypeptide; PSA, prostate-specific antigen; PTH, parathyroid hormone; VIP, vasoactive intestinal peptide.

Table 2
Recommendations of the New Orleans Louisiana Neuroendocrine Tumor group on the use of biomarkers for diagnosis and treatment of neuroendocrine tumors (carcinoid and islet cell)

| Markers | Consensus Recommendation | | Individual Recommendations: Physician/Specialty | | | | | | | | | |
| | Tumor Type | Rec | EAW Surgery/Oncology | | JPB Transplant Surgery | | YZW General Surgery | | SJ HPB Surgery | | LA Medicine/Oncology | |
			Type	Rec	Type	Rec	Type	Rec	Type	Rec	Type	Rec
5-HIAA	C	M	C	M	C	M	C	M	C	M	B	M
CGA	B	M	B	M	B	M	B	M	B	M	B	M
Substance P	B	P	C	P	B	P	B	M	C	P	C	P
Neurokinin A	B	R	C	P	B	R	B	P	C	P	B	M
Secretin	N	NR	N	NR	IC	P	IC	P	N	NR	N	NR
Gastrin	B	P	B	NR	B	P	IC	R	B	P	B	R
Parietal cell Ab	C	R	C	P	C	R	C	P	C	P	B	R
PP	IC	R	IC	P	IC	R	IC	R	IC	P	IC	R
Blood glucose	B	M	B	M	B	M	IC	M	B	M	IC	M
Fasting insulin	IC	R	IC	M	IC	R	IC	M	IC	R	IC	P
Pro-insulin	IC	R	IC	M	IC	R	IC	M	IC	R	IC	P
C-peptide	IC	R	IC	M	IC	P	IC	M	IC	R	IC	P

VIP	IC	R	IC	M	IC	P	IC	P	R	IC	P
Glucagon	IC	R	IC	M	IC	P	IC	P	R	IC	P
Somatostatin	IC	R	IC	M	IC	P	IC	P	R	IC	P
PTH	B	P	B	R	B	P	C	P	P	B	P
Ca++	B	P	B	R	B	P	C	P	P	B	P
Calcitonin	B	P	B	P	B	P	N	P	NR	B	P
Prolactin	IC	P	IC	P	IC	P	N	P	NR	N	NR
ACTH	N	NR	B	P	N	N	N	NR	NR	C	P
PSA	N	NR	N	C	C	P	N	P	NR	N	NR
AFP	N	NR	N	N	N	NR	N	N	NR	N	NR
CEA	N	NR	N	N	N	NR	N	NR	NR	N	NR
Chemistry	B	R	B	C	B	P	IC	P	R	B	B
CBC	B	M	B	B	B	M	B	B	R	B	M

Tumor type: B, both; C, carcinoid; IC, islet cell; N, neither.

Recommendation: M, mandatory; NR, not recommended; P, potentially useful; R, recommended.

Physicians making recommendations: EAW, Eugene Woltering; JPB, J. Philip Boudreau; YZW, Yi-Zarn Wang; SJ, Saju Joseph; LA, Lowell Anthony.

Abbreviations: Ab, antibody (parietal cell antibody); ACTH, adrenocorticotropic hormone; AFP, alpha-fetoprotein; Ca++, calcium ion; CBC, complete blood count; CEA, carcinoembryonic antigen; CGA, chromogranin A; 5-HIAA, 5-hydroxyindoleacetic acid; PP, pancreatic polypeptide; PSA, prostate-specific antigen; PTH, parathyroid hormone; VIP, vasoactive intestinal peptide.

Table 3
Recommendations of the Inter Science Institute Gastrointestinal Council on the use of imaging for diagnosis and treatment of neuroendocrine tumors (carcinoid and islet cell)

| Imaging Study | Consensus Recommendation | | Individual Recommendations: Physician/Specialty | | | | | | | |
| | Tumor Type | Rec | EAW Surgery | | TMO Endocrinology | | AIV Endocrinology | | WG Gastroenterology | |
			Type	Rec	Type	Rec	Type	Rec	Type	Rec
CT	B	M	B	R	B	R	B	M	B	M
MRI/MRA	B	P	B	P	B	P	B	P	B	R
Octreoscan	B	M	B	R	B	M	B	M	B	R
Ultrasound	B	R	B	R	B	R	B	P	IC	M
EUS	IC	P	IC	P	IC	R	IC	P	IC	M
Endoscopy	B	P	B	P	B	R	B	P	B	P
Barium studies	N	NR	N	NR	N	NR	N	NR	N	NR
Angiography	B	P	B	P	B	P	B	P	B	P
Multimodality approach	B	M	B	M	B	M	B	M	B	M
Imaging for metastasis	B	M	B	M	B	M	B	M	B	M
MIBG	B	P	B	P	C	P	B	P	B	P
Bone scan	B	P	B	P	B	P	B	P	B	P
FDG-PET	B	P	B	P	B	P	B	P	B	P
Transthoracic echo	N	NR	NR	NR	NR	NR	NR	NR	NR	NR

Tumor type: B, both; C, carcinoid; IC, islet cell; N, neither.
Recommendation: M, mandatory; NR, not recommended; P, potentially useful; R, recommended.
Physicians making recommendations: EAW, Eugene Woltering; TMO, Thomas O'Dorisio; AIV, Aaron Vinik; WG, Vay Liang (Bill) Go.
Abbreviations: CT, computed tomography; EUS, endoscopic ultrasound; FDG-PET, fluorodeoxyglucose-positron emission tomography; MIBG, meta-iodobenzyl-guanidine; MRA, magnetic resonance angiography; MRI, magnetic resonance imaging.

Table 4
Represents the recommendations of the New Orleans Louisiana Neuroendocrine Tumor group on the use of imaging for diagnosis and treatment of neuroendocrine tumors (carcinoid and islet cell)

Imaging Study	Consensus Recommendation		Individual Recommendations: Physician/Specialty									
	Tumor Type	Rec	EAW Surgery		JPB Transplant Surgery		YZW General Surgery		SJ HPB Surgery		LA Medicine/Oncology	
			Type	Rec	Type	Rec	Type	Rec	Type	Rec	Type	Rec
CT	B	M	B	R	B	M	B	M	B	M	B	M
MRI/MRA	B	P	B	P	B	R	B	P	B	P	B	P
Octreoscan	B	M	B	R	B	M	C	M	B	M	B	M
Ultrasound	B	R	B	R	B	P	B	M	B	R	B	P
EUS	IC	P	IC	P	IC	R	B	P	IC	P	IC	P
Endoscopy	B	P	B	P	C	P	C	P	B	P	B	P
Barium studies	N	NR	N	NR	N	NR	N	NR	N	NR	B	P
Angiography	B	P	B	P	B	P	IC	P	B	P	B	P
Multimodality approach	B	M	B	M	B	R	B	R	B	M	B	M
Imaging for metastasis	B	M	B	M	B	M	B	M	B	M	B	M
MIBG	B	R	B	P	B	R	B	M	B	R	B	R
Bone scan	B	P	B	P	B	R	B	P	B	P	B	P
FDG-PET	B	P	B	P	N	NR	B	P	B	P	B	P
Trans-thoracic Echo	C	R	N	NR	C	M	C	P	C	R	C	R

Tumor type: B, both; C, carcinoid; IC, islet cell; N, neither.
Recommendation: M, mandatory; NR, not recommended; P, potentially useful; R, recommended.
Physicians making recommendations: EAW, Eugene Woltering; JPB, J. Philip Boudreaux; YZW, Yi-Zarn Wang; SJ, Saju Joseph; LA- Lowell Anthony.
Abbreviations: CT, computed tomography; EUS, endoscopic ultrasound; FDG-PET, fluorodeoxyglucose-positron emission tomography; MIBG, meta-iodobenzyl-guanidine; MRI, magnetic resonance angiography; MRI, magnetic resonance imaging.

excellent symptom control in patients with carcinoid syndrome. Similar results have been seen with Somatuline Depot (120 mg every 2 weeks).

Long-acting somatostatin analogs are less effective in the control of hypoglycemia in insulinoma caused by the lack of sst2 receptors on the tumor. Use of somatostatin analogs in patients with insulinomas may actually worsen hypoglycemia because of the relative higher efficacy of these analogs to inhibit glucagon and growth hormone secretion versus insulin secretion.

The control of gastric acid hypersecretion in gastrinoma (Zollinger-Ellison syndrome) is easy to achieve with higher-dose oral proton-pump inhibitors than for treatment of ulcer disease. Proton pump inhibitors effectively control acid, but leave gastrin levels unchanged. Recent studies advocate the early use of somatostatin analogs in patients with metastatic gastrinomas to help control excessive gastrin release and gastric acid secretion.[20,21] Jensen and colleagues,[22] from the National Cancer Institute, believe that somatostatin analog therapy now should be the "front line" therapy rather than chemotherapy in the treatment of patients with metastatic gastrinoma.

Octreotide has been shown to be effective in the control of watery diarrhea for patients with Verner-Morrison syndrome (vasoactive intestinal peptideoma) and for the control of necrolytic migratory erythema in patients with glucagonoma syndrome.[7]

All patients with NETs, except insulinomas, should receive octreotide therapy either with LAR injections or subcutaneous pumps. The goal of this therapy is to control symptoms and keep sst2 receptors saturated to inhibit proliferation of tumor cells. Any patient with worsening symptoms on a stable dose, increasing tumor marker levels, or new patients on treatment should undergo plasma testing for octreotide trough level to ensure the use of appropriate doses. Furthermore, for asymptomatic patients occasional trough levels and tumor marker levels should be checked as part of routine surveillance (**Tables 5** and **6**).

CHEMOTHERAPY

Tumor growth leading to liver failure has emerged as the leading cause of death in patients with NETs, underscoring the need for new systemic therapies. Approximately two thirds of patients present with metastatic disease that is not amenable to surgical resection or biotherapy. In those patients who are not surgical candidates and who do not respond to biotherapy with somatostatin analogs, or in those whose symptoms recur following careful adjustment of analog dosing, chemotherapy should be considered. Cytotoxic therapy is also used in patients with atypical carcinoids that exhibit high proliferation rates, as evidenced by a proliferation index greater than 10% to 20%, determined by Ki-67 staining (MEB-1antibody). In general, patients with pancreatic or duodenal malignant islet cell tumors respond better to systemic chemotherapy than those who suffer from gut-based carcinoid tumors. Recent work by Drs Warner and Woltering suggest that well-differentiated midgut carcinoids with low proliferative indices may still be candidates for chemotherapy.[23]

Responses to single-agent chemotherapy have been disappointing. In patients with pancreatic NETs tumors streptozotocin, chlorozotocin, doxorubicin, 5-fluorouracil, taxol, and dacarbazine have been tested individually and are relatively ineffective. Such monotherapies not only result in poor response rates, but more importantly all induced significant toxicity.[24] Streptozotocin has demonstrated the most activity in pancreatic NETs, with response rates between 36% and 42%.[24,25] Recently, single-agent studies of irinotecan and high-dose paclitaxel have been evaluated but responses continue to be disappointing.[26,27] Combination therapy for pancreatic

Table 5
Recommendations of the Inter Science Institute Gastrointestinal Council on symptomatic treatment of neuroendocrine tumors (carcinoid and islet cell)

| Treatment | Consensus Recommendation | | Individual Recommendations: Physician/Specialty | | | | | | | |
| | Tumor Type | Rec | EAW Surgery | | TMO Endocrinology | | AIV Endocrinology | | WG Gastroenterology | |
			Type	Rec	Type	Rec	Type	Rec	Type	Rec
Somatostatin analog	B	M	B	M	B	M	B	M	B	M
Octreotide	B	M	B	M	B	M	B	M	B	M
Lanreotide	B	M	B	M	B	M	B	M	B	M
Long-acting release	B	M	B	M	B	M	B	M	B	M
Octreotide LAR dose	B	R	B	R	B	R	B	R	C	R
Lanreotide Autogel	B	R	B	R	B	R	B	R	C	R
SSA for symptom control	B	M	B	M	B	M	B	M	B	M
SSA to control tumor progression	B	R	B	R	B	R	B	R	B	R
Interferon	B	P	C	P	IC	R	C	P	B	P
Combination interferon and octreotide	C	P	C	P	IC	R	C	P	C	P
Proton pump inhibitors	IC	R	IC	R	IC	M	IC	R	IC	P
Diazoxide	I	R	IC	R	IC	M	IC	R	N	NR

Tumor type: B, both; C, carcinoid; IC, islet cell; N, neither.
Recommendation: M, mandatory; NR, not recommended; P, potentially useful; R, recommended.
Physicians making recommendations: EAW, Eugene Woltering; TMO, Thomas O'Dorisio; AIV, Aaron Vinik; WG, Vay Liang (Bill) Go.
Abbreviations: LAR, long-acting release; SSA, somatostatin analog.

Table 6
Recommendations of the New Orleans Louisiana Neuroendocrine Tumor group on symptomatic treatment of neuroendocrine tumors (carcinoid and islet cell)

| Treatment | Consensus Recommendation | | Individual Recommendations: Physician/Specialty | | | | | | | | | |
| | | | EAW Surgery/ Oncology | | JPB Transplant Surgery | | YZW General Surgery | | SJ HPB Surgery | | LA Medicine/ Oncology | |
	Tumor Type	Rec	Type	Rec	Type	Rec	Type	Rec	Type	Rec	Type	Rec
Somatostatin analog	B	M	B	M	B	P	B	M	B	M	B	R
Octreotide	B	M	B	M	B	P	B	M	B	M	B	R
Lanreotide	B	M	B	M	B	P	B	M	B	M	B	P
Long-acting release	B	R	B	M	B	P	C	M	B	R	B	R
Octreotide LAR dose	B	R	B	R	B	P	C	M	B	R	B	R
Lanreotide Autogel	B	R	B	R	B	P	C	M	B	M	B	P
SSA for symptom control	B	M	B	M	B	M	B	R	B	M	B	M
SSA to control tumor progression	B	R	B	R	B	P	C	P	B	R	B	R
Interferon	C	P	C	P	B	P	N	NR	C	P	C	P
Combination Interferon & Octreotide	C	P	C	P	B	P	N	NR	C	P	C	P
Proton pump inhibitors	IC	R	IC	R	B	NR	N	NR	IC	R	IC	M
Diazoxide	IC	R	IC	R	IC	P	IC	R	IC	P	IC	P

Tumor type: B, both; C, carcinoid; IC, islet cell; N, neither.
Recommendation: M, mandatory; NR, not recommended; P, potentially useful; R, recommended.
Physicians making recommendations: EAW, Eugene Woltering; JPB, J. Philip Boudreaux; YZW, Yi-Zarn Wang; SJ, Saju Joseph; LA, Lowell Anthony.
Abbreviations: LAR, long-acting release; SSA, somatostatin analog.

NETs most commonly use streptozotocin and 5-fluorouracil, with higher response rates reported than with monotherapy alone. Doxorubicin used in combination with streptozotocin has also been used, but conflicting interpretation of studies has made determination of the efficacy of these regimens difficult. Doxorubicin-streptozotocin combinations have been more effective in patients with metastatic insulinoma and vasoactive intestinal peptideoma than in carcinoid-related tumors. Another indication for chemotherapy is in patients with anaplastic small-cell neuroendocrine carcinomas (atypical carcinoids). These tumors often respond to treatment with etoposide and cisplatin.[24]

Although a two-drug regimen may be more effective than a single-agent regimen, there is no evidence that a three-drug combination, such as streptozotocin, 5-fluoro-uracil, and doxorubicin, is better than a two-drug regimen, and three-drug combinations should not be considered as standard therapy.[28]

Interferon-α, an anticancer therapeutic agent, is active as an immunomodulater secondary to up-regulation of natural killer cells. In addition, interferon demonstrates a cytostatic effect by stalling the (G1-S) phase of the cell cycle and down-regulating genes coding for nuclear proteins involved in cell proliferation. Because of its severe side effects this drug is not commonly used in the United States to treat metastatic NETs. The combined use of interferon and somatostatin has not shown a greater anti-tumor effect that the individual agents alone and the combination is associated with significant side effects.[29]

All patients who require chemotherapy for NETs should be evaluated for clinical trials at expert centers. Although the treatment regimens are quite standard, the rarity of these cases makes it imperative that all eligible patients be involved in clinical trials or tracked for further study (**Tables 7** and **8**).

RADIONUCLIDE THERAPIES AND CHEMOEMBOLIZATION
Radiolabeled Somatostatin Analog Therapy

After somatostatin-receptor binding, a fraction of the ligand-receptor complexes (endosomes) internalize. This internalization process is an effective means of deliv-ering cytotoxic treatments, especially those emitting short-range decay particles, such as Auger or conversion electrons, to the neoplastic cell nucleus. Such short-range therapies include [125]I- and [111]Indium-labeled somatostatin analogs. Unfortu-nately, these short-range agents lack significant ability to kill adjacent non–receptor expressing cells, which has led to the use of higher-energy radionuclides.[30]

In contrast, [177]Lu- and ^{90}Y-labeled somatostatin analogs have significant advan-tages over the short-range therapies because they have significantly higher energy and thus a wider radius of action. Peptide receptor radiotherapy has developed into a critical component of the overall therapeutic strategy in patients with NETs. Even though the more energetic therapies (^{177}Lu and ^{90}Y) are not currently available in the United States, the European nuclear medicine community has been actively treat-ing patients with these agents.[31]

Treatment with radiolabeled somatostatin analogs is a promising new tool in the management of patients who have inoperable or widely metastatic NETs, especially because these treatments are associated with minimal severe side effects. Review of the available literature revealed partial tumor response rates ranging from 9% to 38%.[31] The results obtained with ^{90}Y and ^{177}Lu are encouraging, although a direct, randomized comparison between the various isotopic treatments is unlikely to occur. Tumor remission has been positively correlated with high uptake by tumors during SRS, limited number of metastases, and size of liver metastases. Interestingly,

Table 7
Recommendations of the Inter Science Institute Gastrointestinal Council on the use of chemotherapy for treatment of neuroendocrine tumors (carcinoid and islet cell)

| | Consensus Recommendation | | Individual Recommendations: Physician/Specialty | | | | | | | |
| | | | EAW Surgery | | TMO Endocrinology | | AIV Endocrinology | | WG Gastroenterology | |
Chemotherapeutic Agent	Tumor Type	Rec	Type	Rec	Type	Rec	Type	Rec	Type	Rec
Cisplatin	B	R	C	R	B	R	C	R	B	M
Etopside	B	R	C	R	B	R	C	R	B	R
Cisplatin + etopside	B	R	C	R	B	R	C	R	B	P
5-Fluorouracil	B	R	B	R	B	R	B	R	IC	P
Streptozotocin	IC	P	IC	R	IC	P	IC	R	B	R
5-FU + STZ	IC	P	IC	R	IC	P	IC	R	B	P
Adriamycin	B	P	B	P	N	NR	B	P	N	P
Dacarbazine	N	NR	N	NR	N	NR	N	NR	N	P
Carboplatin	B	P	C	P	B	P	B	P	N	P
Doxorubicin	N	NR	C	P	N	NR	N	NR	N	P
Other combinations	B	P	B	P	B	P	B	P	B	P
5-FU/STZ/Dox	IC	R	IC	R	IC	R	IC	R	N	P

Tumor type: B, both; C, carcinoid; IC, islet cell; N, neither.
Recommendation: M, mandatory; NR, not recommended; P, potentially useful; R, recommended.
Physicians making recommendations: EAW, Eugene Woltering; TMO, Thomas O'Dorisio; AIV, Aaron Vinik; WG, Vay Liang (Bill) Go.
Abbreviations: 5-FU, 5-fluorouracil; Dox, doxorubicin; STZ, streptozotocin.

Table 8
Recommendations of the New Orleans Louisiana Neuroendocrine Tumor group on the use of chemotherapy for treatment of neuroendocrine tumors (carcinoid and islet cell)

Chemotherapeutic Agent	Consensus Recommendation		Individual Recommendations: Physician/Specialty					
			EAW Surgery/ Oncology		SJ HPB Surgery		LA Medicine/ Oncology	
	Tumor Type	Rec	Type	Rec	Type	Rec	Type	Rec
Cisplatin	C	R	C	R	C	P	N	NR
Etoposide	C	R	C	R	C	P	N	NR
Cisplatin + etoposide	C	R	C	R	C	P	N	NR
5-FU	B	P	B	R	B	P	B	P
STZ	IC	P	IC	R	IC	P	IC	P
5-FU + STZ	IC	P	IC	R	IC	R	IC	P
Adriamycin	B	P	B	P	B	P	I	P
Dacarbazine	N	NR	N	NR	N	NR	IC	P
Carboplatin	C	P	C	P	C	P	N	NR
Doxorubicin	B	P	C	P	B	P	IC	P
Other combinations	B	P	B	P	B	P	B	P
5FU/STZ/Dox	IC	P	IC	R	IC	P	IC	P

Tumor type: B, both; C, carcinoid; IC, islet cell; N, neither.
Recommendation: M, mandatory; NR, not recommended; P, potentially useful; R, recommended.
Physicians making recommendations: EAW, Eugene Woltering; SJ, Saju Joseph; LA, Lowell Anthony.
Abbreviations: 5-FU, 5-fluorouracil; Dox, doxorubicin; STZ, streptozotocin.

metastatic gastrinomas often exhibit extremely intense ^{111}In uptake, but have a significantly reduced survival compared with other NETs patients.

In general the "Krenning" scale is used to evaluate the potential for response to these therapies. A "Krenning" Grade II tumor uptake is isodense with the liver, whereas a Grade III tumor uptake is greater than the liver but less that the kidney. A grade IV tumor has equal uptake to the kidney on octreotide scanning.[30] Responses to radiolabeled somatostatin analog therapy are generally proportional to the Krenning scale uptake.

[131]I MIBG Therapy

One of the newest treatment modalities available in the United States is the use of I-MIBG for scanning and treatment for those individuals who exhibit intense tumor uptake. Long-term studies of this therapy are underway and seem to have a reasonable risk–benefit ratio. The newest addition to this therapy is the availability of high specific activity [131]I. The ability to treat patients with higher specific activity iodine should enhance response rates.[32]

Chemoembolization

Early in our clinical experience, chemoembolization was used before surgery to shrink tumors and it was hoped to enhance the effectiveness of resection. It was quickly discovered, however, that subsequent cytoreduction was significantly hindered by the extensive scarring induced by the chemoembolization. Thus, chemoembolization is reserved for patients with advanced NETs involving the liver that are no longer amenable to curative surgery or ablation.[33,34]

On occasion, alternating chemoembolization with systemic chemotherapy may offer an improvement over chemotherapy alone, even when the tumor is not confined to the liver.[32] Because liver disease is often a major source of symptoms and is generally the life-limiting aspect of the disease, aggressive liver-targeted treatment is indicated.

In chemoembolization, doxorubicin, mitomycin C, or cisplatin is combined with iodized oil (lipiodol) or gelatin foam. When Gelfoam (Pfizer Injectables, Pharmacia & Upjohn Co, New York, NY, USA) is used as the embolic material, the chemotherapies are admixed with the Gelfoam until a maple-syrup–like consistency is achieved. Using highly selective hepatic arterial catheterization, the emulsion is injected into the arterial blood supply of the liver metastases. Alternatively, the injection of a lipiodol drug mixture is followed by embolization of the vessels using a gelatin-containing slurry. The process of embolization is continued until a marked degree of vascular occlusion has been obtained. If arterial spasm occurs during embolization the angiographer waits until the spasm clears to ensure that the maximum amount of the embolic agent has been injected.

It has been speculated that the ischemia and resulting hypoxia induced by the embolization component may actually enhance the cytotoxic action of the chemotherapy. The mechanism for this is unclear but may revolve around the metabolic changes induced in tumor cells under hypoxic conditions.

The M.D. Anderson experience suggests that carcinoid tumors have improved outcomes following chemoembolization compared with pancreatic islet cell tumors. The addition of systemic chemotherapy to embolization did not alter treatment effects in patients who had carcinoid tumors but did result in higher response rates in the patients who had pancreatic islet cell tumors. In each tumor type neither chemoembolization nor simple embolization conferred a significant overall survival or progression-free survival advantage over the other.[34]

New techniques for chemoembolization have also enhanced treatment techniques. With the development of microsphere technology, chemoembolization is capable of delivering not only chemotherapeutics but also radiation to the tumor sites. This may represent a new treatment modality that enhances the ability to treat hepatic NETs metastasis.

All patients with metastatic NETs should be evaluated for a multimodality approach. The authors use radiolabeled octreotide for most patients with unresectable metastatic disease. Also, early aggressive treatment of unresectable liver metastasis with chemoembolization and microsphere techniques is recommended. This often allows for symptom reduction, which is a significant morbidity in this patient population. The authors have now begun an aggressive MIBG treatment protocol that is reserved for patients with no surgical options. Any patient with metastatic NETs should be referred to a center with experience in advanced NET treatment techniques including MIBG, microsphere, and chemoembolization procedures. Finally, patients with previous biliary manipulation or reconstruction have a significantly higher incidence of liver abscess after intervention by either chemoembolization or MIBG and these patients should be treated empirically with antibiotics and watched for signs of abscess formation (**Tables 9** and **10**).

SURGERY

NETs are often biologically inert, slow-growing tumors with a prolonged disease course. Their indolent nature makes surgical resection of primary disease, nodal involvement, and metastatic lesions an integral part of both curative and palliative treatment regimens. The slow growth of most NETs and the high incidence of nonfunctional tumors often allow extensive disease to develop undetected. These tumors often manifest themselves by secondary symptoms, such as bowel obstruction or hepatic dysfunction. In general, an aggressive approach should be used to clear the primary tumor, to cytoreduce regional lymph nodes, and to resect or treat appropriate distant metastases, including liver tumors.

Radiofrequency ablation has increased the surgeon's ability to render the liver free of tumor. In addition, for those lesions previously treated with resection or Transarterial chemoembolization, radiofrequency ablation may provide adjunctive treatment after regrowth or recurrence. However, there is still a great deal of controversy as to whether radiofrequency ablation should be used as a primary treatment technique.

The decision to undertake liver cytoreduction is made easier when symptoms of hormone excess are not well controlled medically. Surgical resection of NET liver metastases has, on occasion, seemed to provide a long-term cure and 5-year survival rates have been reported to be 71% to 85%.[35] Resection of the primary tumor and the mesenteric lymph nodes can lead to a significant reduction in tumor-related symptoms and result in a survival advantage.[36]

Cytoreductive surgery, commonly defined as resection of 90% of the tumor, attempts to reduce symptoms and facilitate the effect of nonoperative strategies.[37] Que and colleagues[37] reported a successful control of symptoms in 90% of patients after a debulking of 90% or more of liver-based tumor burden. Givi and colleagues[38] recently showed improved survival in patients whose primary tumors were resected at the time of cytoreductive surgery, despite their having metastatic disease.

In a recent study, mesenteric encasement leading to intestinal ischemia was successfully relieved in 10 of 12 patients.[38] Bowel obstruction secondary to peritoneal carcinomatosis is a major cause of mortality in these patients. Carcinoid tumors of the small intestine typically cause a severe desmoplastic reaction and deeply infiltrate lymph nodes around major vessels of the root of the small bowel. In these circumstances, complete resection is seldom achieved; however, cytoreduction should be

Table 9
Recommendations of the Inter Science Institute Gastrointestinal Council on the use of radionuclide and embolic therapy for the treatment of neuroendocrine tumors (carcinoid and islet cell)

Radionucleotide or Embolic Therapy	Consensus Recommendation		Individual Recommendations: Physician/Specialty							
			EAW Surgery		TMO Endocrinology		AIV Endocrinology		WG Gastroenterology	
	Tumor Type	Rec	Type	Rec	Type	Rec	Type	Rec	Type	Rec
131I-MIBG	C	P	IC	P	C	P	C	P	C	P
90Y Octreotide	B	P	B	P	B	P	B	P	B	P
90Y Lanreotide	B	P	B	P	B	P	B	P	B	P
177Lu-DOTA Try3 Octreotide	B	P	B	P	B	P	B	P	B	P
RFA	B	R	B	R	B	R	B	P	B	P
Chemoembolization	B	R	B	R	B	R	B	R	B	P
CE + doxorubicin	B	R	B	R	B	R	B	R	B	P
CE + cisplatin	B	R	B	R	B	R	B	R	B	P
CE + 5-FU	B	P	B	R	B	R	B	R	N	NR
CE + mitomycin C	B	P	B	R	B	R	B	R	B	NR
Bland HA embolization	N	NR	N	NR	N	NR	B	NR	B	P
CE + IV chemo	N	NR	N	NR	N	NR	N	NR	N	NR
Bisphosphonates	B	P	B	R	B	R	B	R	N	NR
Alcohol injection	B	P	B	P	B	NR	B	P	B	P
Cryotherapy	N	NR	N	NR	N	NR	N	NR	B	P
Laser	N	NR	N	NR	N	R	N	R	B	P
External beam XRT	B	P	B	P	B	R	B	P	B	P
Imatinib	N	NR	N	NR	N	R	N	NR	N	NR

Tumor type: B, both; C, carcinoid; IC, islet cell; N, neither.
Recommendation: M, mandatory; NR, not recommended; P, potentially useful; R, recommended.
Physicians making recommendations: EAW, Eugene Woltering; TMO, Thomas O'Dorisio; AIV, Aaron Vinik; WG, Vay Liang (Bill) Go.
Abbreviations: CE, chemoembolization; HA, hepatic artery; IV, intravenous; 131I-MIBG, iodine-131-meta-iodobenzylguanidine; 177Lu-DOTA Tyr3, Lutecium-177 1,4,7,10-tetraazacyclododecane-1,4,7,10-tetraacetic acid; RFA, radiofrequency ablation; XRT, radiation therapy; 90Y, Yttrium isotope with 90 neutrons.

Table 10

Recommendations of the New Orleans Louisiana Neuroendocrine Tumor group on the use of radionuclide and embolic therapy for the treatment of neuroendocrine tumors (carcinoid and islet cell)

Radionuclide or Embolic Therapy	Consensus Recommendation		Individual Recommendations: Physician/Specialty									
			EAW Surgery		JPB Transplant Surgery		YZW General Surgery		SJ HPB Surgery		LA Medicine/ Oncology	
	Tumor Type	Rec	Type	Rec	Type	Rec	Type	Rec	Type	Rec	Type	Rec
131I-MIGB	B	P	IC	P	B	P	B	P	B	P	C	P
90Y octreotide	B	P	B	P	B	P	B	P	B	P	B	P
90Y lanreotide	B	P	B	P	B	P	B	P	B	P	B	P
177Lu-DOTA Try3 Octreotide	B	P	B	P	B	P	B	P	B	P	B	P
RFA	B	R	B	R	B	P	B	R	B	R	B	R
Chemoembolization	B	R	B	R	B	R	B	R	B	R	B	R
CE doxorubicin	B	R	B	R	B	R	B	P	B	R	B	P
CE cisplatin	B	R	B	R	B	R	B	P	B	R	B	P
CE 5-FU	B	R	B	R	B	R	B	P	B	R*	B	P
CE mitomycin C	B	R	B	R	B	R	B	R	B	R	B	R
Bland HA embolization	N	NR	N/	NR	B	R	N	NR	N	NR	B	P
Combination CE w/IV chemotherapy	N	NR	N	NR	B	P	N	P	N	NR	B	P
Bisphosphonates	B	P	B	R	B	P	IC	P	B	P	B	P
Alcohol injection	B	P	B	P	B	P	N	NR	B	P	B	P
Cryotherapy	N	NR	N	NR	N	NR	N	NR	N	NR	N	NR
Laser	N	NR	N	NR	N	NR	N	NR	N	NR	N	NR
External beam XRT	B	P	B	P	B	P	B	P	B	P	C	P
Imatinib	N	NR	N	NR	B	P	IC	P	N	NR	N	NR

Tumor type: B, both; C, carcinoid; IC, islet cell; N, neither.

Recommendation: M, mandatory; NR, not recommended; P, potentially useful; R, recommended.

Physicians making recommendations: EAW, Eugene Woltering; YZW, Yi-Zarn Wang; SJ, Saju Joseph; LA, Lowell Anthony.

Abbreviations: CE, chemoembolization; HA, hepatic artery; IV, intravenous; 131I-MIBG, iodine-131-meta-iodobenzylguanidine; 177Lu-DOTA Tyr3, Lutecium-177 1,4,7, 10-tetraazacyclododecane-1,4,7,10-tetraacetic acid; RFA, radiofrequency ablation; XRT, radiation therapy; 90Y, Yttrium isotope with 90 neutrons.

attempted by surgical teams with extensive experience in these procedures. Boudreaux and colleagues[39] observed a 50% decrease in 5-HIAA levels during postoperative follow-up and found aggressive surgical exploration and tumor debulking to significantly improve symptomatic outcome with relatively few complications.

The increased incidence of cholelithiasis following chronic administration of somatostatin analog and gallbladder wall necrosis caused by chemoembolization of the liver dictate the routine performance of prophylactic cholecystectomy during the resection of the primary tumor or metastatic lesions. In selected patients, liver transplantation for unresectable neuroendocrine hepatic metastases may provide not only long-term palliation but even cure. There is a severe shortage of donor organs, however, and thus liver transplantation for neuroendocrine metastases should only be considered in patients without evidence of extrahepatic tumor and in whom all other treatment methods are no longer effective. The use of living-related liver transplantation may allow more widespread use of this aggressive approach in patients with extensive liver metastasis.

Patient's tumors are often deemed "unresectable" by clinicians who are not surgeons, or even more disconcerting by physicians who are not familiar with the clinical course and the current array of treatments that have been developed for NETs. In all cases, a surgeon comfortable with advanced surgical techniques, such as repeat liver resection and skeletonizing the mesenteric vasculature at the base of the small bowel mesentery, should view the pertinent radiographs to help the attending physician determine the resectibility of primary, nodal, and metastatic disease.

There are multiple techniques that have been developed to assist surgeons in the operating room dealing with complex NET patients. The authors currently use methylene blue dye injected subserosally to help identify surgical resection margins for midgut carcinoids.[40] They also use radiolabeled octreotide as a guide to identify tumor deposits that are not readily evident on CT or MRI. These lesions are often active on SRS imaging but not visible by standard techniques. By using a gamma-detecting probe similar to that used in sentinel lymph node resection, metastatic deposits can be found in the absence of palpable disease. Furthermore, the authors often use intraoperative chemotherapy-infused Gelfoam for areas of unresected disease. This theoretically provides much higher doses of chemotherapeutic agent in the area of significant disease. They guard against anastomotic leakage or poor healing by protecting the anastamosis using omentum and tacking the Gelfoam to the area of interest to inhibit its movement. Finally, the authors often use multiple operations to address specific areas of metastatic disease after a short healing interval. This allows for better planning and execution on subsequent operations and allows time to assess the biologic behavior of the tumor (**Tables 11** and **12**).

RECOMMENDATIONS

Any patient with suspected NETs either because of symptoms or radiologic findings should undergo a complete history and physical examination. From this the clinician can often discern the location and functionality of the primary tumor.

Patients with NETs should undergo full tumor analysis based on tumor markers. CgA, pancreastatin, and 24-hour urine for 5-HIAA should be checked for all patients with NETs and depending on location other tumor markers should be checked and help guide clinical decision-making.

Imaging of patients with NETs should include attempted visualization of the primary tumor with endoscopy or EUS, evaluation of the lymphatic basins and liver using CT

Table 11
Recommendations of the Inter Science Institute Gastrointestinal Council on the use of surgery for the treatment of neuroendocrine tumors (carcinoid and islet cell)

Surgery	Consensus Recommendation		Individual Recommendations: Physician/Specialty							
			EAW Surgery		TMO Endocrinology		AIV Endocrinology		WG Gastroenterology	
	Tumor Type	Rec	Type	Rec	Type	Rec	Type	Rec	Type	Rec
Preop/periop octreotide to prevent carcinoid crisis	B	M	B	M	B	M	B	M	B	M
Primary resection	B	M	B	M	B	M	B	M	B	M
Debulking of metastasis	B	M	B	M	B	M	B	M	B	M
Resection of metastasis	B	M	B	M	B	M	B	R	B	M
Resection of simultaneous primary and liver metastasis	B	R	B	M	B	R	B	M	B	R
Liver transplantation	B	P	B	R	B	P	B	P	B	P

Tumor type: B, both; C, carcinoid; IC, islet cell; N, neither.
Recommendation: M, mandatory; NR, not recommended; P, potentially useful; R, recommended.
Physicians making recommendations: EAW, Eugene Woltering; TMO, Thomas O'Dorisio; AIV, Aaron Vinik; WG, Vay Liang (Bill) Go.

Table 12
Recommendations of the New Orleans Louisiana Neuroendocrine Tumor group on the use of surgery for the treatment of neuroendocrine tumors (carcinoid and islet cell)

| | Consensus Recommendation | | Individual Recommendations: Physician/Specialty | | | | | | | | | | |
| | | | EAW Surgery | | JPB Transplant Surgery | | YZW General Surgery | | SJ HPB Surgery | | LA Medicine/Oncology | |
Surgery	Tumor Type	Rec	Type	Rec	Type	Rec	Type	Rec	Type	Rec	Type	Rec
Preop/Periop octreotide to prevent carcinoid crisis	B	M	B	M	B	M	C	M	B	M	B	M
Primary resection	B	M	B	M	B	M	B	M	B	M	B	P
Debulking of metastasis	B	M	B	M	B	M	B	M	B	M	B	P
Resection of liver metastasis	B	M	B	M	B	M	B	R	B	M	B	P
Resection of simultaneous primary and liver metastasis	B	R	B	M	B	M	B	R	B	R	B	P
Liver transplantation	B	P	B	R	C	M	B	P	B	P	N	NR

Tumor type: B, both; C, carcinoid; IC, islet cell; N, neither.
Recommendation: M, mandatory; NR, not recommended; P, potentially useful; R, recommended.
Physicians making recommendations: EAW, Eugene Woltering; JPB, J. Philip Boudreaux; YZW, Yi-Zarn Wang; SJ, Saju Joseph; LA, Lowell Anthony.

and MRI, and investigation for metastatic disease not otherwise visible using SRS. SRS should be performed on all patients because this allows for identification of occult disease and evaluation of the receptor status of the tumor for subsequent treatment options.

All patients with NETs, whether or not functional, should be treated with octreotide, initially with short-acting octreotide and then transitioned to a longer-acting agent. Patients should have routine tumor surveillance and any change in symptom control, tumor size, or tumor marker levels, should necessitate trough levels to ensure adequate treatment with somatostatin analogs.

Surgery should be considered for all patients with NETs. Advanced surgical techniques have made large numbers of patients candidates for cytoreductive surgery. These surgical procedures should not be delayed until symptoms occur or tumor causes obstructive symptoms, because this often makes cytoreduction much more difficult. Furthermore, advanced treatment techniques, such as methylene blue lymphatic mapping for surgical margins, gamma probe–guided tumor debulking, and intraoperative chemotherapy, have all been shown to be effective in treatment of these patients.

For patients with unresectable disease, peptide receptor radiotherapy, chemoembolization, microsphere-guided radiation techniques, and MIBG can all be used to reduce tumor burden and help with symptoms. These patients should be evaluated by clinicians with expertise in the advanced treatment of NETs and with a multidisciplinary approach. These patients should be considered for chemotherapy regimens that address the root cause of symptoms and help reduce the chance of death from these tumors. Also, these patients should be considered for clinical trials that might change the future management of such patients.

NETs have become a more common malignancy in recent years. Although the incidence is rising, the treatment of these complex patients has not changed dramatically. However, with better understanding of tumor biology, more aggressive surgical techniques, and significant advances in radiologic techniques, the treatment of patients with NETs has become even more confusing. It is hoped that this article helps clinicians with the decision-making process and surgical management of patients with NETs.

REFERENCES

1. Kloppel G, Perren A, Heitz PU. The gastroenteropancreatic neuroendocrine cell system and its tumors: the WHO classification [abstract]. Ann N Y Acad Sci 2004;1014:13–27.
2. Plockinger U, Rindi G, Arnold R, et al. Guidelines for the diagnosis and treatment of neuroendocrine gastrointestinal tumors. A consensus statement on behalf of the European Neuroendocrine Tumor Society (ENETS). Neuroendocrinology 2004;80:394–424.
3. Woltering EA, Hilton RS, Zolfoghary CM, et al. Validation of serum versus plasma measurements of chromogranin a levels in patients with carcinoid tumors: lack of correlation between absolute chromogranin a levels and symptom frequency. Pancreas 2006;33(3):250–4.
4. Nakakura EK, Venook AP, Bergsland EK. Systemic and regional nonsurgical therapy: what is the optimal strategy for metastatic neuroendocrine cancer? Surg Oncol Clin N Am 2007;16(3):639–51.
5. Sundin A, Vullierme MP, Kaltsas G, et al. ENETS guidelines for the standard of care in patients with neuroendocrine tumours: radiological examination in patients with neuroendocrine tumours. Neuroendocrinology 2009;90:167–83.

6. Oberg K, Ferone D, Kaltsas G, et al. ENETS guidelines for the standard of care in patients with neuroendocrine tumours: biotherapy. Neuroendocrinology 2009;90: 209–13.

7. Ramage JK, Davies AH, Ardill J, et al. Guidelines for the management of gastro-enteropancreatic neuroendocrine (including carcinoid) tumours. Gut 2005; 54(Suppl 4):1–16.

8. Godwin JD II. Carcinoid tumors. An analysis of 2,837 cases. Cancer 1975;36: 560–9.

9. Calhoun K, Toth-Fejel S, Cheek J, et al. Serum peptide profiles in patients with carcinoid tumors. Am J Surg 2003;186(1):28–31.

10. Udupi V, Lee HM, Kurosky A, et al. Prohormone convertase-1 is essential for conversion of chromogranin A to pancreastatin. Regul Pept 1999;83(2–3):123–7.

11. Niederhuber JE, Fojo T. Treatment of metastatic disease in patients with neuroendocrine tumors. Surg Oncol Clin N Am 2006;15:511–33.

12. Oberg K, Astrup L, Eriksson B, et al. Guidelines for the management of gastroenteropancreatic neuroendocrine tumours (including bronchopulmonary and thymic neoplasms). Part II – specific NE tumour Types. Acta Oncol 2004;43(7):626–36.

13. Morton KM, Kamel I, Hofmann L, et al. Carcinoid tumors of the small bowel: a multitechnique imaging approach. AJR Am J Roentgenol 2004;182:559–67.

14. Graham GW, Unger BP, Coursin DB. Perioperative management of selected endocrine disorders. Int Anesthesiol Clin 2000;38:31–67.

15. Woltering EA, Mamikunian PM, Zietz S, et al. Effect of octreotide LAR dose and weight on octreotide blood levels in patients with neuroendocrine tumors. Pancreas 2005;31:392–400.

16. Woltering EA, Salvo VA, O'Dorisio TM, et al. Clinical value of monitoring plasma octreotide levels during chronic octreotide long-acting repeatable therapy in carcinoid patients. Pancreas 2008;37(1):94–100.

17. Luo Q, Peyman GA, Conway MD, et al. Effect of a somatostatin analog (octreotide acetate) on the growth of retinal pigment epithelial cells in culture. Curr Eye Res 1996;15(9):909–13.

18. Ducrux M, Ruszniewski P, Chayvialle JA. The antitumoral effect of the long acting somatostatin analog lanreotide in neuroendocrine tumors. Am J Gastroenterol 2000;95:3276–81.

19. Rinke A, Muller HH, Schade-Brittinger C, et al. Placebo-controlled, double blind, prospective, randomized study of the effect of octreotide LAR in the control of tumor growth in patients with metastatic neuroendocrine midgut tumors: a report from the PROMID study group. J Clin Oncol 2009;27(28):4635–6.

20. Mozell E, Woltering EA, O'Dorisio TM, et al. Effect of somatostatin analog on peptide release and tumor growth in the Zollinger-Ellison syndrome. Surg Gynecol Obstet 1990;170:474–84.

21. Mozell EJ, Cramer AJ. Long term efficacy of octreotide acetate in the treatment of Zollinger-Ellison syndrome. Arch Surg 1992;127:1019–26.

22. Shojamanesh H, Gibril F, Louie A, et al. Prospective study of the antitumor efficacy of long-term octreotide treatment in patients with progressive metastatic gastrinoma. Cancer 2002;94(2):331–43.

23. Lyons JM, Abergel J, Thomson J, et al. In vitro chemoresistance testing in well-differentiated carcinoid tumors. Ann Surg Oncol 2009;16(3):649–55.

24. O'Toole D, Hentic O, Corcos O, et al. Chemotherapy for gastro-enteropancreatic endocrine tumors. Neuroendocrinology 2004;80(Suppl 1):79–84.

25. Broder LE, Carter SK. Pancreatic islet cell carcinoma. results of therapy with streptozotocin in 52 patients. Ann Intern Med 1973;79:108–18.

26. Baker J, Schnirer II, Yao JC, et al. Phase II trial of irinotecan in patients with advanced carcinoid tumors. Proc Am Soc Clin Oncol 2002;21:662.
27. Ansell SM, Pitot HC, Burch PA, et al. A phase II study of high-dose paclitaxel in patients with advanced neoriendocrine tumors. Cancer 2001;91:1543–8.
28. Oberg K. Chemotherapy and biotherapy in the treatment of neuroendocrine tumors. Ann Oncol 2001;12(Suppl 2):S111–4.
29. Kolby L, Persson KJ, Franzen S, et al. Randomized control trial of the effect of interferon alpha on survival in patients with disseminated midgut carcinoid tumors. Br J Surg 2003;90:687–93.
30. Kwekkeboom DJ, Teunissen JJM, Kam BL, et al. Treatment of patients who have endocrine gastroenteropancreatic tumors with radiolabeled somatostatin analogues. Hematol Oncol Clin North Am 2007;21:561–73.
31. Kwekkeboom DJ, Teunissen JJM, Bakker WH, et al. Treatment with radiolabeled somatostain analogue [^{177}Lu-DOTA, Tyr^3] octreotate in patients with gastroenteropancreatic (GEP) tumors. J Clin Oncol 2005;23:2754–62.
32. Nobels FR, Kwekkeboom DJ, Coopmans W, et al. Chromogranin a as serum marker for neuroendocrine neoplasia: comparison with neuron-specific enolase and the alpha-subunit of glycoprotein hormones. J Clin Endocrinol Metab 1997;82:2622–8.
33. Garrot C, Stuart K. Liver-directed therapies for metastatic neuroendocrine tumors. Hematol Oncol Clin North Am 2007;21:545–60.
34. Ahlman H, Westbert G, Wangberg B, et al. Treatment of liver metastases of carcinoid tumors. World J Surg 1996;20:196–202.
35. Norton JA. Surgical treatment of neuroendocrine metastases. Best Pract Res Clin Gastroenterol 2005;9(4):577–83.
36. Hellman P, Lundstrom T, Ohrvall U, et al. Effect of surgery on the outcome of midgut carcinoid disease with lymph node and liver metastasis. World J Surg 2002;26(8):991–7.
37. Que FG, Nagorney DM, Batts KP, et al. Hepatic resection for metastatic neuroendocrine carcinomas. Am J Surg 1995;169:36–42.
38. Givi B, Pommier SJ, Thompson AK, et al. Operative resection of primary carcinoid neoplasms in patients with liver metastases yields significantly better survival. Surgery 2006;140:891–7.
39. Boudreaux JP, Putty B, Frey DJ, et al. Surgical treatment of advanced-stage carcinoid tumors: lessons learned. Am Surg 2005;241(6):839–45 [discussion: 845–6].
40. Wang YZ, Joseph S, Lindholm E, et al. Lymphatic mapping helps determine surgical margins in midgut carcinoids. Surgery 2009;146(6):993–7.

Index

Note: Page numbers of article titles are in **boldface** type.

A

Abdominal pain, in neuroendocrine tumor syndromes, 20, 25–26
Acromegaly, as neuroendocrine tumor presentation, 38
ACTH suppression studies, 38–39
ACTH-secreting tumors, 26, 29–30, 33, 38
   in children and young adults, 69–70
   surgery for, 165
Activities of daily living, neuroendocrine tumor syndromes and, QOL
   measurement of, 100–107
Adenocarcinomas, chromogranin A elevation with, 119–120
Adiponectin, obesity and, 83
Adiposity. See also *Obesity.*
   visceral, cardiometabolic risk syndrome and, 82
Adrenal tumors, chromogranin A and, 121
   in children and young adults, 66
Amines, neuroendocrine tumors and, chromogranin A secretion and, 112, 114, 120
     current recommendations for, 207, 210–213
     quantitative and qualitative analysis of, **135–151**
        evolutionary advances in, 135, 143
        glossary for, 147
        history of, 143–147
        methodological differences in, 136
        serotonin and tryptophan techniques, 136–143, 146
        standardization in laboratories, 135–136
Angiography, of neuroendocrine tumors, 49, 51
     current recommendations for, 208, 214–215
Antibodies, insulin-binding, 143
   to chromogranin A, immunoassays of, 115–116
     immunohistochemical staining and, 117
Appendiceal neuroendocrine tumors, in children and young adults, 69, 72–73
   surgery for, 168
Appetite, bariatric surgery and, 85
   obesity and, 82–83
Asymptomatic primary neuroendocrine tumors, surgery indications for, 167

B

Bariatric surgery, metabolic and cardiovascular consequences of, **81–96**
     CMRS benefits of weight loss and, 85–86
     CMRS-specific, 86–87
     compared to non-surgical therapies, 84–85

Endocrinol Metab Clin N Am 40 (2011) 233–263
doi:10.1016/S0889-8529(11)00021-1
0889-8529/11/$ – see front matter © 2011 Elsevier Inc. All rights reserved.

W

Y

Z

Moving?

Make sure your subscription moves with you!

To notify us of your new address, find your **Clinics Account Number** (located on your mailing label above your name), and contact customer service at:

Email: journalscustomerservice-usa@elsevier.com

800-654-2452 (subscribers in the U.S. & Canada)
314-447-8871 (subscribers outside of the U.S. & Canada)

Fax number: 314-447-8029

Elsevier Health Sciences Division
Subscription Customer Service
3251 Riverport Lane
Maryland Heights, MO 63043

*To ensure uninterrupted delivery of your subscription, please notify us at least 4 weeks in advance of move.

Printed and bound by CPI Group (UK) Ltd, Croydon, CR0 4YY

03/10/2024

01040448-0007